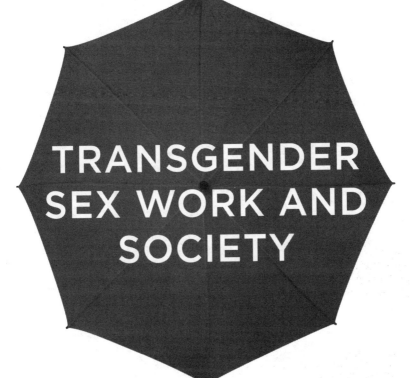

TRANSGENDER SEX WORK AND SOCIETY

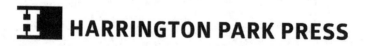

HARRINGTON PARK PRESS

NEW YORK, NY • USA

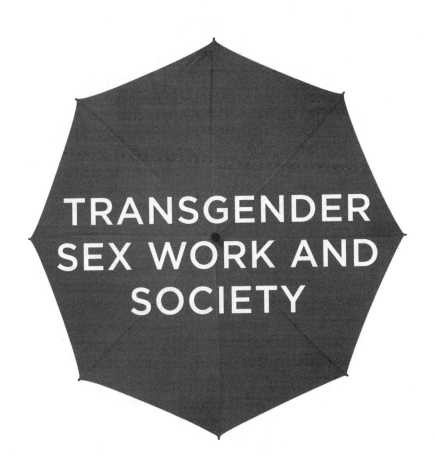

TRANSGENDER SEX WORK AND SOCIETY

EDITED BY

LARRY NUTTBROCK

Harrington Park Press
Box 331
9 East 8th Street
New York, NY 10003

http://harringtonparkpress.com

Libray of Congress Cataloging-in-Publication Data
Names: Nuttbrock, Larry A., 1946– editor.
Title: Transgender sex work and society / edited by Larry A. Nuttbrock.
Description: New York, NY : Harrington Park Press, [2018] | Includes
    bibliographical references and index.
Identifiers: LCCN 2017039041| ISBN 9781939594228 (hardcover : alk. paper) |
    ISBN 9781939594235 (ebook)
Subjects: LCSH: Prostitution. | Transgender people.
Classification: LCC HQ115 .T73 2018 | DDC 306.74086/7—dc23
LC record available at https://lccn.loc.gov/2017039041

Manufactured in the United States of America

Dedicated to all the gender-nonconforming individuals who participated in the studies reported throughout this volume.

CONTENTS

Foreword

Social stigma is an overarching theme in the challenges and vulnerabilities faced by transgender and gender-nonconforming people around the world. Stigma attached to gender nonconformity results in minority stress that negatively affects health and well-being. Transwomen who engage in sex work face a double whammy: stigma attached to gender nonconformity is compounded by stigma attached to sex work. However, there is a third force that plays an important role in the health and well-being of transgender individuals, and that is the dysphoria many may experience as a result of incongruence between their gender identity and their sex assigned at birth, and the corresponding heightened need to affirm identity. Sex work, at least initially, may provide such affirmation for transgender women, which, combined with economic hardship, may explain why a relatively high proportion of transwomen report a history of sex work. This book explores the role of sex work in the lives of transwomen and the hazards that come with this type of work, revealing a complex interplay between sex and gender, survival and validation, desire and love, social justice and health.

Dr. Nuttbrock, the editor of this book, is a sociologist with a long track record of research on the intersection of social stigma, substance use, and mental health among marginalized populations. In 2003 Dr. Nuttbrock invited me to join his team of investigators to conduct a groundbreaking study of HIV and other sexually transmitted infections among transwomen in New York City, the first longitudinal study of its kind, funded by the National Institute on Drug Abuse. This gave me the opportunity to bring my expertise as a clinical psychologist specializing in transgender health to the design and implementation of this HIV-prevention research study. From the very beginning, Dr. Nuttbrock recognized the importance of involving transgender community members in every aspect of the study; he recruited transgender-identified investigators and staff to ensure the relevance and success of

Nuttbrock, Larry, *Transgender Sex Work and Society*
dx.doi.org/10.17312/harringtonparkpress/2017.11.tsws.00a
© 2018 by Harrington Park Press

the project. Dr. Nuttbrock brought his high standards of scientific rigor and analytic skills to this study and, as a result, contributed greatly to an empirical understanding of the vulnerabilities and resilience found among transwomen. One of the consistent findings of this work is the relationship among gender-related abuse, depression, and HIV/STI. In *Transgender Sex Work and Society*, Dr. Nuttbrock and his team disseminate unique findings from this study on the challenges facing transwomen sex workers, highlighting the influence of sexual development, poverty and racism, social marginalization, and violence on substance use, depression, and sexual health. As the book's editor, he invited experts from around the world to add their contributions, the result being a comprehensive overview of what we know today.

What does this compendium of research findings and insights tell us about the current status and needs of transgender sex workers? What is calling out to be investigated further, and what are the work's implications for interventions and services, education and advocacy?

We learn that transgender sex workers suffer abuse and violence. Compared to nontransgender female and male sex workers, they are paid less for their services; face more violence from clients, partners, family members, and law enforcement; are more likely to be HIV-positive; and are less likely to be reached by HIV prevention and other service programs. Research findings presented in this book begin to illuminate the mechanisms of how gender-based stigma and power inequities contribute to health disparities. For example, findings indicate that gender-related abuse and substance use mediate the relationship between sex work and depression, and that in turn, depression predicts HIV risk and infection. Findings also indicate that felt stigma negatively affects safer sex self-efficacy. Clinical interventions are needed to address these mental health concerns and increase self-efficacy. Moreover, social and educational interventions are needed to reduce stigma in society and improve working conditions to prevent psychological distress.

Findings presented in this book indicate that transgender sex workers are a diverse group; that not all sex work is the same, but rather varies greatly in setting, autonomy and power, risks and rewards; and that factors such as race or ethnicity and socioeconomic status are related to the likelihood of sex work and the type of sex work transwomen do. A number of structural factors make sex work risky and marginalize transgender sex workers. These include those that apply to sex workers of any gender, such as criminalization, violence, sexism, racism, and ageism. They also include some that are more common specifically to transgender sex workers, such as discrimination in housing, education, and employment, and a lack of access to gender-affirming and general healthcare. Confronting these structural factors is key to promoting the health of transgender sex workers, their families, and their clients.

A greater understanding is needed of developmental trajectories of transwomen who engage in sex work. Among nontransgender sex workers, substance use is known to contribute to entrance into sex work. Is this equally true for transgender sex workers? Or is substance use for transwomen more often a way to cope with the hazards of sex work? Factors contributing to transwomen's entrance into sex work include social stigma, rejection, homelessness, and the need for economic survival. In addition, the heightened need for affirmation and community connectedness may contribute to engagement in sex work, particularly in the beginning. Transwomen may find a community of similar others on the street or in other sex work settings. Being admired and desired by male clients may serve as a powerful affirmation of their femininity. However, once they are engaged in sex work, the hazards of additional layers of stigma, marginalization, and gender-based violence take their toll on self-esteem and self-efficacy. Peer support then has its limits, owing to internalized oppression and competition for the attention of clients and other partners. Transwomen may also enter sex work aware of these hazards, with clear goals in mind (e.g., to cover the cost of gender-affirming medical interventions; to pay for college), and once these goals are achieved, some continue sex work to supplement their incomes or meet other needs.

We also learn that transgender women sex workers have lives and relationships that we know little about yet are critical to their health and well-being. This conclusion is well documented in the findings presented in this book on sexually risky behavior. It turns out that transgender sex workers most of the time do use condoms with their clients. Two circumstances may interfere: (1) the client's offering more money for sex without a condom, and (2) substance use immediately before or during sex. However, condom use is more inconsistent with casual partners and least likely with primary partners. Thus, from an HIV/STI-prevention perspective, we need to understand and address the issues different types of partners bring to the equation, as well as relationship dynamics that may produce risk or offer opportunities for affirmation and resilience. This book's chapter about transwomen sex workers' primary relationships indicates that their male partners are diverse in sexual orientation, and that they may conceal their attractions to transwomen to avoid stigma. Transwomen may enact traditional gender roles in these relationships and may forgo condom use both to express trust in and commitment to their primary partners and in an effort to meet their own often neglected needs for intimacy and love. Interventions are needed to address these relationship dynamics; male partners can be successfully reached through referrals from transgender sex workers.

To move the evidence to inform interventions forward, future research on transgender sex work and society can benefit from theory-derived questions and hypotheses. A number of theoretical frameworks are suggested in this volume, ranging from the social-ecological, minority-stress, and gender-affirmation models to approaches that take into account nonbinary gender identities, life stages, and the role of society in providing social protections. The last is well illustrated in Chapter 14, on sex work among the *hijras* in India. Cultural differences notwithstanding, future efforts should address the universal themes of stigma attached to nonconformity in gender and in sexuality, its negative effect on the health of transgender sex workers and their loved ones, and the multipronged approach necessary to make things better.

In conclusion, this volume provides a comprehensive and rich overview of what we know about the situation of transgender sex workers and the challenges we face in ensuring their safety and promoting their health and well-being. It offers numerous opportunities for future research, intervention, and advocacy to reduce stigma and promote resilience. The book is a must-read for any researcher and health provider working with transwomen as well as for policy makers concerned with sex work and the health and well-being of transgender and sexual minority populations around the world.

Walter Bockting, PhD
Professor of Medical Psychology (in Psychiatry and Nursing)
Research Scientist, New York State Psychiatric Institute
Codirector, Program for the Study of LGBT Health at
Columbia University Medical Center

Introduction

Toward a Better Understanding of Transgender Sex Work

Larry A. Nuttbrock[1]

1 Previously affiliated with the National Development and Research Institutes (NDRI) and now a private consultant living in New York City.

Small but significant numbers of individuals in the United States and worldwide experience or present themselves in ways that challenge cultural norms about sexuality and gender.[1] Sex assigned at birth for these individuals is inadequate or inappropriate for describing their feelings and sense of self. Some surgically alter their sexual anatomy and transition to the gender opposite their birth sex; some become committed to a gender different from their natal sex and dress in ways expressive of that gender; some derive personal and perhaps sexual satisfaction from wearing the apparel appropriate for a different sex; some define themselves along a continuum from maleness to femaleness; and some totally reject the binary gender system, and the very concept of gender, as applying to themselves. Those born as males who later experience or present themselves in feminine ways are often described as transgender women, or transwomen; those born as females who later experience or present themselves in masculine ways are often described as transgender men, or transmen.[2]

In the United States and increasingly around the world, all these individuals are now collectively described as transgender. The term arose in a political context to reflect the fact that these individuals, while diverse, nonetheless share histories of social oppression (Feinberg, 1996). Since the 1990s the term has been used by service providers to

Nuttbrock, Larry, *Transgender Sex Work and Society*
dx.doi.org/10.17312/harringtonparkpress/2017.11.tsws.00b

incorporate gender-nonconforming populations within a single mechanism for federal funding (Valentine, 2007); transgender studies have become a recognized field of study (Stryker, 2008); and the term is now embedded in popular culture.

Transgender has typically been defined and measured as incongruence between sex—understood as a biologically determined division of humans into males and females—and gender identity, understood as a psychologically determined division of humans into boys (men) and girls (women).[3] This formulation, while often used in research studies, is conceptually elusive (Thurer, 2005). The assumption that there are two mutually exclusive sexes that map (or fail to map) onto two mutually exclusive genders has been questioned in anthropological studies (Herdt, 1996; Nanda, 1999, 2014; Sinnott, 2004), and some scholars have described both sex and gender as socially constructed (Seidman, 2010) and historically variable (Foucault, 1990; Laqueur, 1990). Transgender and gender-nonconforming individuals may, indeed, be defined and understood in different ways around the world, but (following Feinberg) there is nonetheless considerable uniformity in the ways all these individuals are misunderstood and socially marginalized (Feinberg, 1996; Nanda, 2014).

Small but significant numbers of individuals in the United States and worldwide provide sexual services for material compensation as well as selling erotic performances and products (Weitzer, 2012).[4] Sex work includes direct physical contact between a buyer and seller as well as indirect sexual stimulation and may include emotional intimacy and companionship. Sex work may be negotiated and occur in different venues and social contexts, including streets and public spaces, parlors or residences known as places where sex may be purchased, hookups through message boards and the Internet, and various informal arrangements (Sanders, O'Neill, & Pitcher, 2009).

Terminology and social understanding about sex work (like transgender) vary across cultures and have been historically variable. At the turn of the twentieth century, for example, *sex work* was understood in moralistic terms as "prostitution" and often vaguely defined to include marital infidelity and other violations of monogamous sex in the context of marriage (Connelly, 1980). In the twenty-first century, this exchange is increasingly understood in economic terms as a transaction of sex for money among consenting adults. In contrast to prostitution, the term *sex work* points to the skills, labor, emotional work, and physical presentation of sellers in the context of a commercial relationship.

Small but significant numbers of individuals in the United States and worldwide are both transgender and sex workers.[5] Given the diversity in transgender and sex work noted above, transgender sex workers should be regarded as highly heterogeneous populations that include different identities, modalities of operation, and provided services.

Numerous studies of transgender persons have been conducted that incorporate (primarily street-based) sex work as a correlate of mental health issues or HIV, but very few of these studies have focused on sex work as the primary variable of interest. The current volume is an initial attempt to systematically examine transgender sex work, and the issues associated with it, in the United States and around the world.

The first three chapters provide detailed descriptions of sex work among transwomen in New York City, in conjunction with theory that includes socioeconomic disadvantages, sexual orientation, ethnicity, and issues associated with urban poverty. Special issues associated with transgender sex work during adolescence and early adulthood are then described and compared across the United States and United Kingdom. Qualitative data pertaining to high-risk sexual behavior between transwomen and their cisgender partners are presented, followed by a current review of substance use among transgender sex workers. Issues associated with different forms of gender-related abuse are examined from different methodological perspectives and in different subpopulations. The extent to which observed associations of sex work with major depression and HIV/STI are mediated by abuse is investigated in some detail.

Subsequent chapters provide glimpses of transgender populations from around the world, including discussions of the extent to which these populations, in different cultural contexts, experience social adversity and health issues that may reflect this adversity. Approaches to the care and treatment of transgender sex workers are then discussed, with an emphasis on integrating multiple factors, including abuse, in these regimens. This volume concludes with examinations of public health compared to criminal justice perspectives on transgender sex work that include discussions bearing on the hotly debated topic of decriminalization.

All the contributors to this volume were confronted with conceptual and methodological challenges that include clearly defining the populations under study and obtaining samples representative of broader transgender populations. Most of the chapters define transgender as a mismatch between natal sex and current gender identity, but this definition, while at the moment standard in research studies, may exclude those who totally reject the binary gender system. Probability samples of transgender populations are beginning to appear in the literature, but analytic studies examining the lifestyles and health of transgender populations have thus far been based on convenience or nonprobability community samples.

The book is divided into sections that reflect important themes and issues. Most of the chapters focus on transwomen sex workers, though there are some discussions, when relevant, pertaining to transgender male sex workers. Additional study is needed about the level of HIV risk in the latter population. There is some overlap in content, but the chapters may be read and understood independently.

NOTES

1. The size of this population is largely unknown, but a household probability sample of adults in Massachusetts found that .5% of them could be described as transgender (Conron et al. 2012). This may be an undercount and may not reflect the full range of transgender as described here.

2. Such terminology may not include individuals who experience or present themselves in gender-neutral ways.

3. Current guidelines from the American Psychological Association (2015) define transgender as a mismatch between sex assigned at birth and gender identity, but these individuals are now described more broadly as transgender and gender-nonconforming people. The *Diagnostic and Statistical Manual of Mental Disorders* (5th edition) has likewise replaced Gender Identity Disorder, understood as a mismatch between assigned sex and gender identity, with Gender Dysphoria, understood as incongruence between gender expression and the gender that would be assigned by others (American Psychiatric Association, 2013).

4. Estimates of female sex workers in different parts of the world range from .2% to 2.6% in Asia and .2% to 7.4% in Latin America (Vandepitte et al., 2006).

5. The size of this population is largely unknown; however, as is discussed throughout this book, significant numbers of transgender women are involved in the sex trade, and a significant percentage of sex workers appears to be transgender. In the red-light districts of Antwerp, Belgium, for example, 10% of the window workers have been described as transgender (Weitzer, 2012).

REFERENCES

American Psychiatric Association. (2013). *Diagnostic and statistical manual of mental disorders* (5th ed.). Arlington, VA: American Psychiatric Association.

American Psychological Association. (2015). Guidelines for psychological practice with transgender and gender nonconforming persons. *American Psychologist, 70* (9), 832–864.

Connelly, M. T. (1980). *The response to prostitution in the Progressive Era.* Chapel Hill: University of North Carolina Press.

Conron, K. J., Scott, G., Stowell, G. S., & Landers, S. J. (2012). Transgender health in Massachusetts: Results from a household probability sample of adults. *American Journal of Public Health, 102* (1), 118–122.

Feinberg, L. (1996). *Transgender warriors: Making history from Joan of Arc to Dennis Rodman.* Boston: Beacon Press.

Foucault, M. (1990). *The history of sexuality: An introduction* (vol. 1). New York: Random House.

Herdt, G. (ed.). (1996). *Third sex/third gender: Beyond sexual dimorphism in culture and history.* New York: Zone Books.

Laqueur, T. (1990). *Making sex: Body and gender from the Greeks to Freud.* Cambridge: Harvard University Press.

———. (2014). *Gender diversity: Crosscultural variations* (2nd ed.). Long Grove, IL: Waveland Press.

Nanda, S. (1999). *Neither man nor woman: The hijras of India* (2nd ed.). Belmont, CA: Wadsworth.

Sanders, S., O'Neill, M., & Pitcher, J. (2009). *Prostitution: Sex work, policy, and politics.* Los Angeles: Sage.

Seidman, S. (2010). *The social construction of sexuality* (2nd ed.). New York: Norton.

Sinnott, M. J. (2004). *Toms and dees: Transgender identity and female same-sex relationships in Thailand.* Honolulu: University of Hawaii Press.

Stryker, S. (2008). *Transgender history.* Berkeley, CA: Seal Press.

Thurer, S. L. (2005). *The end of gender: A psychological autopsy.* New York: Routledge.

Valentine, D. (2007). *Imaging transgender: An ethnography of a category.* Durham, NC: Duke University Press.

Vandepitte, J., Lyerla, R., Dallabetta, G., Crabbe, F., Alary, M., & Bave, A. (2006). Estimates of the number of female sex workers in different regions of the world. *Sexually Transmitted Infections, 82* (suppl. 3), iii18–iii25.

Weitzer, R. (2012). *Legalizing prostitution: From illicit vice to lawful business.* New York: New York University Press.

SECTION I

EMPIRICAL DESCRIPTIONS AND A CONCEPTUAL FORMULATION FOR SEX WORK AMONG TRANSWOMEN IN THE UNITED STATES

Sex work has frequently been included as a covariate in studies of HIV risk and mental health among transgender persons, but there have been few attempts to describe the dimensions and correlates of sex work in these populations. In this section, we provide two empirical descriptions of sex work among transwomen in New York City. Two interrelated themes run through these chapters: (1) transwomen sex workers in New York City, and perhaps in other large metropolitan areas, are highly diverse, with major differences across levels of sex work (number of partners) and socio-economic factors, including ethnicity; and (2) different communities of transwomen sex workers are highly stratified with regard to income, power, and other forms of social advantage.

Building on these empirical descriptions and the broader existing literature, an attempt is made to provide a conceptual formulation for the factors that lead transwomen to enter the sex trade and cause subsets of these individuals to experience psychological problems and an array of social and economic disadvantages.

CHAPTER 1

Qualitative Description of Sex Work among Transwomen in New York City

Sel J. Hwahng[1]

1 Adjunct associate professor in the Women and Gender Studies Department at
Hunter College – City University of New York.

SUMMARY

This chapter provides a qualitative description of transwomen sex
workers in New York City. Sex work occurs largely in "ethnocultural
communities" that are distinct with regard to ethnicity and other variables. These include African American or black and Latina(o) and
transgender people involved in the House Ball community, Asian sex
workers, and white cross-dressers. Variation across these communities in
the frequency and motivations for sex work, working conditions, typi-
cal clients, and power dynamics with clients were examined. The communities have little in common with one another and are economically
and culturally structured along a hierarchy of power and privilege.

KEY TERMS

cross-dresser; ethnicity; ethnography; House Ball community; power
dynamics; sex worker

For reasons examined throughout this volume, significant numbers of
male-to-female (MTF) transgender persons are involved in the sex trade.
Motivations for sex work in this population, and the lifestyle, socioeconomic, and cultural factors associated with it, have been described in ethnographic studies in South America (Kulick, 1998) and Mexico (Prieur,
1998); a few qualitative studies have been conducted in the United States

Nuttbrock, Larry, *Transgender Sex Work and Society*
dx.doi.org/10.17312/harringtonparkpress/2017.11.tsws.001
© 2018 by Harrington Park Press

(Nadal, Davidoff, & Fujii-Doe, 2014; Sausa, Keatley, & Operario, 2007; Weinberg, Shaver, & Williams, 1999; Wilson & Garofalo, 2009).

This chapter selectively incorporates and discusses data obtained in conjunction with an in-depth qualitative study of sex work among MTF persons in New York City (Hwahng & Nuttbrock, 2007). An orienting premise of that study, supported by the data, is that the experience and practice of sex work in this population are shaped by everyday interactions in a community of peers and structured by broader economic and cultural forces, especially ethnicity. Sex work among MTF persons in New York City, I suggest, occurs in the context of relatively distinct "ethnocultural communities" that have little in common with one another and are economically and culturally structured along a hierarchy of power and privilege.

METHOD

The institutional review board at National Development and Research Institutes Inc. approved this study. Data collection included twelve months of participant observation at venues where transgender persons congregate in New York City. The research included 35 informal interviews, 15 formal in-depth interviews, and interviews with researchers. The in-depth interviews with transgender participants lasted from 60 to 90 minutes and started with questions about each participant's general background, including race, ethnicity, socioeconomic status, age, and immigration or citizenship status.

Participants who were or had been involved with sex work answered additional questions about their initial involvement in sex work, solicitation, negotiating power with clients, and their attitudes toward intimate partners versus clients. These participants were also asked to provide information about the drug use and sexual behaviors of those in their social groups and communities. I analyzed field notes and interviews using open coding and grounded theory (Strauss & Corbin, 1990).

It should be noted that I identify as a transmasculine gender-variant person of color and have been involved in transgender social, political, and cultural organizing and academic research on local, national, and international levels since 1995. I was also on the staff at a community-based organization, the Asian/Pacific Islander Coalition on HIV/AIDS, during the time of this research.

RESULTS

I recognized three distinct ethnocultural contexts: (1) African American or black, Latina(o), and transgender people involved in the House Ball community; (2) Asian sex workers; and (3) white cross-dressers. Other groups of transgender sex workers were observed, such as immigrant trans Latinas; however, in this chapter I focus on comparisons of these three groups. The House Ball and Asian communities were both low-income populations. House Ball members were mostly in their teens and twenties, and Asian sex workers were mostly in their twenties and thirties. Members of the white cross-dressing community were middle-class and mostly in their forties and fifties.

General Descriptions

Members of the House Ball community were primarily nonimmigrant African American or black, Caribbean, Puerto Rican, and Dominican ethnicities and lived in Harlem, Spanish Harlem, the Bronx, Queens, Brooklyn, and cities in New Jersey such as Newark. They congregated uptown in the Bronx, Harlem, and East Harlem; at the clubs Esquelita and Opaline in midtown Manhattan; and attended balls in Manhattan, Brooklyn, and the Bronx. They often referred to themselves as fem queens, nu women, or girls, and they usually did not use terms such as transvestite, transgender, or transsexual.

The Asian sex worker community appeared to be exclusively immigrant and often undocumented; comprised several ethnicities, including Thai, Vietnamese, Filipina(o), Malaysian, and Chinese; and lived in areas such as Jackson Heights in Queens, Chinatown in Manhattan, and Hoboken in New Jersey. Members of this community congregated in their own neighborhoods at after-work events organized by these transgender people in private homes, at sex work solicitation clubs in Manhattan, and at designated areas in Manhattan and Queens at places such as diners. They often referred to themselves as transvestites, women, or girls.

White cross-dressers were nonimmigrant and generally lived in white middle-class enclaves such as areas of Manhattan, Long Island, Yonkers, White Plains, and Poughkeepsie in New York; the New Jersey suburbs; and Bethlehem, Pennsylvania. They tended to congregate at local meeting places such as motel conference rooms for events organized by local chapters of organizations such as Tri-ESS (Society for the

Second Self) or the Mid-Hudson Transgender Society as well as clubs in Manhattan such as Silver Swans and Karolyn's.

House Ball Community

Members of the House Ball community often participated as streetwalkers and engaged in sex work in cars, on the streets, and in abandoned parking lots. As marginalized transgender members of an ethnocultural community with very little economic capital, many of the transgender people in the House Ball community felt compelled to go into sex work. Because African American or black and Latina(o) transgender people were ascribed lower social status within an ethnocultural community of already low socioeconomic status, often the only options seemingly available to them were the riskiest forms of sex work.

House Ball members were forced into prostitution because of drug addiction, poverty, or lack of education. Because of the long history of extreme stigma experienced by members of the House Ball community, sex work, along with drug use as a coping mechanism for sex work, has become internalized within the community as a rite of passage. Young MTF members of the House Ball community must go through this rite of passage because of the perception that there is no alternative for them other than sex work and drug use—a finding similar to that of a study conducted in San Francisco on MTF people of color (Nemoto, Operario, et al., 2004).

One member of the House Ball community stated, "You know, when you first experience the transgender life, you want to see what they're [the streetwalkers] all about, where they hang out, what do they do." Because of the type of sex work they were involved in, House Ball members appeared to have the lowest negotiating power in relation to safe sex with sexual partners. As indicated by the normalization of multiple rapes and drug use voiced by several members in this community, House Ball members were more vulnerable to random acts of violence as streetwalkers, and these harsh conditions seemed to push many into drug use. Members gave accounts of numerous deaths occurring regularly in this community through overdose and homicide. A House Ball member related: "I never had an experience, but I know a lot of the girls that have, where they've been cut in the face, [the clients] give them the money, then they drive them away somewhere and then they beat them and take the money back."

One House Ball member reported that 90% of the clients who cruise the areas in Manhattan and the Bronx are white, middle-class, married men, and the remaining 10% are African American or black men and Latinos. The authors confirmed the racial mix of these clients with participant-observation. This House Ball member also stated that when she was a streetwalker, she found the African American or black and Latino clients to be more rough sexually and physically than white clients; thus, she preferred white clients, whom she characterized as submissive, over men of color. In describing her experiences as a sex worker, another member stated that many of her clients were married and lived public lives as heterosexual, monogamous men. What really surprised her was that many of the clients wanted to be anally penetrated.

She stated that over 90% of her clients are white: "Most, almost all of them are married. And a lot of them who are married like to—how could I put this in a way that's not so vulgar—they prefer to bend over. . . . Yes." A lot of the clients do like to be penetrated. One group of clients that made an impression on another member was Hasidic Jewish men, who would often drive up asking for sexual services, including anal penetration, from the House Ball members.

As one member articulated: "Most of [the clients] are white men and Jewish men. . . . Jewish men, with their outfits on . . . those are the ones that like to pay the girls two–three hundred dollars. . . . They're Hasidic Jews. Isn't it funny? On 14th Street and the Bronx." Another member stated that encounters with clients were almost always quick and rarely built into long-term, sustained relationships, even as client–sex worker relationships. When asked if she would have liked to have a long-term attachment, such as a sugar daddy relationship, with one of her clients as a way to gain more economic stability and thus reduce the number of different clients, she said she would, but her clients were all married. Furthermore, it appeared that the clients themselves often did not initiate or propose long-term agreements with these streetwalkers.

Transgender people in the House Ball community appeared to often procure body modifications, such as silicone injections and surgery, and hormones within both the legal and underground body-modification markets. These transgender people engaged in sex work, then, to pay for these modifications, not just to finance survival needs such as clothing, food, and shelter. They often experienced the financial expenses of body modifications as additional burdens within lifestyles for which survival itself was often a struggle.

Because of the harsh conditions of sex work, study participants did not idealize such work. One House Ball member stated: "I think it's degrading that I have a man slobbering all over me for fifty bucks, you know? You'll find a lot of, it's a lot of [clients] that are really weird. It's a lot of weird things that they want. . . . That's why I stopped. I mean, from the beginning I was disgusted with it, and I said this is not really me. But sometimes I did what I had to do to survive."

As a research associate explained: "These girls go through a lot of stuff, a lot of them have to turn to lifestyles and do things that they don't want to do because they have no other choice . . . sex working and selling drugs and stuff like that. . . . But they don't have any opportunities." In fact, some House Ball members as they get older will actually transition back to men or present as more masculine. A member stated that one reason for this reverse transition is that as transgender sex workers start to age, they are perceived as losing their youth and beauty, so economic survival may become too difficult for them as fem queens or nu women.

Thus, transwomen may be able to find work more easily if they appear masculine. A House Ball member confirmed this idea in comparing older transgender people who present as feminine and those who transition back to masculine presentations: "A lot of [older transgender] were just surviving as sex workers, actually, a lot of them have changed their ways. And it's being, I guess, a lot of them have woken up, and some of them don't want to compete with the new generation or they woke up and said, you know what . . . They change their name, they become legal, they marry a husband who will take care of them for the rest of their lives, you know?"

When the interviewer asked, "They stay trans though, right?" the House Ball member replied:

> Yeah, a lot of them do. [But] a lot of them become men again, I don't understand that. . . . I've heard cases where they went and got their implants done, they went and got cheekbones done, they went and got ass done, and then the next thing you know it's like they're men again. I met this one guy like that. . . . He had titties, he had

implants, he had, you know, taken hormones, soft face, and now it's like he removed the titties, he started building muscles, and he got built and he left his cheekbones so now he's a [male] stripper.

Asian Sex Workers

As a group with moderate HIV risk, Asian sex workers appeared to engage solely in club and online solicitation and apartment- and hotel-based sex work. With this type of solicitation, Asian MTF people seemed to be able to screen their clients more thoroughly and engage in sex work with fewer clients because they got paid more per client. Although they were engaged in sex work to finance survival needs such as food, shelter, and clothing, Asians often did not incur large financial expenses in relation to body modifications and thus did not have this added financial burden.

According to both a member of this community and an MTF outreach worker from an Asian American HIV organization, many Asian sex workers transition sometime between their teenage and early adult years solely through clothing and behavior. Some Asian "girls" may also start taking hormones at puberty, but this practice has a fairly low cost compared with other body modifications. According to the outreach worker, Asian "girls" pass as au naturel females without costly or uncomfortable body modifications such as surgery or silicone injections.

Like the clients of House Ball community members, those of Asian sex workers appeared to be primarily white. Asian sex workers have estimated their client base to consist on average of 94% white, married, middle-class men; 3% Latino men; 2% Asian men; and 1% African American or black men, percentages that the researchers substantiated by participant-observation.

According to one member of the Asian sex worker community, clients searching for transgender sex workers at transgender bars always chose the Asians first, preferring them over African Americans or blacks and Latinas(os). This member maintained that because Asians possessed natural femininity and had not undergone major surgical or other body-modification enhancements, they appeared more feminine — and thus more desirable — to customers than African Americans or blacks and Latinas(os).

An additional likely factor is that Asians were considered more high class than other sex workers soliciting in places such as bars — a notion corroborated by another member, who related her own experiences of clients taking her to elite establishments such as the Park Plaza Hotel, where she was treated with respect by the hotel service workers. Several other Asian sex workers confirmed the assertion that Asians were paid more for their sex work than African Americans or blacks and Latinas(os). Like House Ball members, sex workers in this community were often asked to sexually penetrate their male clients.

Members of both the Asian and the House Ball communities frequently referred to the importance of remaining anatomically functional in order to continue to be seen as desirable by clients and to fulfill clients' requests. According to one member of the Asian community, many Asian transgender people viewed any type of modification, including hormones and surgery, as potentially inhibitory of their functionality. Furthermore, many Asian sex workers wanted to retain their functionality not only as a way to generate more money but also sometimes to satisfy their own desires. An interview with a member of this community illustrated the importance of functionality. When the interviewer asked, "But you didn't take hormones?" the Asian sex worker replied, "No, I don't, I love my dick. . . . It doesn't work [on hormones]. . . . Also [it's] my job, too, to make the client happy, so I have to keep it hard, you know. So, I don't get hormones."

The interviewer then asked, "Because a lot of the times the clients want to be penetrated?" The Asian sex worker replied, "They want to feel . . . functional."

> *Interviewer:* In your experience, most of the time you were the giver [penetrator]?
> *Asian sex worker:* Yeah, because these were supposedly heterosexual guys. And then I hate the guy when they asked me, it totally turned me off. . . . I don't like to be asked. It's like, my god, they're so macho, they're like, "Honey, will you fuck me?" And I'm so feminine! I like to be like, you know, just do it. . . . Just happened, I prefer that. I don't like them to ask me. Big muscle and open the leg [sic], you know . . . don't ask, either have a good time, don't ask me, I do it if I do it. But don't ask me.
> *Interviewer:* Do you think that that's what they wanted: [to be penetrated] most of the time?
> *Asian sex worker:* Exactly, they want to feel it, how to be. . . .

They want to feel this. All their lives they've been giving. . . .
Exactly, they want to feel this . . . they want to feel how it's like
to have . . . in the end they always ask [to be penetrated].

Clients may use a smoke-and-mirrors approach in which they ask to
engage in a series of different sexual acts, including sexually penetrating the sex worker or engaging in mutually penetrative sex acts, in
order to mask what they really want: to be anally penetrated. When the
client engages in a variety of sex acts with the sex worker, his desire for
anal-receptive intercourse does not come across as blatantly obvious,
even though, according to the outreach worker, that had been the client's goal from the outset. A refined sexual experience with a femi-
nized Asian sex worker, however, sometimes did not even include
actual sex.

One member described how middle-class businessmen often sought
emotional and psychological pampering in the form of soothing dia-
logue, compliments, and physical touch and caresses, and sex workers
were often paid for these services rather than for actual sex. Another
member described her own experiences of clients paying her for other
nonsexual services, such as putting on a private fashion show as a run-
way model, an activity that entailed her putting on different outfits and
posing in them without any sexual exchange taking place. Even when
sex did take place, Asian transgender people often exhibited greater
negotiating power than members of the House Ball community.

For instance, members of the Asian community often stated that
their using condoms with clients was nonnegotiable and absolutely mandatory, a principle that the House Ball members did not observe. Many
members of the Asian sex worker community, particularly those who
were undocumented in the United States, also did not seek or have access
to social and medical services. In addition, members of this community also exhibited a distrust of the medical and healthcare systems,
feared deportation, and were concerned about adequate language and
translation provisions, which is consistent with findings in other studies
of Asians in the United States.

Members of the Asian sex worker community also seemed less
likely to use drugs than those in the House Ball community. The type
of sex work Asians engaged in was not as stressful as streetwalking, so
drugs did not appear to be needed as a coping mechanism for daily sur-

vival. One Asian member noted that, when drugs were used, the drug of choice was often cocaine. She also stated that many male clients who were snorting or using cocaine would encourage the sex workers to join them in using the drug. Asian sex workers, however, reported that they would often pretend to be snorting or using cocaine along with their male clients while actually covertly discarding the drug; because these male clients were intoxicated, they would not notice.

The type of sex work that Asians engaged in thus allowed members more leverage in negotiating safe sex and staving off threats of violence and coerced drug use.

WHITE CROSS-DRESSERS

Unlike members of the other two communities, white, middle-class cross-dressers often maintained or had maintained traditional masculine gender roles as husbands and fathers and were or had been closeted from their wives and families. Study data showed that these cross-dressers held jobs as businessmen, real estate brokers, and other white-collar occupations. Even if they did come out of the closet—an action that often resulted in loss of marriage and family—these white cross-dressers were able to remain legally employed, either in the jobs and professions they had held before the domestic breakups or in new occupations.

White cross-dressers who had to find new jobs usually ended up with lower socioeconomic status but still could work within the legal economy as salesclerks at department stores and novelty shops, for example, or in other pink-collar (woman-dominated) professions. At a local chapter of Tri-ESS in Poughkeepsie, New York, comprising white middle-class MTF people in their forties and fifties, the authors observed that several cross-dressers had jobs as salesclerks and that some had been mid-level executives before they displayed their cross-dressing or transgender identities more publicly.

Members of this community often benefited from having access to a white, middle-class network. At Silver Swans, a nightclub located in the Gramercy district of Manhattan and often frequented by white, middle-class, and middle-aged cross-dressers, researchers observed that several cross-dressers, who mentioned their occupations, were all working within the legal economy and even assisting other cross-dressers. For instance, one cross-dresser, who passed as a male real estate broker by day, was helping several other cross-dressers find housing in white, middle-class, suburban neighborhoods that was relatively safe or private to accommodate their cross-dressing lifestyle.

Additionally, cross-dressers living in suburban enclaves outside New York City stated that Cross Dresser's International, a New York City–based cross-dressing organization, rented dressing rooms and lockers to cross-dressers. Members explained that cross-dressers would come to the organization's site as men and then change into femme to go out on the town in New York City, storing their clothes in the lockers. When it was time to go home, they would change back into their men's clothes and leave their women's clothes at Cross Dresser's International.

Even though members of this group were in many ways the most secretive about their transgender status compared with the other two communities, white cross-dressers were often able to retain legal jobs, housing, and some economic security by pooling their resources as white and middle-class people. This double life of secrecy, however, also led to emotional and psychological confusion and stress. These cross-dressers explained that because of their desire to maintain a traditional masculine gender role and hide their transgender status, they often did not undergo transition, hormonal supplementation, or surgery until well into their forties or fifties. Transition often occurred after a domestic breakup, when they could be more out as transgender. According to one member, however, starting transition this late in life had some costs: "For the most part, starting hormones at an earlier age is a great advantage in transitioning; for those who wait until we are in our forties and fifties and have accumulated all the traditional American male baggage that we've accumulated along the road, trying to be what we're supposed to be with all this crap that we drag along with us, taking hormones at an earlier age is . . . I certainly wish I had started hormones then."

So, although cross-dressers experienced job security and social privilege by maintaining a traditional white, masculine role, the sacrifice they made for the benefit of this economic and social security was not being out as transgender until much later in their lives, including not feminizing at an earlier age. Because many transgender people in this community were already employed within the legal economy, when white cross-dressers did engage in sex work, it was almost always for recreational purposes. In fact, recreational sex work seemed to fit within an overall schema of recreational sexual exploration and experimentation for these people when dressed in femme.

The atmosphere in white cross-dressing clubs was flirtatious, light, and playful compared with the survival sex work clubs frequented by Asian and Latina(o) transgender sex workers. For instance, when the author's research team conducted outreach and interviews with members of the white cross-dressing community, cross-dressers often openly flirted with members of the research team and seemed to desire and enjoy any type of positive attention.

In the survival sex work clubs, the atmosphere was often serious and heavy despite the fact that overt displays of sexuality also occurred. Sex workers in these clubs did not engage in light banter and flirtations; conversation often centered on financial and sex act negotiations. Even when acting sexy, such as when they were dancing with and caressing clients, Asian and Latina(o) sex workers still often appeared wary. They did not seem to pay attention to anyone who was not a potential paying client. Because cross-dressers often experienced their transgender sexuality as exploratory, light, and playful, and did not have to depend on sex work for their survival needs, they often eroticized sex work. A research associate explained:

> And I think it's interesting to see the difference in ages and ethnicities, like how people answer questions. I find that so fascinating. Like even just talk about sex work, there's some older white people that I've interviewed that talk about this sex work as like this, like, great kind of fantasy, like I've had some people kind of brag about it, you know, when we go through the Life Chart Interview there's no sex work, and then later on, there was one person who was like, "Oh, yeah, well, you know, I get $20 for blow jobs now," and was really excited and proud of it, and there was someone . . . who when we got to the sex work part was, "I've really been thinking about that, I really want to do that now, I bet people will pay me because you know I've had all this work done and I look great."

The ability to choose to engage in recreational sex work, then, also allowed white cross-dressers great negotiating power with sexual partners. For the most part, white cross-dressers' paying sexual partners tended to be white, middle-class, and legally employed. Thus, relationships between cross-dressers and their clients seemed to be more equitable than those between clients and survival sex workers in the other two communities.

Because most cross-dressers were not involved in body modification, cross-dressers also did not have this financial burden. Some cross-dressers did, however, transition through body modifications, and they usually also transitioned out of the cross-dressing community as a result. In those cases, members had often been able to accrue personal savings from their legal employment to finance body modifications and so did not have to rely on sex work to finance their modifications.

In terms of drug use, it appeared that illegal drug use was minimal for the white cross-dressing population. Because cross-dressers engaged in sex work for recreational purposes, they felt little pressure from clients regarding coercive or persuasive drug use: their survival did not depend on placating clients. Furthermore, many cross-dressers seemed to be invested in staying within the legal and acceptable limits of society, their only so-called transgression being their expression of gender identity.

DISCUSSION

This study revealed that MTF people in New York City are often more connected to their ethnocultural community than to a gender or sexual minority community. Depending on their ethnocultural context, transgender people can vary widely in terms of their employment, socioeconomic status, and education.

Significance of Economic Issues

Economic survival was a main priority for all the MTF communities we studied. Concerns over economic survival often structured their gender expression, type of work, day-to-day schedules, social activities, choice of sexual partners, and, ultimately, their HIV vulnerabilities. Because of their precarious positions in society, MTF people must place economic survival at the center of their existence while also managing a multitude of other survival and gender-identity needs such as obtaining food, shelter, and clothing and dealing with immigration, gender identity and expression, and gender transition. These ethnocultural communities, then, were often organized to maximize scarce or moderately available resources. What was noticeably apparent was that white, middle-class cross-dressers were usually employed in legal occupations. If they engaged in sex work, it was always as a recreational pursuit. On the other hand, many of the House Ball community members also did sex work, but they, like the Asian sex workers (who were immigrants and also often undocumented), for the most part engaged in survival sex work, even if just temporarily.

A division thus appeared between those engaged in recreational sex work and those who did survival sex work. Recreational sex work could be described as sex work in which the participant engaged for purposes of sexual experimentation or to act out erotic fantasies. The participant did not have to engage in sex work for her survival and was usually not a full-time sex worker, but may have used sex work to supplement her income. In comparison, those who engaged in survival sex work often needed to obtain monetary compensation for clothing, food, shelter, and other essentials of life and so usually worked full-time as sex workers. However, even the realm of survival sex work offered different types of sex work. Street-based sex workers, for example, had experiences vastly different from those of apartment- and hotel-based sex workers.

Significance of Ethnicity

What accounted for House Ball members often engaging in street-based sex work and Asian MTF people engaging in apartment- and hotel-based sex work? These choices were not arbitrary; they filled specific sexual markets. Markets for survival sex work in particular were often adapted according to the desires of white, middle-class male clients. In relation to HIV and STI vulnerabilities, violence, and rape, House Ball community members seemed to engage in the riskiest form of survival sex work, whereas Asian sex workers seemed to be involved in moderate-risk survival sex work, and white cross-dressers seemed to engage in very low-risk recreational sex work with the most negotiating power.

Interestingly, the levels of risk inversely correlate with the economic hierarchy between general racial groups in the United States, where African Americans or blacks and Latinos have the least amount of economic capital; followed by Asians, who have moderate capital; and then whites, who have the most economic resources. Although it may seem obvious why white cross-dressers would exhibit low HIV risk behaviors, it is not as evident why the House Ball members, who are a nonimmigrant group, would exhibit higher HIV risk behaviors than the Asian sex workers, who are immigrants and often undocumented.

REFERENCES

Hwahng, S. J., & Nuttbrock, L. A. (2014). Adolescent gender-related abuse, androphilia, and HIV risk among transgender people of color in New York City. *Journal of Homosexuality, 61,* 691–713.

———. (2007). Sex workers, fem queens, and cross-dressers: Differential marginalizations and HIV vulnerabilities among three ethnocultural male-to-female transgender communities in New York City. *Sex Research and Social Policy, 4* (4), 36–59.

Kulick, D. (1998). *Travesti: Sex, gender, and culture among Brazilian transgendered prostitutes.* Chicago: University of Chicago Press.

Nadal, K. L., Davidoff, B. S., & Fujii-Doe, W. (2014). Transgender women and the sex work industry: Roots in systemic, institutional, and interpersonal discrimination. *Journal of Trauma and Dissociation, 15,* 169–183.

Nemoto, T., Iwamoto, M., Wong, S., Lem, M. N., & Operario, D. (2004). Social factors related to risk for violence and sexually transmitted infections/HIV among Asian massage parlor workers in San Francisco. *AIDS and Behavior, 8,* 475–483.

Nemoto, T., Operario, D., Keatly, J., Han L., & Somo, T. (2004). HIV risk behaviors among transgender women of color in San Francisco. *American Journal of Public Health, 94* (7), 1193–1199.

Prieur, A. (1998). *Mema's house, Mexico City: On transvestites, queens, and machos.* Chicago: University of Chicago Press.

Sausa, L. A., Keatley, J., & Operario, D. (2007). Perceived risks and benefits of sex work among transgender women of color in San Francisco. *Archives of Sexual Behavior, 36,* 768–777.

Strauss, A. L., & Corbin, J. M. (1990). *Basics of qualitative research: Grounded theory procedures and techniques.* Newbury Park, CA: Sage.

Weinberg, M. S., Shaver, F. M., & Williams, C. J. (1999). Gendered sex work in the San Francisco Tenderloin. *Archives of Sexual Behavior, 3,* 503–521.

Wilson, E. C., & Garofalo, R. (2009). Transgender female youth and sex work: HIV risk and comparisons of life factors related to engagement in sex work. *AIDS and Behavior, 13,* 902–913.

CHAPTER 2

Quantitative Description of Sex Work among Transwomen in New York City

Larry A. Nuttbrock[1]

1 Previously affiliated with the National Development and Research Institutes
(NDRI) and now a private consultant living in New York City.

SUMMARY

This chapter provides quantitative analysis of sex work among transwomen in New York City. Levels of sex work were shown to range from
low (fewer than 5 partners a month) to moderate (5 – 49 partners a
month) to high (50 – 400 partners a month); different demographic
and lifestyle factors were associated with these different levels. This
analysis, following Hwahng, highlights nonwhite ethnicity and its association with an early entry into the sex trade as strong predictors of
moderate and high levels of sex work. Early entry into the sex trade, in
turn, reduces the odds of completing high school and of being employed
during early adulthood, which further increase the odds of later life
involvement in sex work.

KEY TERMS

adolescent sex work: ethnicity; sexual orientation; transgender women;
unemployment

Chapter 1 provided a qualitative description of sex work among transgender women across three communities in New York City. In this
chapter I describe the antecedents and correlates of sex work among
transgender women in New York City using quantitative techniques.

Nuttbrock, Larry, *Transgender Sex Work and Society*
dx.doi.org/10.17312/harringtonparkpress/2017.11.tsws.002
© 2018 by Harrington Park Press

BACKGROUND

The analysis is guided by a selective review of the literature pertaining to factors that predispose or cause transwomen to become involved in the sex trade. Sex work among transwomen has been much discussed in the literature, and there have been a few qualitative studies, but quantitative specifications of factors associated with transgender sex work are rare. The rationale for selecting variables, and including them in the analysis, was based in part on the broader sex work literature and relevant theory.

SELECTIVE REVIEW OF THE LITERATURE

Background Variables

AGE As transgender women grow older, the physical capacity for sex work and the physical attributes necessary to attract paying partners may decline (Dalla, 2002). The younger generation, in particular, may be more inclined to engage in sex work (Reback et al., 2005).

ETHNICITY Because of their nonconforming gender presentation, combined with their status as ethnic minorities, transwomen of color are thought to be doubly disadvantaged in finding legitimate employment (Weinberg, Shaver, & Williams, 1999). Issues in finding employment are assumed to prompt these individuals to seek sex work instead (Boles & Elifson, 1994). Cultural traditions and permissive attitudes toward sex work in certain subgroups of transwomen of color may further increase their numbers in the sex trade. Two quantitative studies specifically analyzed ethnicity and sex work in this population. Among transwomen seeking social work services in Los Angeles, Hispanics were more likely than whites to report sex work (Reback et al., 2005). In a comparative study of transwomen and biological females arrested for sex work in Phoenix, Arizona, the latter were more likely to be white (Schepel, 2011).

NATIVITY Because of language barriers or other factors, transwomen born outside the United States may experience additional difficulties finding employment, and they may seek out sex work instead (Howe, Zaraysky, & Lorentzen, 2008). Immigrants from cultural contexts with long traditions of sex work among transwomen may drift into the sex trade regardless of economic factors (Infante, Sosa-Rubi, & Cuadra, 2009).

SEXUAL ORIENTATION According to Blanchard (1985), transwomen sexually attracted to men only (androphilic) are developmentally distinct from those attracted only to women, both men and women, or neither men nor women. Those who are androphilic are more likely to recall nonconforming gender behavior during childhood. As a result, they may enter adolescence with a greater tendency to present themselves as sex or gender nonconforming (Blanchard, 1985), which may potentially include an early debut of sexual behavior and perhaps sex work.

In some South American subcultures, almost all the transwomen sex workers (*travestis*) report preadolescent histories of erotic attraction to men (Kulick, 1998). After adolescence, they may engage in commercial sex, in part because they enjoy sex with men and, in the context of these sexual encounters, they may also affirm their sexual attractiveness and femininity (Kulick, 1998; Prieur, 1998).

SEX WORK DURING ADOLESCENCE While seldom specifically analyzed, it is frequently assumed that sex work during adolescence leads almost invariably to sex work during adulthood. This assumption resonates with a broader theory suggesting that problem or nonnormative behavior during adolescence, which would include sex work, interferes with early academic achievement and undermines socialization for involvement in mainstream society (Jessor, Donavon, & Costa, 1991).

FAILURE TO GRADUATE FROM HIGH SCHOOL Transgender women with low levels of education, in particular those who fail to complete high school, may lack the skills and credentials to compete for legitimate employment, which may then motivate them to become involved in the sex trade (Reback et al., 2005; Wilson & Garofalo, 2009).

UNEMPLOYMENT DURING ADULTHOOD A basic factor, assumed in much of this literature, is a lack of overlap between employment in the legitimate economy and sex work. Difficulties in finding or keeping employment and earning income legitimately are widely regarded as instigating factors for entry into the sex trade (Bockting, Robinson, & Rosser, 1998;

Grant, Mottel, & Tanis, 2011; Nadal, Davidoff, & Fujii-Doe, 2014; Sausa, Keatley, & Operario, 2007; Weinberg, Shaver, & Williams, 1999).

Alternatively, those earning an income in the sex trade may be less financially compelled to seek legitimate employment. The overlap (or lack of it) between employment and sex work, at a given time, probably depends on the volume of sex partners, there being less overlap among those with numerous partners.

Data Analytic Model
The above variables were conceptually organized as a causal sequence of factors whereby background variables lead to sex work during adolescence, which then leads to a failure to graduate from high school, subsequent unemployment, and ultimately sex work during adulthood.

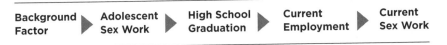

FIGURE 2.1
Causal model of factors leading to sex work among transwomen

My objective was to estimate the effects of predictor variables on current sex work, independent of the antecedent variables (if any) that may significantly bias or confound theses estimates. Age, ethnicity, nativity, and androphilic orientation were posited as intercorrelated exogenous variables; they have no antecedent effects. The effects of these background variables on current sex work were analyzed first. The effect of adolescent sex work on current sex work was then estimated with controls for the antecedent background factors. The effect of education on current sex work was then estimated with controls for current sex work and background variables. Finally, the association of employment and current sex work was estimated with controls for education, adolescent sex work, and the background variables.

METHOD
Transgender or gender-variant individuals were actively involved in all aspects and phases of this project, including the design of the instrument, data collection, data analysis, and dissemination of the findings.

The Institutional Review Board (IRB) of the National Development and Research Institutes (NDRI) approved all the research protocols.

Selection of Study Participants

From an initial pool of 571 transwomen recruited for the baseline component of the New York Transgender Project, 230 were randomly selected to further participate in a prospective study. The analysis reported here is based only on the initial follow-up interviews with these 230 individuals.

All those admitted to the study were medically assigned as male at birth but subsequently did not regard themselves as "completely male" in all situations or roles (reflecting an MTF/transfeminine spectrum). Eligibility criteria also included age of 19 through 59 and absence of psychotic ideation (e.g., gender-related delusions, such as seeing oneself as potentially becoming pregnant).

The study participants were initially recruited through transgender organizations in the New York metropolitan area, newspaper advertisements, the streets, clubs, referrals of other participants, and paid assistants from transgender communities who worked on a day-to-day basis with the field staff. Because one specific aim of this funded research was to identify incident cases of HIV, all the individuals selected for the prospective component were initially HIV-negative. Individuals determined to be HIV-negative were randomly selected for the prospective study, including an oversampling for younger age (under 30) and recent high-risk sexual behavior for HIV (unprotected receptive anal intercourse).

Statistical Technique and Modeling

The data were analyzed with multinomial logistic regression (Hosmer, Lemeshow, & Sturdivant, 2013) as implemented with version 9 of Stata. This is an extension of ordinary logistic regression that estimates the effects of predictor variables across categories of an outcome variable, one of the outcome categories being used as a reference category. The effects were expressed as relative risk ratios (RRR), which may be broadly interpreted as percentage differences (Hosmer, Lemeshow, & Sturdivant, 2013). The variables identified as causes or correlates of sex work among transwomen were used to predict low, moderate, and high levels of current sex work; no current sex work was used as the reference category.

Associations between the predictors shown in Figure 2.1 and levels of current sex work were estimated with controls for all those predictors (if any) posited as causally antecedent to the predictor variable under analysis. In much of this analysis, control variables were entered in a hierarchical manner. The basic association between employment and current sex work, for example, was recomputed with cumulative controls for (a) background variables, (b) background variables plus adolescent sex work, and (c) background variables plus adolescent sex work plus education. The effects of these sets of controls, as posited antecedent factors to a basic association, were judged by changes in the strength of the basic association as a result of including these controls (see Anashensel, 2013).

Measurements

Participants completed face-to-face interviews in conjunction with the Life Review of Transgender Experiences (LRTE). The English version of the LRTE was fully translated to Spanish, and 19% (44/230) were interviewed in Spanish with a fluent interviewer. The study participants were compensated $40 for completing the interview.

BACKGROUND VARIABLES

AGE was included as a continuous variable from 19 through 59. *Ethnicity* was coded using preestablished census categories. In some of the analysis, this was classified as non-Hispanic black (Black), Hispanic, or all other categories (Other), using non-Hispanic white (White) as a reference category. In most of the analysis, ethnicity was classified as non-white versus white. *Nativity* was measured by reports of being born outside the United States as compared to being born in the United States. *Sexual orientation* was assessed with queries about sexual attraction to different types of partners (males only; females only; both males and females; and neither males nor females). Those attracted to males only were coded as "androphilic"; those otherwise attracted were coded as "non-androphilic."

ADOLESCENT SEX WORK

In conjunction with the life chart interview (Lyketsos et al., 1994; Nuttbrock et al., 2010), participants were asked about paying sexual partners (if any) during early adolescence (ages 10 through 14) and during late adolescence (ages 15 through 18). Respondents indicating any such partners during either stage of adolescence were coded positive; those not reporting such a partner during early or late adolescence were coded as negative.

COMPLETION OF HIGH SCHOOL This factor was coded as completion of high school or higher, as compared to not completing high school.

CURRENT EMPLOYMENT This factor was assessed as working full- or part-time on any regular job (on or off the books) in the legitimate economy during the previous six months.

CURRENT SEX WORK Respondents were asked if they traded sex for money, drugs, or gifts during the previous month, and if they answered in the affirmative, they were asked about the number of different sexual partners. The responses were coded as "none" (no paying partner); "low" (1 through 4 partners); "moderate" (5 through 49 partners); and "high" (50 through 400 partners).

RESULTS

More than half (54.5%) of the participants were 19 through 30 years of age; 45.5% were 31 through 59 years of age. Reports of ethnicity were White (35.2%); Hispanic (35.7%); Black (17.4%); and Other (11.7%). About two-thirds (64.8%) were classified as nonwhite (which included Hispanics, Blacks, and Other). Fewer than one-fourth (22.4%) were foreign-born; 58.9% were classified as androphilic; and 24.1% reported engaging in sex work during adolescence. More than half (57.8%) graduated from high school, and a similar percentage (53.0%) indicated current employment. More than half (60.9%) reported no sex work during the previous six months; 12.2%, 16.5%, and 10.4%, respectively, were classified as engaging in low, moderate, or high levels of current sex work.

Bivariate Associations of Study Variables

Pairwise correlations among the study variables are presented in the appendix to this chapter. Ethnicity was associated with most of the other variables. Nonwhite ethnicity was positively associated with nativity, androphilia, and sex work during adolescence and adulthood. Being nonwhite was negatively associated with high school education and current employment. To better specify how combinations of ethnicity and other variables affect adult sex work, a sequence of analyses was conducted taking advantage of theory and the causal model shown in Figure 2.1.

Background Variables with Current Sex Work

Associations of the background variables and current levels of sex work are summarized in Table 2.1. A low level of sex work was associated with being younger (RRR = .96), black (RRR = 6.08), Hispanic (RRR = 6.09), and androphilic (RRR = 3.17) in a bivariate analysis. This level of sex work was associated with being black (RRR = 5.32) and Hispanic (RRR = 5.29) in a multivariate analysis (with all background variables included simultaneously).

A moderate level of sex work was associated with being younger (RRR = .96), Hispanic (RRR = 10.48), foreign-born (RRR = 2.90), and androphilic (RRR = 7.85) in a bivariate analysis. This level of sex work was associated with being Hispanic (RRR = 6.91) and androphilic (RRR = 3.61) in a multivariate analysis.

A high level of sex work was associated with being younger (RRR = .91), black (RRR = 10.29), Hispanic (RRR = 20.57), foreign-born (RRR = 2.59), and androphilic (RRR = 8.87) in a bivariate analysis. This level of sex work was associated with being younger (RRR = .94) and Hispanic (RRR = 11.98) in the multivariate analysis.

With the exceptions of age and androphilia as predictors of high and moderate levels of sex work, respectively, nonwhite ethnicity (especially Hispanic) was the dominant predictor of all levels of sex work. To improve interpretation of the results, ethnicity (coded as Nonwhite versus White) was included and controlled as the sole indicator of the background variables in the remainder of the analysis.

Adolescent Sex Work with Current Sex Work

The uncontrolled and controlled associations of adolescent sex work and current sex work are displayed in Table 2.2. Adolescent sex work was associated with low (RRR = 3.89), moderate (RRR = 5.60), and high (RRR = 5.92) levels of current sex work. Controlling for ethnicity, these associations were reduced by approximately 50%. These numbers suggest that the association between adolescent sex work and adult sex work largely reflects the antecedent effects of ethnicity.

TABLE 2.1

Background Variables with Current Sex Work

	CURRENT SEX WORK		
	LOW	MODERATE	HIGH
BIVARIATE			
Age	.96*	.96**	.91**
Ethnicity			
White (reference)	—	—	—
Black	6.08**	3.38	10.29**
Hispanic	6.09**	10.48**	20.57**
Other	2.42	3.55	3.55
Foreign-born	1.81	2.90**	2.59*
Androphilic	3.17*	7.85**	8.87**
MULTIVARIATE			
Age	.99	.99	.94*
Ethnicity			
White (reference)	—	—	—
Black	5.32*	1.25	4.79
Hispanic	5.29*	6.91**	11.98**
Other	2.66	2.02	1.52
Foreign-born	1.18	.98	1.25
Androphilic	1.35	3.61*	2.23

NOTE: Relative risk ratios based on multinomial logistic regression. No sex work is the reference category. Base N = 230.
*$p < .05$. **$p < .01$.

TABLE 2.2

Adolescent Sex Work with Current Sex Work

	CURRENT SEX WORK		
	LOW	MODERATE	HIGH
Adolescent sex work	3.89*	5.60**	5.92**
Ethnicity controlled	2.19	2.95**	2.09

NOTE. Relative risk ratios based on multinomial logistic regression. No current sex work is the reference category. Base N = 230.
*$p < .05.$ **$p < .01.$

Completion of High School with Current Sex Work

The uncontrolled and controlled associations of education and current sex work are shown in Table 2.3. Completion of high school was associated with a reduced likelihood of a moderate level of current sex work (RRR = .29). This basic association was reduced by approximately 40% (RRR increased toward the null value of 1.00) with ethnicity included; only a small further reduction in the basic association resulted from adding adolescent sex work to the controls. Completion of high school, according to these data, significantly reduces the likelihood of engaging in a moderate level of sex work during adulthood, but this association partially reflects the prior effect of ethnicity.

TABLE 2.3

Completion of High School with Current Sex Work

	CURRENT SEX WORK		
	LOW	MODERATE	HIGH
Completion of high school	.56	.29**	1.11
Hierarchical controls			
Ethnicity	.71	.38**	2.05
Adolescent sex work	.79	.40*	2.36

NOTE. Relative risk ratios based on multinomial logistic regression. No sex work is the reference category. Base N = 230.
*$p < .05.$ **$p < .01.$

Current Employment with Current Sex Work

The uncontrolled and controlled associations of current employment with current sex work are shown in Table 2.4. In the uncontrolled analysis, current employment was strongly associated with moderate (RRR = .10) and high (RRR = .12) levels of current sex work (i.e., the employed were about 90% less likely to be involved with these levels of sex work). These associations were reduced (RRR increased toward the null value of 1.00) with ethnicity included as a control; only small further reductions in the basic association resulted from including adolescent sex work and high school completion as controls. Current employment, according to these data, strongly reduces the likelihood of engaging in moderate or high levels of sex work, but this association is partially the result of the antecedent effect of ethnicity.

TABLE 2.4

Current Employment with Current Sex Work

	CURRENT SEX WORK		
	LOW	MODERATE	HIGH
Current unemployment	.46	.10**	.12**
Hierarchical controls			
Ethnicity	.64	.14**	.19**
Adolescent sex work	.62	.13**	.19**
High school completion	.63	.14**	.17**

NOTE. Relative risk ratios based on multinomial logistic regression. No sex work is the reference category. Base N = 230.
$*p < .05. **p < .01.$

DISCUSSION

This chapter set out to identify and statistically evaluate key demographic, economic, and lifestyle factors associated with sex work among transwomen in New York City. A basic finding was that predictors of sex work in this population varied by level of sex work. A low level of sex work (1 through 4 partners a month) may be characterized as "recreational." A few paying partners a month may reflect situational or motivational factors largely independent of demographic or economic issues. A high level of sex work (50 through 400 partners), in contrast, while strongly linked to ethnicity and current employment, was not a function of educational attainment. Having many paying sex partners a month may be driven by factors not included in the analysis (e.g., substance use).

These data consistently highlight the significance of ethnicity as a fundamental factor leading to sex work among transgender women in New York City. Very few of the white respondents reported a moderate level of sex work, and almost none of them reported a high level of sex work. On the other hand, Hispanic individuals in particular were much more likely to report moderate (RRR = 10.48) or high levels (RRR = 20.57) of sex work (see Table 2.1).

The strength of ethnicity as a risk factor for sex work reflects, in large part, its association with most of the variables identified in the literature as correlates or causes of sex work among transwomen. Nonwhite ethnicity was associated with sex work during adolescence, failure to graduate from high school, and current unemployment, all of which combined to affect current sex work.

The extent to which these findings regarding ethnicity and sex work among transgender women can be generalized to areas other than New York City is unknown. The sample of transgender women analyzed here was 35.7% Hispanic, 65.8% of whom were born in a foreign country, primarily Mexico or a country in South America.[2] Prior ethnographic studies of transgender women in Mexico and South America suggest that they may have been socialized in early life to engage in sex work and pursue economic life outside mainstream institutions (Kulick, 1998; Parker, 1991; Preiur, 1998). These and related issues pertaining to ethnicity and sex work among transgender women will be further developed in the next chapter.

Intercorrelation Matrix of Study Variables

	1	2	3	4	5	6	7	8
1. Age	1.00							
2. Nonwhite ethnicity	−49**	1.00						
3. Foreign-born	−.06	.29**	1.00					
4. Androphilic	−.39**	.66**	.27**	.1.00				
5. Adolescent sex work	−.39**	.40**	−.03	−.30**	1.00			
6. H.S. education	.21**	−.21**	−.02	−.12	−.26	1.00		
7. Current employment	.25**	−.35**	−.14*	−.33**	−.18**	.15**	1.00	
8. Current sex work[a]	−.29**	.40**	.19**	37**	.33**	−.16**	−.39**	1.00

[a] Measured here as any level of sex work.
$*p < .05$. $**p < .01$.

NOTES

Support for the research described in this chapter was obtained in conjunction with grant R01 DA018080 from the National Institute on Drug Abuse.

1. Specific countries of origin were not determined, but field researchers indicated that most of the Hispanics emigrated from Mexico or South America.

REFERENCES

Anashensel, C. S. (2013). *Theory-based data analysis for the social sciences* (2nd ed.). Thousand Oaks, CA: Sage.

Blanchard, R. (1985). Typology of male-to-female transexualism. *Archives of Sexual Behavior, 14,* 247–261.

Bockting, W. O., Robinson, B. E., & Rosser, B. R. S. (1998). Transgender HIV prevention: A qualitative needs assessment. *AIDS Care, 10,* 505–526.

Boles, J., & Elifson, K. W. (1994). Transvestic prostitution and AIDS. *Social Science and Medicine, 39,* 85–93.

Dalla, R. (2002). Night moves: A qualitative assessment of street-level sex work. *Psychology of Women Quarterly, 26* (1), 63–73.

Grant, J. M., Mottel, L. A., & Tanis, J. (2011). *Injustice at every turn: A report of the National Transgender Discrimination Survey.* Washington, DC: National Center for Transgender Equality and National Gay and Lesbian Task Force.

Hosmer, D. W., Lemeshow, W., & Sturdivant, R. X. (2013). *Applied logistic regression* (3rd ed.). Hoboken, NJ: John Wiley & Sons.

Howe, C., Zaraysky, K., & Lorentzen, L. (2008). Transgender sex workers and sexual transmigration between Guadalajara and San Francisco. *Latin American Perspectives, 35,* 31–50.

Hwahng, S. J., & Nuttbrock, L. A. (2014). Adolescent gender-related abuse, androphilia, and HIV risk among transgender people of color in New York City. *Journal of Homosexuality, 61,* 691–713.

———. (2007). Sex workers, fem queens, and cross-dressers: Differential marginalizations and HIV vulnerabilities among three ethnocultural male-to-female transgender communities in New York City. *Sex Research and Social Policy, 4* (4), 36–59.

Infante, C., Sosa-Rubi, S. G., & Cuadra, S. M. (2009). Sex work in Mexico: Vulnerability of male, *travesti,* transgender and transsexual sex workers. *Culture, Health & Sexuality, 11* (2), 125–137.

Jessor, R., Donavon, J. E., & Costa, F. M. (1991). *Beyond adolescence: Problem behavior and young adult development.* Cambridge: Cambridge University Press.

Kulick, D. (1998). *Travesti: Sex, gender, and culture among Brazilian transgendered prostitutes.* Chicago: University of Chicago Press.

Lyketsos, C., Nestadt, G., Cwi, J., Heithoff, K., & Eaton, W. W. (1994). The life chart interview: A structured method to describe the course of psychopathology. *International Journal of Methods in Psychiatric Research, 4,* 133–145.

Nadal, K. L., Davidoff, B. S., & Fujii-Doe, W. (2014). Transgender women and the sex work industry: Roots in systemic, institutional, and interpersonal discrimination. *Journal of Trauma and Dissociation, 15,* 169–183.

Nuttbrock, L. A., Bockting, W. O., Mason, M., Hwahng, S., Rosenblum, A., Macri, M., & Becker, J. (2011). A further analysis of Blanchard's homosexual versus nonhomosexual or autogynephilic gender dysphoria. *Archives of Sexual Behavior, 44,* 247–257.

Nuttbrock, L. A., Bockting, W. O., Rosenblum, A., Hwahng, S., Mason, M., Macri, M., & Becker, J. (2010). Psychiatric impact of gender-related abuse across the life course of male-to-female transgender persons. *Journal of Sex Research, 47,* 12–23.

Parker, R. G. (1991). *Bodies, pleasures, and passions: Sexual culture in contemporary Brazil.* Boston: Beacon Press.

Prieur, A. (1998). *Mema's house: On transvestites, queens, and machos.* Chicago: University of Chicago Press.

Reback, C. J., Lombardi, E. L., Simon, P. A., & Frye, D. M. (2005). HIV seroprevalence and risk behaviors among transgender women who exchange sex in comparison with those who do not. *In* J. D. Parsons (ed.), *Contemporary research on sex work* (pp. 5–22). New York: Haworth Press.

Sausa, L. A., Keatley, J., & Operario, D. (2007). Perceived risks and benefits of sex work among transgender women of color in San Francisco. *Archives of Sexual Behavior, 36,* 768–777.

Schepel, E. (2011). A comparative study of adult transgender and female prostitution. Master's thesis, Arizona State University.

Weinberg, M. S., Shaver, E. M., & Williams, C. J. (1999). Gendered sex work in the San Francisco Tenderloin. *Archives of Sexual Behavior, 3,* 503–521.

Wilson, E. C., & Garofalo, R. (2009). Transgender female youth and sex work: HIV risk and comparisons of life factors related to engagement in sex work. *AIDS and Behavior, 13,* 902–913.

CHAPTER 3

Why Are So Many Transwomen in the Sex Trade, and Why Are So Many of Them Ethnic Minorities?

Larry A. Nuttbrock[1]
Sel J. Hwahng[2]

1 Previously affiliated with the National Development and Research Institutes (NDRI) and now a private consultant living in New York City.
2 Adjunct associate professor in the Women and Gender Studies Department at Hunter College – City University of New York.

SUMMARY

Building on the qualitative and quantitative descriptions of sex work in Chapters 1 and 2, the two of us (LN and SH) collaborate here in a further analysis of two fundamental issues: the high proportion of transwomen who engage in sex work and the high proportion of transwomen sex workers who are ethnic minorities.

KEY TERMS

androphilia; cumulative disadvantages; ethnic minorities; racism; transgender sex workers; underground economy; urban poverty

Prior studies have reported extremely high numbers of transwomen with histories of involvement in the sex trade, but these numbers have seldom been the focus of inquiry, and alternative explanations for sex work in this population have seldom been delineated and examined. To understand the high prevalence of transgender women in the sex trade, the life course model developed in Chapter 2 will be expanded to include a predisposition for sex work in a subgroup of transwomen (androphilics) and factors

Nuttbrock, Larry, *Transgender Sex Work and Society*
dx.doi.org/10.17312/harringtonparkpress/2017.11.tsws.003
© 2018 by Harrington Park Press

associated with urban poverty that may further perpetuate sex work across the life course and perhaps across generations.

Understanding the high numbers of transgender sex workers who are ethnic minorities will be approached in terms of how the above explanations for sex work are intertwined with ethnicity. Both of us, in Chapters 1 and 2, suggested a type of "double jeopardy" in which being transgender and an ethnic minority may combine to produce socioeconomic disadvantages across the life course, which may partially account for the higher levels of sex work among nonwhites compared to whites. This perspective will be broadened to include ethnic differences in a tendency for sex work as a result of androphilia and the overlay of racism with social class in American society.

HIGH PREVALENCE OF SEX WORK AMONG TRANSWOMEN

Current estimates suggest that less than 1% to 7% of women in the United States and worldwide have engaged in some type of sex work; available estimates of male sex work approach one-half of those for female sex work (Vandepitte et al., 2006; ProCon.org, 2013). The proportions of transwomen who engage in sex work (as summarized below) are, by comparison, several times higher.[1]

The six-month prevalence of sex work was 37.4% in our study of transwomen from the New York metropolitan area (Nuttbrock et al., 2013). Lifetime histories of sex work in this population have been estimated as 80% in San Francisco (Clements-Nolle et al., 2001); 25%–75% in a meta-analysis across geographic areas mostly in the United States (Operario, Soma, & Underhill, 2008); 54%–80% in Asia and the Pacific region (Winter, 2012). Even in some cultural settings that recognize sexes other than male and female, such as the *hijras* in India, reports of sex work exceed 50% (Nanda, 1999).

Cumulative Disadvantages across the Life Course

Informed by theory (Jessor, Donavon, & Costa, 1991), Chapter 2 presented data suggesting that sex work during adolescence leads to a reduced likelihood of graduating from high school, which then leads to unemployment during adulthood, followed by a continuation of sex work. We will broaden this perspective to include sexual selection into the sex trade and issues associated with urban poverty.

Selection of Androphilics into the Sex Trade

Most studies of transwomen suggest that they are diverse with regard to sexual orientation. In our study of 571 transgender women from the New York City area (Nuttbrock et al., 2010), 69.4% were sexually attracted to men only (androphilic); 16.1% were attracted to both men and women (androphilic/gynephilic); 12.4% were attracted to women only (gynephilic); and 2.1% were attracted to neither men nor women (asexual).[2] The proportion of transwomen (biological men) attracted solely to men in this study (androphilics), 69.4%, far exceeds estimates of the proportion of men sexually attracted to men in the US adult population (estimates typically range from 3% to 6%) (see, for example, Laumann et al., 1994).

Other researchers have suggested that biological males who are sexually attracted to other males (androphilics) may present themselves as women (cross-dress), and perhaps become transwomen, in an attempt to gain sexual access to other men. Some of these writers further suggest that androphilics may enter the sex trade as a way of further increasing their sexual access to men.[3]

Since the early nineteenth century, according to Bullough and Bullough (1993), one of the motivations for cross-dressing by males has been to solicit other males for sexual encounters. This proposition has been elaborated on in Bailey's (2003) much-read albeit highly controversial work.[4] He suggested that androphilic males present themselves as women, and perhaps undergo sexual-reassignment surgery, because it is only by "being a woman" that their desire for other (heterosexual) men can be adequately met (p. 146). Because of their erotic attraction to other males and their desire for a large number of sexual encounters with them, the subset of transwomen attracted only to men (androphilic or "homosexual") was characterized as "well-suited for sex work" (Bailey, 2003, p. 211).

Ethnographies of transwomen in Brazil (Kulick, 1998) and Mexico City (Prieur, 1998) and a later study in New York City by the two of us (Hwahng & Nuttbrock, 2014) suggest that androphilia and sex work may be intertwined as a result of early development. When Kulick (1998, p. 24) queried Brazilian *travestis* about early experiences regarding gender identification, they invariably described being anally penetrated during childhood or early adolescence by an older boy or man. These early sexual encounters, while initially traumatic, were followed by urges to repeat them, a growing sense of themselves as feminine, and a need to be seen as such by others. During puberty, childhood experiences of sexuality and gender coalesced to form an identity as a *viado* ("homosexual")[5] and a commitment to feminize one's body, mostly using silicone implants. These early-life experiences, termed developmental homosexuality, were invariably intertwined with a life trajectory of oneself as a travesti (feminine-appearing sex worker). Early experiences of being penetrated by a man and experiencing oneself as a desirable "female" were seen as fundamentally intertwined with sex work.

This model of early-life anal penetration by a male followed by perception of oneself as a homosexual (*joto*) and involvement in the sex trade has been largely replicated in Mexico City by Prieur (1998), and aspects of it have been observed among transwomen of color in New York City (many of whom were Hispanic) (Hwahng & Nuttbrock, 2014). The study participants in New York City, like those in Brazil and Mexico, recalled early-life encounters of being penetrated by an older boy or man, and these experiences were construed as one of the factors causing them to become sex workers. These qualitative findings from different geographic areas, and the earlier works by Bullough and Bullough (1993) and Bailey (2003), broadly point to androphilia as a factor underlying sex work among transwomen.

To quantitatively assess this general hypothesis, we examined the association between sexual orientation (as categorized above) and levels of current sex work. The data were obtained in conjunction with the study of transwomen from the New York City area that was introduced in Chapter 2 (Nuttbrock et al., 2010, 2013). Methodological details for the current analysis are presented in Chapter 11. The analysis here excluded individuals classified as asexual and those indicating an ethnicity other than white, Hispanic, or black (N = 505). Level of sex work was scaled as none (0 partners), low (1 through 4 partners), moderate (5 through 49 partners), and high (50 or more partners).

As Table 3.1 shows, a significant minority of those classified as androphilic were currently involved in low (13.4%), moderate (17.6%), and high (15.6%) levels of sex work. These percentages were reduced by more than 50% among those classified as androphilic/gynephilic, and by more than 75% among those classified as gynephilic.

To evaluate the specific hypothesis that androphilia during adolescence further escalates life-course disadvantages, the association between

TABLE 3.1

Sexual Orientation with Levels of Current Sex Work (Percentages)

	LEVELS OF SEX WORK			
	NONE	LOW	MODERATE	HIGH
Androphilic (N = 358)	53.4	13.4	17.6	15.6
Androphilic/gynephilic (N = 83)	77.1	7.2	7.2	8.4
Gynephilic (N = 64)	95.3	3.1	1.6	0.0

NOTE: Total N = 505 (no missing cases). Chi-square = 50.32; p < .001.

androphilia and recollection of sex work during adolescence was examined. As Table 3.2 shows, sex work during adolescence was reported by 41.1% of those classified as androphilic, by 16.9% of those classified as androphilic/gynephilic, and by 1.6% of those classified as gynephilic. These data suggest that the life-course model of sex work, where sex work in adolescence leads to socioeconomic disadvantages and continued sex work in adulthood, applies primarily to those with an androphilic sexual orientation.

Underground Economy and Urban Poverty

Transwomen are diverse in terms of occupation, education, and income (Institute of Medicine, 2011), but socioeconomic inequality and marginalized lifestyles were nonetheless major themes running through the qualitative studies of transwomen reviewed above (Kulick, 1998; Prieur, 1998; Hwahng & Nuttbrock, 2007, 2014). Many of those involved in sex work may reside in or drift into urban areas characterized by an underground economy, a lack of nearby employment opportunities, and perhaps a culture of poverty that emphasizes survival needs and short-term interests at the expense of long-term goals and planning (Gilbert, 2015; Small, Harding & Lamont, 2010; Wacquant, 2008).

An underground economy typically occurs in the context of urban poverty, where opportunities for mainstream employment are scarce (Wilson, 1987, 1996). The jobs that do exist are typically low-paying, and transwomen may rationally choose to engage in illegal activities, including sex work, because of its comparatively higher income potential (Charles, 2008). In the context of unavailable employment, traditions of

TABLE 3.2

Sexual Orientation with Sex Work during Adolescence (Percentages)

	ADOLESCENT SEX WORK
Androphilic (N = 353)	41.1
Androphilic/gynephilic (N = 83)	16.9
Gynephilic (N = 64)	1.6

NOTE: Total N = 500; 5 missing cases for adolescent sex work. Chi-square = 56.0; $p < .001$.

obtaining income illegally, including sex work, may be legitimated and perhaps socially encouraged (Young, 2004).[6]

In sum, the high numbers of transwomen in the sex trade may arise from multiple factors, including cumulative disadvantages across the life course, sexual selection into the sex trade as a result of androphilia, and (for some) issues associated with urban poverty.

HIGH NUMBERS OF ETHNIC MINORITY TRANSWOMEN IN THE SEX TRADE

Associations of ethnicity and current sex work were presented in Chapter 2 using a sample of 230 transwomen from the New York Transgender Project (Nuttbrock et al., 2010, 2013) and multinomial logistic regression. Cross-tabulations of ethnicity with level of sex work during the previous six months are presented here for the broader sample of 505 transgender women.

As Table 3.3 shows, only small percentages of whites were currently involved in low (5.0%), moderate (2.8%), or high (.7%) levels of sex work. Significant percentages of Hispanics were involved in low (12.7%), moderate (20.5%), and high (20.1%) levels of sex work. Significant, albeit somewhat lower, percentages of blacks were involved in low (15.0%), moderate (13.3%), and high (10.8%) levels of sex work.

Double Jeopardy for Cumulative Disadvantages across the Life Course
In Chapter 2 we presented data suggesting that sex work during adolescence may lead to a failure to graduate from high school, unemploy-

TABLE 3.3

Ethnicity with Level of Sex Work (Percentages)

	LEVELS OF SEX WORK			
	NONE	LOW	MODERATE	HIGH
White (N = 141)	91.5	5.0	2.8	.7
Hispanic (N = 244)	46.7	12.7	20.5	20.1
Black (N = 120)	60.8	15.0	13.3	10.8

NOTE: Total N = 505 (no missing cases). Chi-square = 83.05; $p < .001$.

ment during adulthood, followed by continued sex work. Nonwhite transwomen may be doubly disposed to this sequence of events because a higher proportion of them engaged in sex work during adolescence.

Data shown in Table 3.4 indeed suggest that ethnicity is strongly associated with sex work during adolescence. Only a few of the whites (2.8%) recalled sex work during adolescence, compared to almost one-half of the Hispanics (43.4%) and blacks (44.4%). Data presented in Chapter 2 suggested that, independent of sex work, ethnicity is associated with a failure to graduate from high school and unemployment during early adulthood.

TABLE 3.4

Ethnicity with Sex Work during Adolescence (Percentages)

	SEX WORK DURING ADOLESCENCE
White (N = 141)	2.8
Hispanic (N = 244)	43.4
Black (N = 120)	44.4

NOTE:. Total N = 505 (no missing cases). Chi-square = 77.6; $p < .001$.

Ethnicity and Selection of Androphilics into the Sex Trade

Ethnicity is associated not just with sex work during adolescence, which then sets in motion life-course disadvantages; it is also associated with androphilia, which further escalates these processes. As Table 3.5 shows, 19.9% of the whites were classified as androphilic, compared with 91.0% of the blacks and 90.0% of the Hispanics who were so classified. In contrast, 40.4% of the whites were classified as gynephilic, compared to 1.6% of the blacks and 2.5% of the Hispanics who were so classified.

TABLE 3.5

Ethnicity with Sexual Orientation

	SEXUAL ORIENTATION		
	ANDROPHILIC	ANDROPHILIC/ GYNEPHILIC	GYNEPHILIC
White (N = 141)	19.9	39.7	40.4
Hispanic (N = 244)	90.0	7.5	2.5
Black (N = 120)	91.0	7.4	1.6

NOTE: Total N = 505 (no missing cases). Chi-square = 255.3; $p < .001$.

To compare the independent effects of sexual orientation and ethnicity on sex work, multinomial logistic regression models (Hosmer, Lemeshow, & Sturdivant, 2013) were estimated to predict low (1 through 20 partners) and high (21 or more partners) levels of sex work, using no sex work (0 partners) as the reference category for this outcome variable. As Table 3.6 shows, when androphilia was used as the reference category (for a predictor variable), androphilia/gynephilia and gynephilia were associated with lower likelihoods of low (relative risk ratios of −.97 and −2.43) and high (relative risk ratios of −1.11 and −3.36) levels of sex work. When white was used as the reference category, Hispanics and blacks were associated with increased likelihoods of low (relative risk ratios of 1.98 and 1.65) and high (relative risk ratios of 3.40 and 2.50) levels of sex work.

A multivariate analysis of both sexual orientation and ethnicity as predictors of sex work (lower section of Table 3.6) showed that ethnicity remained statistically significant, and the effects of sexual orientation were no longer statistically significant. This finding suggests that sexual

TABLE 3.6

Sexual Orientation and Ethnicity with Levels of Sex Work

	LEVELS OF SEX WORK[a]	
	LOW	HIGH
BIVARIATE		
Sexual orientation		
Androphilic (reference)	—	—
Androphilic/gynephilic	-.97**	-1.11**
Gynephilic		-3.36**
Ethnicity		
White (reference)	—	—
Hispanic	1.98**	3.40**
Black	1.65**	2.50**
MULTIVARIATE		
Sexual orientation		
Androphilic (reference)	—	—
Androphilic/gynephilic	-.17	.09
Gynephilic	-1.36	-1.56
Ethnicity		
White (reference)	—	—
Hispanic	1.54*	3.06**
Black	1.21*	2.16**

NOTE: Base N = 505 ("other" ethnic category and asexuals not included). Relative risk ratios based on multinomial logistic regression.

[a] No sex work is the reference category. Low sex work was defined as 1–20 paying partners during the previous six months; high sex work was defined as 21 or more paying partners during the previous six months.

* $P<.05.$**$P<.01.$

orientation is an intervening variable between ethnicity and sex work (i.e., ethnicity leads to sexual orientation, which then leads to sex work). For the logic underlying such an analysis, see Anashensel (2013).

Urban Poverty and Racism in American Society

Studies of inequality and poverty in large American inner cities show that these areas disproportionately comprise ethnic minorities (Wilson, 1987). Issues associated with urban poverty that perpetuate sex work in these areas (as reviewed above) should therefore be viewed as intertwined with racism. Racism in American society may function as an overarching factor that compounds socioeconomic disadvantages, selection into the sex trade, especially during adolescence (perhaps because involvement in mainstream institutions is not seen as realistic), and issues associated with urban poverty.

Race is a fundamental element in structuring and representing the social world in which racial formations organize and distribute resources along particular racial lines (Omi & Winant, 2015). Racism is indeed crucial to understanding the United States: the colonization of America did not create race; instead, race and racialization produced America. Racism is not only a fundamental cultural structure but also the foundation of class structure (Martinot, 2003).

NOTES

1. The supply of transwomen's sex work is by definition matched by the demand for these services, and various explanations have been suggested about why certain individuals may be inclined to seek these services (and transwomen more generally). Some men may be drawn to the idea of sex with another man but are reluctant to choose a male partner and instead seek out a partner who appears to be female (Prestage, 1994). Other reasons for sexual interest in gender-ambiguous or transgender persons have been suggested, including the possibility that this attraction may be a variant of autogynephilia (Blanchard & Collins, 1993). Recent research suggests that such attraction may represent a distinct form of sexual desire (Hsu et al., 2015; Weinberg & Williams, 2010).
2. In an early study in San Francisco (Clements-Nolle et al., 2001), sexual orientation was assessed from the standpoint of the respondent's adopted gender (presumably female). The majority (69%) of these transwomen identified themselves as "heterosexual," suggesting a sexual attraction to men.
3. Although a small number of women buy sex, the vast majority of individuals who pay for sex are males (ProCon.org, 2016).

4. Bailey's research has been widely criticized on both methodological and ethical grounds, but some of his concepts and predictions may nonetheless have scientific merit (Dreger, 2008).

5. In parts of Brazil and in some other countries, homosexuality has been understood as what one does sexually (being sexually penetrated), not an underlying disposition or identity (Kulick, 1998).

6. It is noteworthy that Lewis's (1961) classic study of the culture of poverty took place in a suburb of Mexico City that was later the location for Prieur's (1998) ethnography.

REFERENCES

Anashensel, C. S. (2013). *Theory-based data analysis for the social sciences* (2nd ed.). Thousand Oaks, CA: Sage.

Bailey, J. M. (2003). *The man who would be queen: The science of gender-bending and transsexualism*. Washington, DC: Joseph Henry Press.

Blanchard, R., & Collins, P. I. (1993). Men with sexual interest in transvestites, transsexuals, and she-males. *Journal of Nervous and Mental Disease, 181,* 570–573.

Bullough, V. L., & Bullough, B. (1993). *Cross dressing, sex, and gender*. Philadelphia: University of Pennsylvania Press.

Charles, M. (2008). Culture and inequality: Identity, ideology, and difference in "postascriptive society." *Annals of the American Academy of Political and Social Science, 619,* 41–58.

Clements-Nolle, K., Marx, R., Guzman, R., & Katz, M. (2001). HIV prevalence, risk behaviors, health care use, and mental health status of transgender persons: Implications for public health intervention. *American Journal of Public Health, 91,* 915–921.

Dreger, A. D. (2008). The controversy surrounding *The Man Who Would Be Queen*: A case history of the politics of science, identity, and sex in the Internet age. *Archives of Sexual Behavior, 37,* 361–422.

Gilbert, D. (2015). *The American class structure in an age of growing inequality* (9th ed.). Thousand Oaks, CA: Sage.

Hosmer, D. W., Lemeshow, W., & Sturdivant, R. X. (2013). *Applied logistic regression* (3rd ed.). Hoboken, NJ: John Wiley & Sons.

Hsu, K. J., Rosenthal, A. M., Miller, D. I., & Bailey, J. M. (2015, October 26). Who are gynandromorphophilic men? Characterizing men with sexual interest in transgender women. *Psychological Medicine,* published online (9 pp.). Retrieved from http://d-miller.github.io/assets/HsuEtAl2015.pdf.

Hwahng, S. J., & Nuttbrock, L. (2014). Adolescent gender-related abuse, androphilia, and HIV risk among transgender people of color in New York City. *Journal of Homosexuality, 61,* 691–713.

———. (2007). Sex workers, fem queens, and cross-dressers: Differential marginalizations and HIV vulnerabilities among three ethnocultural male-to-female transgender communities in New York City. *Sex Research and Social Policy, 4* (4), 36–39.

Institute of Medicine. (2011). *The health of lesbian, bisexual, and transgender persons: Building a foundation for understanding.* Washington, DC: National Academy of Science.

Jessor, R., Donavon, J. E., & Costa, F. M. (1991). *Beyond adolescence: Problem behavior and young adult development.* Cambridge: Cambridge University Press.

Kulick, D. (1998). *Travesti: Sex, gender, and culture among Brazilian transgendered prostitutes.* Chicago: University of Chicago Press.

Laumann, E. O., Gagnon, J. H., Michael, R. T., & Michaels, S. (1994). *The social organization of sexuality: Sexual practices in the United States.* Chicago: University of Chicago Press.

Lewis, O. (1961). *The children of Sanchez: Autobiography of a Mexican family.* New York: Random House.

Martinot, S. (2003). *Rule of racialization: Class, identity, governance.* Philadelphia: Temple University Press.

Nanda, S. (1999). *Neither man nor woman: The* hijras *of India* (2nd ed.). Belmont, CA: Wadsworth.

Nuttbrock, L. A., Bockting, W. O., Rosenblum, A., Hwahng, S., Mason, M., Macri, M., & Becker, J. (2013). Gender abuse, depressive symptoms, and HIV and other sexually transmitted infections among male-to-female transgender persons: A three-year prospective study. *American Journal of Public Health, 103,* 300–307.

Nuttbrock, L. A., Hwahng, S., Bockting, W. O., Rosenblum, A., Mason, M., Macri, M., & Becker, J. (2010). Psychiatric impact of gender-related abuse across the life course of male-to-female transgender persons. *Journal of Sex Research, 47,* 12–23.

Omi, M., & Winant, H. (2015). *Racial formation in the United States* (3rd ed.). New York: Routledge.

Operario, D., Soma, T., & Underhill, K. (2008). Sex work and HIV status among transgender women: Systematic review and meta-analysis. *Journal of Acquired Immunodeficiency Syndrome, 48* (1), 97–103.

Prestage, G. (1994). Male and transsexual prostitution. *In* R. Perkins (ed.), *Sex work and sex workers in Australia* (pp. 58–92). Sydney: University of New South Wales Press.

Prieur, A. (1998). *Mema's house: On transvestites, queens, and machos.* Chicago: University of Chicago Press.

ProCon.org. (2016, July 20). Percentage of men (by country) who paid for sex at least once. Retrieved from http://prostitution.procon.org/view.resource.php?resourceID=004119.

———. (2013, August 25). How many prostitutes are there in the United States and the rest of the world? Retrieved from http://prostitution.procon.org/view.answers.php?questionID=000095.

Slaman, K. (1998). Transgenders and sex work in Malaysia. *In* K. Kempadoo and J. Doezema (eds.), *Global sex workers* (pp. 210–214). New York: Routledge.

Small, M. L., Harding D. J., & Lamont, M. (2010). Reconsidering culture and poverty. *Annals of the American Academy of Political and Social Science, 629,* 6–29.

Vandepitte, J., Lyerla, R., Dallabetta, G., Crabbe, F., Alary, M., & Bave, A. (2006). Estimates of the number of female sex workers in different regions of the world. *Sexually Transmitted Infections, 82* (suppl. 3), iii18–iii25.

Wacquant, L. (2008). *Urban outcasts: A comparative sociology of advanced marginality.* Malden, MA: Polity Press.

Weinberg, M. S., & Williams, C. H. (2010). Men sexually interested in trans women: Gendered embodiments and constructions of sexual desire. *Journal of Sex Research, 47,* 374–383.

Wilson, W. J. (1996). *When work disappears: The world of the new urban poor.* New York: Random House.

———. (1987). *The truly disadvantaged: The inner city, the underclass, and public policy.* Chicago: University of Chicago Press.

Winter, S. (2012). *Lost in transition: Transgender people, rights, and HIV vulnerability in the Asia-Pacific region.* Bangkok, Thailand: Asia Pacific Transgender Network.

Young, A. A. (2004). *The minds of marginalized black men: Making sense of mobility, opportunity, and future life chances.* Princeton: Princeton University Press.

SECTION II

SURVIVAL SEX AMONG YOUNG TRANSGENDER PERSONS IN THE UNITED STATES AND THE UNITED KINGDOM

The issue of "survival sex" among adolescents and young adults has been much discussed, but there have been few attempts to systematically examine and integrate this literature. This section consists of a single chapter that aims to review this literature as it relates to young trans people in the United States and the United Kingdom.

CHAPTER 4

Compound Harms

What the Literature Says about Survival Sex among Young Trans People in the United Kingdom and the United States

Lorna C. Barton[1]

1 PhD candidate in the Humanities, Arts, and Social Sciences Graduate School at the University of Strathclyde in Glasgow, UK.

SUMMARY

Survival sex is defined as the exchange of sex for food, shelter, drugs, money, or other items. Young trans people engaging in survival sex in the United States and the United Kingdom constitute a major research gap, and this literature review focuses on a selection of compound harms gleaned from an interdisciplinary literature review. It highlights, first, young trans people and homelessness; second, access to services for the homeless; third, young trans people's recruitment into the street economy and survival sex; and last, young trans people's public visibility to law enforcement.

KEY TERMS:

homelessness; public visibility; street economy; survival sex; young trans people

In the United States young trans people experiencing homelessness are marginalized by structural and institutional inequalities concerning gender, race, and class (Snapp et al., 2015). Trans youth of color are

Nuttbrock, Larry, *Transgender Sex Work and Society*
dx.doi.org/10.17312/harringtonparkpress/2017.11.tsws.004

disproportionately represented within the research in terms of economic inequalities and involvement in the juvenile justice system (Reck, 2009; Rosario, 2009; Talburt, 2010). Research states that young trans people of color come from low-economic, working-class households in poorer areas of cities and towns (Reck, 2009; Noga-Styron, Reasons, & Peacock, 2012). They are also reported to experience some of the highest levels of adversity in their daily lives owing to the intersection of transphobia, poverty, and racism (Peterson, 2013).

Unlike their nontransgender[1] counterparts, young trans people experiencing homelessness have greater levels of social invisibility, having adopted gender classifications that fall outside societal binary norms of male and female (Grossman & D'Augelli, 2006). Studies have reported that young trans people contend with all the issues that their nontransgender and LGB counterparts encounter, including being "thrown away"—that is, forced to leave the family home (Building, 1998; Oparah, 2012; Rosario et al., 2012). The main motivators for family rejection involve young trans people being caught "trying out" or revealing their identified gender, frequently facing physical and sexual violence at the hands of their families in the process of leaving (Ray, 2006; Mottet & Ohle, 2008; Reck, 2009; Rosario et al., 2012; Hussey, 2015; Yu, 2010; Albert Kennedy Trust [AKT], 2014). Studies from the United States suggest that young trans people can be "thrown away" when they are as young as 12 years old (Building 1998; Ray 2006).

Studies additionally report that young trans people and LGB youth in the United States are more likely than young nontrans people to mobilize and migrate toward larger cities such as New York, Chicago, and San Francisco, and, in the United Kingdom, Glasgow, Edinburgh, Manchester, London, and Brighton, where they hope to find acceptance in established gay communities (Stevenson & Jardine, 2009; Gibson 2011). Anecdotal evidence from the United Kingdom reports that young trans people may additionally migrate to larger cities to access gender identity clinics and support services (Stevenson & Jardine, 2009). Kovats-Bernat (2006), in his research involving street children in Port-au-Prince, Haiti, refers to the street children's experience of being thrown away from home and from their community as a form of "displacement." I believe the term *displacement* can also be applied to young trans people being rejected and having to become involved in mobilization, which often involves rural-to-urban migration, from a fear of further victimization or abuse from their families or communities, but also to seek out a place of safety and solidarity, and to figure out and come to terms with who they are.

Some young trans people experience a unique state of liminality: a space in which normative gender conventions are temporarily suspended as their sense of self is redefined and they navigate their place on the "transgender map" (Wilson, 2002). In this liminal state, young trans people are also evaluating and establishing their place in a heteronormative society and at times in the gay community (Wilson, 2002; Reck, 2009). As a consequence of this combination of factors, young trans people experience elevated levels of discrimination and disparities in health and well-being. These disparities span family, peers, community, education, healthcare, employment, and the law enforcement and justice systems (Cochran et al., 2002; Ray, 2006; Winn, 2011; Hussey, 2015).

ACCESS TO HOMELESSNESS SERVICES

Youth homelessness in the United Kingdom and United States today is a pressing political and social issue as a result of young people's level of vulnerability, the complexity of their needs, and the social stigma surrounding homelessness (Kidd, 2007). In recent research studies from the United States, numbers of homeless youths ages 12–25 are estimated to be anywhere between 575,000 and 2.8 million nationwide (Quintana et al., 2010; Walsh & Donaldson, 2010; Hein, 2011; Winn, 2011; Hussey, 2015). Furthermore, studies report that up to 40% of homeless youths in the United States are LGBT (Ray, 2006; Quintana et al., 2010; Winn, 2011; Hussey, 2015). According to some UK reports, LGBT young people make up between 24% and 30% of the general youth homelessness population (Stevenson & Jardine, 2009; AKT, 2014).

What proportion of these numbers is specifically young trans people is unknown, but speculative statistics suggest that they are overrepresented within the LGB demographic of homeless youths (Stevenson & Jardine, 2009; AKT, 2014; Hussey, 2015). Additionally, some studies state that numbers are approaching epidemic proportions, but this phenomenon is US-specific (Ray 2006; Durso & Gates, 2012; Hussey, 2015). Within the United Kingdom, there is limited research into young trans people experiencing homelessness, as non-LGBT youth homelessness reports tend to retain a normative gender split of male and female, possibly leading to inaccuracies in the data. Also, young people may not declare their gender or their gender identity to homelessness services, to avoid the possible resulting discrimination and stigma.

Research from the United States and United Kingdom further demonstrates that young trans people can be wary of social services, as a result of negative past experiences, including involvement in the foster care system and children's or juvenile homes (Gwadz et al., 2004; Irvine, 2010). Studies report that the levels of need of young trans people at times surpass those of LGB youths, because of their health, well-being, and social needs. These include coping with familial rejection, reduced peer support, acceptance of trans identity, access to adequate healthcare, increased feelings of depression, and suicidal ideation. Recent studies suggest that social workers and hostel workers do not have adequate training, awareness, or understanding of these needs and are therefore unable to fulfill their duties, thereby letting young trans people down.

Social workers admit that when young trans people are housed with foster caregivers who are not themselves trans or do not have an understanding of trans needs, the young people frequently run back to the streets or are thrown away when their gender identity becomes clear (Ray, 2006). According to Ray (2006) and Yu (2010), this is also the case for youth homelessness units and shelters in the United States, which are predominantly federally funded and run by religious groups. These groups are required to provide a safe, protected space for all young people, not just nontransgender youths. However, young trans people, on the whole, receive stigmatizing, transphobic, discriminatory, and exclusionary reactions by shelter staff because of a lack of training or understanding, which makes the young trans people feel safer on the streets (Mottet & Ohle, 2008; Yu, 2010).

Service provision for youth homeless differs between the United Kingdom and the United States. Despite US law, which states that state social services are required to intervene and protect young people until they are 18 years old, research reports that the United States has people as young as 12 living in youth homeless shelters and on the streets (Wauchope, 2010; Unites States Interagency Council on Homelessness, 2010). This could be a result of the high number of homeless youths in the United States and the limited resources available to the welfare system. UK law, in comparison, has social work services intervening in young people's lives until they are 18 years old, but this intervention is dependent on other factors, such as the young person's having been previously placed in state care (Crisis.org, 2012; Fitzpatrick et al., 2013). UK youth homelessness reports do not feature legitimate or recorded numbers of those under 16 who approach homelessness services; it is not known whether this lack of reliable information is due to "the statutory responsibility of local authorities for children under the age of 16," or the fact that those under 16 are remaining hidden from services.

Young trans people can face immediate discriminatory barriers in attempting to secure a shelter bed, especially if they are minors, as they face the threat of being reported to law-enforcement officers or social services (Hussey, 2015). Moreover, they face being placed in gender-segregated wings by their birth sex or "anatomic sex" and forced to change their gender presentation or expression to retain that bed (Mottet & Ohle, 2008; Spicer, 2010; Yu, 2010; Hussey, 2015). According to Spicer (2010), this policy denies young trans people both their internal gender identity and their dignity, affecting their overall well-being and mental health. Additional issues of young trans people experiencing harassment as well as physical and sexual assault by shelter clients during their stays are also reported (Quintana et al., 2010; Hussey, 2015).

One report found these problems to be significantly higher for young trans people of color than for white young trans people and higher for transwomen than for transmen (Hussey, 2015). If a young trans person already has an established "gender dysphoria" status on arrival at a shelter, he or she should be assigned to the correct gender wing. However, some shelter policies acknowledge that nontransgender individuals, especially women, do not want young transwomen or transmen sharing their space or facilities. Spade (as cited in Sycamore, 2006) states that this type of policy under US law is referred to as the "bigot's veto" and is "a policy that allows the misunderstandings or biases of a general population in an institution to excuse the exclusion of a person with characteristics that marks hir as different" (p. 670). Spade (as cited in Sycamore, 2006) goes on to argue that the choice to shape policy around society's "presumed" beliefs or the biases of people who stay in these facilities confirms for bureaucracies and policy makers that transwomen and transmen are in fact not real women and men and therefore do not deserve access to services. This type of discrimination only reinforces young trans people's belief that they are neither accepted nor protected in hostels and therefore are safer on the streets.

RECRUITMENT INTO THE STREET ECONOMY AND SURVIVAL SEX

Young trans people become quickly acquainted with and inducted into the street-level economy as a method of survival. One current study found that homelessness is one of the most common catalysts to engaging in survival sex for young trans people (Dank et al., 2015). One US-based study reported that of 51 trans youths of color interviewed, 59% were involved in regular sex work (Singh, 2013). The street economy is also referred to as the "informal economy," in which people do not earn their money through legitimate and legally regulated avenues (Gwadz et al., 2004). With specific regard to sex work, the underground economy can be referred to as the "shadow economy" (Sanders, 2008). However, this term encapsulates all forms of sex work, from pornography to high-class escorts, under what Sanders (2008) refers to as a "four-point continuum": legal formal, legal informal, illegal informal, illegal criminal.

In this case, young trans people under the age of 18 involved in survival sex would fall under the "illegal criminal" point of the continuum, according to laws in the United Kingdom and United States, because of their status as minors. They are not viewed by the law or society as being old enough to have agency or give consent (Musto, 2013). I believe that this approach in itself is a harmful contradiction that sees laws, systems, and policies designed to protect young people from having to engage in sex work denigrate them further by forcing them into a cycle of survival, arrest, incarceration, homelessness, criminal (in)justice, and progressively lower social standing and life trajectories.

Research studies on LGBTQ homeless young people in New York City found that a large number of those interviewed were recruited into the street economy, and specifically survival sex, by their peers (Curtis et al., 2008; Dank et al., 2015). The majority of young people observed how peers made money quickly and, in their view, relatively easily, which encouraged them, in their desperation for basic needs, to try survival sex. Peer recruitment involving LGBTQ young people is confirmed and verified in past studies; only a small proportion of young people were recruited directly by exploiters. In Dank and colleagues' (2015) study, exploiters took the form of peers who did not engage in sex work themselves but took the role of a "peer recruiter" for someone else. In addition, a small number of young people began engaging in survival sex after having been approached and propositioned by a client, which is highlighted in other studies on youth homelessness and survival sex (Walls & Bell, 2011). Interestingly, a large proportion of LGBTQ young people who engaged in survival sex preferred this method of earning money for basic needs over theft or pickpocketing because they felt it was less harmful to others and more honest on their part (Dank et al., 2015).

Survival sex is viewed by governments, agencies, and young trans people themselves as a high-risk activity; research indicates that they are more likely to be involved in sex work and take greater physical risks, such as unprotected sex with clients, than LGB young people (Ray, 2006; Walls & Bell, 2011; Hussey, 2015). It also provides some homeless young trans people with emotional, social, and economic needs (Hussey, 2015). Young transwomen especially are reported to have a need to be affirmed in their gender identity by their clients (Poteat et al., 2014). Young trans people in sex work are at risk of being "found out" if they have not previously advertised themselves to clients as trans, or are not physically "passing" as the gender they are expressing.

Research indicates that young trans people experience high rates of physical and sexual violence while involved in sex work and that the perpetrators include law enforcement officers and clients (Stotzer, 2009). This violence probably intersects with transphobia and racism, as some violent attacks end in murder. According to Trans Europe's Trans Murder Monitoring Project (2014), in the year preceding September 30, 2014, 226 trans individuals had been murdered worldwide, and a total of 1,612 since January 1, 2008. In North America 104 trans individuals were murdered between January 2008 and November 2014, and 90 in Europe within the same time frame (Trans Europe, 2014). A large proportion of these murders were of transwomen, many of whom were women of color (Peterson, 2013). Research does not confirm whether a proportion of the victims were involved in sex work. A young trans person's need to survive, to be affirmed in his or her gender identity, and potentially to use sex work to earn money to transition (which will be discussed next), seems to outweigh the risks associated with engaging in survival sex.

According to some studies, young transwomen are more likely to engage in survival sex to make money to access "street hormones" (unregulated, illicit hormone injections), as well as silicon injections, for the purposes of facial feminizing and bolstering their gender identity (Ray, 2006; Grossman & D'Augelli, 2006; Spicer, 2010; Dank et al., 2015). Unlike those in the United Kingdom, where a young trans person can theoretically transition for free through the National Health Service, US treatment policies are varying but unanimous, stating that young trans people have to pay for hormones and gender-reassignment surgery. As there is a high probability that they will not be in employment that allows them to access clinical care or insurance coverage that supports their transition (American Psychiatric Association, 2013), street hormones are for some young trans people the only viable choice.

The risk in using street hormones in contracting HIV is moderately high as a result of needle sharing among young trans people (Poteat et al., 2014). In addition, the unregulated nature of the injections can also cause long-term health and organ damage because of the unknown quantities or quality of the hormones they are injecting, as well as the accuracy of the hormone dosage in the syringe to counteract the body's natural secretion of estrogen or testosterone (Hussey, 2015). There is a research gap regarding street or illicit hormones and access to them for young trans people in the United States and the United Kingdom—involving not just their long-term physical effects, but also their prices, availability, and relationship to young trans people and survival sex.

PUBLIC VISIBILITY

Young trans people are at risk of being involved with law enforcement officers and the juvenile justice system (JJS) in the United States as a consequence of personal bias and policies that criminalize sex work and homelessness (Hussey, 2015). Young trans people use their peers to glean advice on how to reduce risk and remain safe when engaging in survival sex. They often pair up to walk the streets, or "stroll," for clients. Strolling is defined as walking around a specific circuit or area of communities and neighborhoods to find clients (Shaver, 2005; Dank et al., 2015). In one study, young trans people viewed certain areas and communities in which they strolled as places of safety, such as the East Village in Manhattan, owing to the level of acceptance and tolerance of people in them (Dank et al., 2015). However, strolling was also viewed as dangerous depending on the area, and could also be competitive and territorial if they were to walk on streets controlled by exploiters or gangs. At times, trans youths in the study were targeted by the police and arrested for loitering and prostitution despite not being engaged in either activity at the time of arrest, a result confirmed in similar studies (Marksamer, 2008; Hussey, 2015).

Transwomen, particularly transwomen of color, are reported to be regularly profiled as sex workers, which results in frequent harassment, arrests, and violence perpetrated by law enforcement officers (Hussey, 2015). Dwyer (2011a) calls this phenomenon "over policing." On the other hand, engaging in the street economy results in high rates of violent crime, physical assault, violent robbery, and sexual assault (Ventimiglia, 2012). As a result of their distrust of the police, and of most authorities and adults in general, young trans people are unlikely to report themselves as victims of crimes to the police for fear of not being taken seriously or being arrested themselves (Dwyer, 2011a).

It has been established that young people experience a much higher rate of victimization and violence while homeless, especially young trans people, who may not "pass" as the gender they identify with. This makes them not only a target while engaging in survival sex but also a target of other homeless youths, the public, law enforcement officers, and the JJS. Police in the United Kingdom and United States target homeless young people for what are known as "quality of life crimes": trespassing, loitering, panhandling, public urination, and prostitution (Marksamer, 2008; Hussey 2015). Young trans people are not only overrepresented in youth homelessness statistics but are also overrepresented in the demographics for young people involved in the JJS in the United States (Marksamer, 2008; Squatriglia, 2008; Ventimiglia, 2012; Graham, 2014).

There is a major gap in the research regarding young trans people involved in the youth justice system in the United Kingdom. However, causal factors for involvement in the US JJS include a combined result of the regulating and increased policing of public spaces, which highlights the presence and visibility of all young people, not just trans people (Dwyer, 2011a, 2014; Gibson, 2011). The transgressing of heteronormative gender roles through the "non-heteronormative body" and representation of queerness results in police profiling young trans people (Dwyer, 2011b). This in turn makes them more visible and guarantees frequent police attention and harassment (Ventimiglia, 2012). It is important to acknowledge that before becoming involved with the police and JJS while experiencing homelessness, many young trans people initially become involved while they are still living at home and attending school (Marksamer, 2008; Squatriglia, 2008).

Squatriglia (2008) states that there is a direct connection to young trans people's gender identity or nonconformity and entry into the JJS. In dressing to convey and expressing their gender-nonconforming identities publicly, young trans people cause friction in their heteronormative and gender-conforming environments of community and school. They are flagged as being troublesome, rebellious, and delinquent in not abiding by school dress codes or policies (Squatriglia, 2008). According to Marksamer (2008), 90% of trans youth across the United States describe feeling unsafe at school; their need to express their gender identity leaves them open to discrimination, perpetrated through school policy by teachers and students alike, as well as vulnerable to being verbally and physically harassed or assaulted.

Furthermore, in a study undertaken by the Gay, Lesbian, and Straight Education Network (GLSEN) (Greytak, Kosciw, & Diaz, 2009) involving principals' perspectives of bullying, safety, and harassment in US public schools, principals admitted that their antibullying strategies, educational resources, and support systems were the least inclusive of young trans people among all minority identities recorded in their schools. Marksamer (2008) additionally found 55% of trans youths in the United States reported experiencing physical harassment at the hands of their peers, which can have an effect on self-esteem and mental health and reduce the likelihood of continuing or succeeding at school.

Similarly, within a UK context, LGBT Youth Scotland (Dennell & Logan, 2012) undertook an educational survey using questionnaires sent out to Scottish schools, colleges, and universities regarding the experiences of LGBT young people. They found that 76.9% of young trans people involved in the study experienced homophobic, biphobic, or transphobic bullying in school at the hands of their peers, and only one in four schools has an awareness of transphobic bullying. In addition, fewer than 50% of young trans people reported feeling confident enough to approach school staff for help when being bullied. It was also found that young trans people were more likely to experience bullying throughout their educational experience, spanning school, college, and university, unlike LGB young people. Moreover, it was found that 88.8% of young trans people reported that transphobic bullying in school had a negative effect on their education, and 42.3% stated that it caused them to leave education altogether (Dennell & Logan, 2012).

Research from the United States reports that family rejection, problems at school, and harassment within their community can increase the risk of young trans people's being arrested and held in a locked youth-detention facility by their birth sex, unless diagnosed with gender dysphoria, for the duration of delinquency proceedings (Marksamer, 2008). Much like the young trans people who live in homeless shelters, young trans people in detention facilities experience discrimination, transphobic or homophobic abuse, and physical harassment from their peers and the staff charged with their care. They may also experience sexual assault and violence (Feinstein et al., 2001; Marksamer, 2008; Squatriglia, 2008; Irvine, 2010). The duration of detention is entirely dependent on the age of the young trans person and the viewed severity of the offending behavior or "vulnerability" by the JJS. Therefore, young trans people could begin their involvement at 14 years old and be held in detention until they are released at 18 for defying dress codes or standing up to their bullies in their communities and schools.

It must be highlighted that young trans people's involvement in the youth justice system in the United Kingdom is a major gap in the literature. This discrimination makes young trans people even more of a regular target for a repeated cycle of survival through the street economy, visibility in public places, arrest, incarceration, and homelessness.

CONCLUSION

It is clear from the research discussed that young trans people engaging in survival sex are vulnerable, marginalized, and discriminated against on a structural level and are essentially set up to fail from the outset. However, the research also reports that they are limited agents who are resilient and take control of their lives as best they can in order to survive.

NOTES

1. Individuals who identify with their birth gender (Spicer, 2010; Graham, 2014).

REFERENCES

Albert Kennedy Trust (AKT). (2014). *LGBT youth homelessness: A UK national scoping of cause, prevalence, response, and outcome.* Retrieved from www.akt.org.uk/webtop/modules/_repository/documents/AlbertKennedy_ResearchReport_FINALInteractive.pdf.

American Psychiatric Association. (2013). *Gender dysphoria DSM-5.* Retrieved from www.dsm5.org/documents/gender%20dysphoria%20fact%20sheet.pdf.

Building, H. (1998). Familial backgrounds and risk behaviors of youth with thrownaway experiences. *Journal of Adolescence, 21,* 241–252.

Cochran, B. N., Stewart, A. J., Ginzler, J. A., & Cauce, A. M. (2002). Challenges faced by homeless sexual minorities: Comparison of gay, lesbian, bisexual, and transgender homeless adolescents with their heterosexual counterparts. *American Journal of Public Health, 92* (5), 773–777. doi:10.2105/AJPH.92.5.773.

Crisis.org. (2012). *Research briefing: Young, hidden, and homeless.* Retrieved from www.crisis.org.uk/data/files/publications/Crisis%20briefing%20-%20youth%20homelessness.pdf.

Curtis, R., Terry, K., & Dank, M. (2008). *The commercial sexual exploitation of children in New York City: Executive summary.* Center for Court Innovation. Retrieved from www.courtinnovation.org/sites/default/files/CSEC_NYC_Executive_Summary.pdf.

Dank, M., Yahner, J., Madden, K., Bañuelos, I., Yu, L., Ritchie, A., . . . & Conner, B. (2015). *Surviving the streets of New York: Experiences of LGBTQ youth, YMSM, and YWSW engaged in survival sex.* Retrieved from www.urban.org/Uploaded PDF/2000119-Surviving-the-Streets-of-New-York.pdf.

Dennell, B. L. L., & Logan, C. (2013). *Life in Scotland for LGBT young people: Community & identity.* Retrieved from www.lgbtyouth.org.uk/files/documents/Research_/LGBTYS_Life_-_Community_and_Identity_-_new_version.pdf.

———. (2012). *Life in Scotland for LGBT young people: Education report.* Retrieved from https://www.lgbtyouth.org.uk/files/documents/Life_in_Scotland_for_LGBT_Young_People_-_Education_Report_NEW.pdf.

Durso, L. E., & Gates, G. J. (2012). *Serving our youth: Findings from a national survey of services providers working with lesbian, gay, bisexual and transgender youth who are homeless or at risk of becoming homeless.* Retrieved from http://williamsinstitute.law.ucla.edu/wp-content/uploads/Durso-Gates-LGBT-Homeless-Youth-Survey-July-2012.pdf.

Dwyer, A. (2014). "We're not like these weird feather boa–covered AIDS-spreading monsters": How LGBT young people and service providers think riskiness informs LGBT youth-police interactions. *Critical Criminology, 22* (1), 65–79. doi:10.1007/s10612-013-9226-z.

———. (2011a). Policing lesbian, gay, bisexual, and transgender young people: A gap in the research literature. *Current Issues in Criminal Justice, 22* (3), 415–433.

———. (2011b). "It's not like we're going to jump them": How transgressing heteronormativity shapes police interactions with LGBT young people. *Youth Justice, 1* (3), 203–220. doi:10.1177/1473225411420526.

Feinstein, R., Greenblatt, A., Hass, L., Kohn, S., & Rana, J. (2001). *Justice for all? A report on lesbian, gay, bisexual and transgendered youth in the New York juvenile justice system.* Retrieved from http://njjn.org/uploads/digital-library/resource_239.pdf.

Fitzpatrick, S., Pawson, H., Bramley, G., Wilcox, S., & Watts, B. (2013). *The homelessness monitor, England 2013.* Retrieved from www.crisis.org.uk/data/files/publications/HomelessnessMonitorEngland2013.pdf.

Gibson, K. E. (2011). *Street kids: Homeless youth, outreach, and policing New York's streets.* New York: New York University Press.

Graham, L. F. (2014). Navigating community institutions: Black transgender women's experiences in schools, the criminal justice system, and churches. *Sexuality Research and Social Policy, 11* (4), 274–287. doi:10.1007/s13178-014-0144-y.

Greytak, E. A., Kosciw, J. G., & Diaz, E. M. (2009). *Harsh realities: The experiences of transgender youth in our nation's schools.* Retrieved from www.glsen.org/sites/default/files/Harsh%20Realities.pdf.

Grossman, A. H., & D'Augelli, A. R. (2006). Transgender youth: Invisible and vulnerable. *Journal of Homosexuality, 51* (1), 111–128. doi:10.1300/J082v51n01.

Gwadz, M. V., Clatts, M. C., Leonard, N. R., & Goldsamt, L. (2004). Attachment style, childhood adversity, and behavioral risk among young men who have sex with men. *Journal of Adolescent Health, 34* (5), 402–413. doi:10.1016/j.jadohealth.2003.08.006.

Hein, L. C. (2011). Survival strategies of male homeless adolescents. *Journal of the American Psychiatric Nurses Association, 17* (4), 274–282. doi:10.1177/1078390311 407913.

Hussey, H. (2015). *Beyond 4 walls and a roof: Addressing homelessness among transgender youth.* Retrieved from http://static1.squarespace.com/static/54873880e4b028ad7a710b0e/t/5513f2dce4b053108e5da8dd/1427370716570TransHomeless.pdf.

Irvine, A. (2010). "We've had three of them": Addressing the invisibility of lesbian, gay, bisexual, and gender non-conforming youths in the juvenile justice system. *Columbia Journal of Gender and Law, 19* (3), 675–701.

Kidd, S. (2007). Youth homelessness and social stigma. *Journal of Youth and Adolescence, 36*, 291–299. doi:10.1007/s10964-006-9100-3.

Kovats-Bernat, J. C. (2006). *Sleeping rough in Port-au-Prince: An ethnography of street children and violence in Haiti.* Gainesville: University Press of Florida.

Marksamer, J. (2008). And by the way, do you know he thinks he's a girl? The failures of law, policy, and legal representation for transgender youth in juvenile delinquency courts. *Sexuality Research and Social Policy, 5* (1), 72–92. doi:10.1525/srsp.2008.5.1.72.

Mottet, L., & Ohle, J. (2008). Transitioning our shelters : Making homeless shelters safe for transgender people. *Journal of Poverty, 10* (2), 77–101. doi:10.1300/J134v10n02.

Musto, J. (2013). Domestic minor sex trafficking and the detention-to-protection pipeline. *Dialectical Anthropology, 37* (2), 257–276. doi:10.1007/s10624-013-9295-0.

Noga-Styron, K. E., Reasons, C. E., & Peacock, D. (2012). The last acceptable prejudice: An overview of LGBT social and criminal justice issues within the USA. *Contemporary Justice Review, 15,* 369–398.

Oparah, J. C. (2012). Feminism and the (trans)gender entrapment of gender-nonconforming prisoners. *UCLA Women's Law Journal, 18,* 239–271.

Peterson, N. (2013). *The health and rights of transgender youth.* Retrieved from www.advocatesforyouth.org/publications/publications-a-z/2282-the-health-and-rights-of-Trans-youth.

Poteat, T., Wirtz, A. L., Radix, A., Borquez, A., Silva-Santisteban, A., Deutsch, M. B., . . . & Operario, D. (2014). HIV risk and preventive interventions in transgender women sex workers. *Lancet, 6736* (14). doi:10.1016/S0140-6736(14)60833-3.

Quintana, N. S., Rosenthal, J., & Krehely, J. (2010). *On the streets: The federal response to gay and transgender homeless youth.* Retrieved from https://www.americanprogress.org/wp-content/uploads/issues/2010/06/pdf/lgbtyouthhomelessness.pdf.

Ray, N. (2006). *Lesbian, gay, bisexual, and trans youth: An epidemic of homelessness.* Retrieved from www.thetaskforce.org/static_html/downloads/reports/reports/Homeless Youth_ExecutiveSummary.pdf.

Reck, J. (2009). Homeless gay and transgender youth of color in San Francisco: "No one likes street kids"—even in the Castro. *Journal of LGBT Youth, 6* (2–3), 223–242. doi:10.1080/19361650903013519.

Rosario, M., Schrimshaw, E. W., & Hunter, J. (2012). Risk factors for homelessness among lesbian, gay, and bisexual youths: A developmental milestone approach. *Children and Youth Services Review, 34* (1), 186–193. doi:10.1016/j.childyouth.2011.09.016.

Rosario, V. A. (2009). African-American transgender youth. *Journal of Gay & Lesbian Mental Health, 13* (4), 298–308. doi:10.1080/19359700903164871.

Sanders, T. (2008). Selling sex in the shadow economy. *International Journal of Social Economics, 35* (10), 704–716. doi:10.1108/03068290810898927.

Shaver, F. M. (2005). Sex work research: Methodological and ethical challenges. *Journal of Interpersonal Violence, 20* (3), 296–319. doi:10.1177/0886260504274340.

Singh, A. A. (2013). Transgender youth of color and resilience: Negotiating oppression and finding support. *Sex Roles, 68* (11–12), 690–702. doi:10.1007/s11199-012-0149-z.

Snapp, S. D., Hoenig, J. M., Fields, A., & Russell, S. T. (2015). Messy, butch, and queer: LGBTQ youth and the school-to-prison pipeline. *Journal of Adolescent Research, 30* (1), 57–82. doi:10.1177/0743558414557625.

Spicer, S. S. (2010). Healthcare needs of the transgender homeless population. *Journal of Gay & Lesbian Mental Health, 14* (4), 320–339. doi:10.1080/19359705.2010.505844.

Squatriglia, H. (2008). Lesbian, gay, bisexual, and transgender youth in the juvenile justice system: Incorporating sexual orientation and gender identity into the rehabilitative process. *Cardozo Journal of Law and Gender, 14,* 793–817.

Stevenson, T., and Jardine, L. (2009). *Understanding the housing needs and homeless experiences of LGBT people in Scotland.* Retrieved from https://www.south ayrshire.gov.uk/documents/stone%20wall%20lgbt%20guidance.pdf.

Stotzer, R. L. (2009). Violence against transgender people: A review of United States data. *Aggression and Violent Behavior, 14* (3), 170–179. doi:10.1016/j.avb.2009.01.006.

Sycamore, J. B. (2006). *Nobody passes: Rejecting the rules of gender and conformity.* Emeryville, CA: Seal Press.

Talburt, S. (2010). Constructions of LGBT youth: Opening up subject positions. *Theory into Practice, 43* (2), 116–121. doi:10.1207/s15430421tip4302.

Trans Europe. (2014, November 15). TDOR press release. Retrieved from http://trans respect.org/en/transgender-europe-tdor-2014/.

Unites States Interagency Council on Homelessness. (2010). *Supplemental document to the Federal Strategic Plan to Prevent and End Homelessness: June 2010: Background paper—Youth homelessness.* Retrieved from http://usich.gov/resources/uploads/asset_library/BkgrdPap_Youth.pdf.

Ventimiglia, N. (2012). LGBT selective victimization: Unprotected youth on the streets. *Journal of Law and Society, 13* (2), 439–453.

Walls, N. E., & Bell, S. (2011). Correlates of engaging in survival sex among homeless youth and young adults. *Journal of Sex Research, 48* (5), 423–436. doi:10.108 0/00224499.2010.501916.

Walsh, S. M., & Donaldson, R. E. (2010). Invited commentary: National Safe Place: Meeting the immediate needs of runaway and homeless youth. *Journal of Youth and Adolescence, 39* (5), 437–45. doi:10.1007/s10964-010-9522-9.

Wauchope, B. (2010). *Homeless teens and young adults in New Hampshire.* Retrieved from http://scholars.unh.edu/cgi/viewcontent.cgi?article=1108&context=carsey.

Wilson, M. (2002). "I am the prince of pain, for I am a princess in the brain": Liminal transgender identities, narratives, and the elimination of ambiguities. *Sexualities, 5* (4), 425–448. doi:10.1177/1363460702005004003.

Winn, L. (2011). *U.S. State Department of Health and Human Services: Learning from the field: Programs serving youth who are LGBTQ2-S and experiencing homelessness.* Retrieved from https://www.samhsa.gov/sites/default/files/programs_cam paigns/homelessness_programs_resources/learning-field-programs-serving-youth-lgbtqi2s-experiencing-homelessness.pdf.

Yu, V. (2010). Shelter and transitional housing for transgender youth. *Journal of Gay & Lesbian Mental Health, 14* (4), 340–345. doi:10.1080/19359705.2010.504476.

SECTION III

PERSONAL RELATIONSHIPS AND HEALTH RISK BEHAVIOR

A major omission of much of the research on sex workers is a failure to look beyond sex work per se and examine other types of relationships, such as long-term or main sexual partners. This section also consists of a single chapter, which aims to examine relationships of transwomen with their cisgender partners, and how these relationship dynamics affect health risk behavior. Chapter 5, by Tiffany R. Glynn and Don Operario, presents qualitative data bearing on this largely neglected issue.

CHAPTER 5

Relationship Dynamics and Health Risk Behavior among Transwomen and Their Cisgender Male Partners

Tiffany R. Glynn[1]
Don Operario[2]

1 PhD student in clinical health psychology at the University of Miami.
2 Professor of public health in the Department of Behavior and Social Sciences at Brown University.

SUMMARY

This chapter looks into the relationships between transwomen and their cisgender male partners, with a focus on sex work as a specific variable that shapes these relationships. This chapter examines health risk behaviors within these relationships and how sexual behaviors vary in the context of primary (i.e., emotionally committed) partnerships versus commercial exchange partnerships between transwomen and cisgender men. The aims of this chapter are threefold. First, we will review research on the complexity related to identities and sexual dynamics within these dyads, with specific focus on cisgender men. Second, we will explore health risk behaviors within this relationship context, including the role of sex work and psychological motives that might contribute to partners' health behaviors. Third, we will examine implications of this research for guiding health-promotion interventions for these populations.

KEY TERMS

cisgender; gender presentation; health risk behavior; sexual dynamics; sexual identity

Nuttbrock, Larry, *Transgender Sex Work and Society*
dx.doi.org/10.17312/harringtonparkpress/2017.11.tsws.005
© 2018 by Harrington Park Press

INTRODUCTION

Partnerships between transwomen and cisgender men are highly complex owing in part to the dynamic identities that constitute these dyads. As is noted elsewhere in this volume, transwomen often have complex identities stemming from the intersections of gender identity, sexual identity, race or ethnicity, gender presentation, and socioeconomic status (including sex work history). Few studies have examined the identities, patterns of sexual attraction, and health concerns of cisgender men who are attracted to transwomen. Historically, this population has not signified a socially coherent or scientifically accepted category in the way other sexual identity populations (e.g., homosexual, heterosexual, bisexual men or women) are understood. To begin the discussion of the relationship issues among transwomen and cisgender men, we explore some of the fluidity and complexity related to cisgender male partners, including their sexual orientations, attractions, and experiences of discrimination.

Evidence does not support the presence of a single sexual orientation identity for male partners of transwomen, and an uncritical application of conventional categories to these men can create challenges and frustration. This is due in large part to the historical construction of sexual orientation identities on a binary notion of gender-based attraction (i.e., toward either cisgender males or females). In previous research from our lab, we conducted interviews with cisgender males who were engaging in sex with transwomen in order to explore how these men defined their behaviors and attractions (Operario et al., 2008). Overall, the men did not describe their sexual orientation uniformly. Rather, their definitions were quite diverse. Some men identified as straight or heterosexual, some as bisexual, some as gay, and some chose not to identify themselves as belonging to any category, or they endorsed situational sexual orientation identities depending on their current partner. A common theme for all the men interviewed was an awareness of the inconsistencies between conventional classifications of sexual orientation and their own sexual preferences and behaviors, which led to frustrations with the inability to label their identity as a discrete category. One man in this study commented: "I'm a try-sexual. I'll try anything. I don't label myself. I used to. I used to label myself as being straight, but then, since I find myself attracted to the transgender, I'm like, 'Well okay, so I can't use straight. Am I gay? Am I this? Am I that?' So I just say I don't need to label myself" (Operario et al., 2008, p. 22).

Although some participants in the study were able to identify with a specific identity label, they articulated an initial resistance, as is reflected by the following two men: "Society got to label everybody, so I guess I'll go for gay" (Operario et al., 2008, p. 22); "[The terms] . . . they're irrelevant. Like I said, I'm a man, that's all. . . . Well, I guess if you want to go by the labels, you know, I guess you'd have to call me bisexual, I would imagine" (Operario et al., 2008, p. 21).

Within the same interviews, Operario and colleagues further explored how these men described their sexual attractions to transwomen. Three themes emerged. Some men described their attraction to an individual who happened to be transgender, in such a way that their attraction was specific to the person and not to anatomy or gender identity or expression. Other men explained that they were attracted to transwomen in general because these women represented something "exotic" because of their challenge of the gender binary. Finally, some men said that they were attracted to the transwoman's physical body and appearance (e.g., "There's something about me knowing that physically they have the physical characteristics of a man. I always date pre-op. There's something that just turns me on," p. 23). Given this diversity in narratives regarding both sexual orientation and attraction, it is important to note that male partners of transwomen are not a homogeneous group.

It is also important to acknowledge the experiences of discrimination and relationship stigma among cisgender men and transwomen. As the previous chapters noted, transwomen, especially those involved in sex work, experience high rates of stigma and discrimination attributed to their gender minority status (Operario et al., 2014). However, there has been less research on experiences of relationship stigma targeted at cisgender men and transwomen couples. One study examining this issue involved surveys of 191 couples comprising transwomen and their cisgender male primary partners. The study found that transwomen reported significantly higher levels of relationship stigma (e.g., having friends and family disapprove of the relationship, feeling uncomfortable holding hands in public) compared to their cisgender male partners (Gamarel et al., 2014).

This finding suggests that male partners may experience relationship stigma differently from transwomen, perhaps owing to the ability of men to conceal their attraction toward transwomen. By contrast, some transwomen report more frequent discrimination that is due in part to the visibility of their gender identity or inability to "pass." Notably, relationship stigma was associated with lower levels of relationship quality among both transwomen and cisgender men, which indicates the deleterious effects of stigma on relationship satisfaction and functioning for both partners. These findings align with the Minority Stress Model (Hendricks & Testa, 2012; Meyer, 2003), which posits that prolonged exposure to prejudice and discrimination experienced by members of minority and marginalized groups is associated with adverse psychological outcomes.

HEALTH RISK BEHAVIORS IN THE CONTEXT OF PAYING AND PRIMARY PARTNERSHIPS

A range of health risk outcomes has been documented among transwomen who engage in sex work and their cisgender male partners. Most notably, research has documented alarmingly high HIV prevalence among transwomen, particularly those who engage in sex work (Poteat et al., 2015). Research has shown that transwomen who engage in sex work are nearly 50% more likely to be infected with HIV than cisgender male and female sex workers (Operario et al., 2008). HIV infection among transwomen occurs primarily through condomless anal sex in the context of relationships with cisgender male partners (both paying and nonpaying). Transgender women typically take the receptive role (anal or neovaginal) in sex with cisgender men. Interestingly, the greatest HIV risk for transwomen who engage in sex work occurs with primary, noncommercial male partners. Studies have shown transwomen report more frequently engaging in high-risk sexual behaviors (e.g., condomless sex, substance use) in the context of these relationships than in the context of commercial partnerships (Melendez & Pinto, 2007; Nemoto, Operario, Keatley, & Villegas, 2004). Research on men who have sex with transwomen has also found high HIV prevalence (as high as 40%, as reported in Gamarel et al., 2014), inconsistent condom use, and diverse sexual networks (Operario et al., 2008; Operario et al., 2011). Frequent use of illicit drugs and sex under the influence of drugs have been reported in both transwomen and their cisgender male partners (Reisner et al., 2014).

These behavioral risk factors must be understood in the context of the lived experiences of these populations. We consider four psychosocial factors that contribute to sexual and substance use behaviors among partners within these dyads: gender affirmation (for transwomen), intimacy motives, economic pressure, and role strain.

Gender Affirmation

According to Sevelius (2013), gender affirmation is the process by which transgender individuals interact with their environment in ways that recognize and value their gender expression. Gender affirmation can manifest itself through social processes (e.g., "passing," correct pronoun use), medical processes (e.g., hormone use, surgery), legal processes (e.g., ability to legally change one's name), or psychological processes (e.g., feeling comfortable with one's personal gender expression) (Glynn et al., 2016). However, sometimes individuals may seek gender affirmation in ways that might pose risks to health, such as having sex to affirm one's femininity (Bockting et al., 1998; Melendez & Pinto, 2007; Sevelius et al., 2009). The gender-affirmation framework proposes that social oppression increases psychological distress and decreases access to gender affirmation among transgender populations (Sevelius, 2013). Consequently, when a transwoman's need for gender affirmation is high but her access to affirmation is low, she will seek out opportunities to receive affirmation. In support of this idea, some research has suggested that experiences of discrimination among transwomen may lead to greater HIV risk behaviors (e.g., condomless sex) because of a desire to feel validated in their sexual partnerships with cisgender men (Melendez & Pinto, 2007; Nemoto, Operario, Keatley, & Villegas, 2004; Rodríguez-Madera & Toro-Alfonso, 2005).

The disparate levels of condom use reported by transwomen between primary and commercial partners could be explained by this need for gender affirmation. Qualitative studies of transwomen have explored some of the psychological and interpersonal factors that motivate condomless sex in the context of primary relationships. In focus-group discussions conducted by Bockting and colleagues (1998), transwomen described the need for gender affirmation and feeling validated as a woman, which can operate as motivations for condomless sex with cisgender male primary partners. In the context of these primary relationships, transwomen feel wanted and loved, and sex with primary partners can affirm their sense of femininity. Thus, difficulties arise in negotiating condom use within primary relationships; introducing condom use poses a risk for rejection (of sex or of the entire relationship), which would undermine the sense of gender affirmation. Gender affirmation may also manifest itself in the desire to take on traditional female gender roles (e.g., being subservient to the male primary partner), which also contributes to the difficulty in negotiating condom use (Melendez & Pinto, 2007).

Notably, sex work may serve as a source of gender affirmation for some transwomen. Qualitative research has described how sex work can affirm their feeling of desirability and attractiveness, insofar as men seek out and pay transwomen for their sexual services (Nemoto, Operario, Keatley, & Villegas, 2004). Some transgender women have described how sex work serves as a "rite of passage" for entrance into a transgender community network and thus can validate their sense of belonging in the community (Sausa et al., 2007).

Intimacy

Condomless sex with primary partners can also be attributed to the desire for intimacy and connectedness, which manifests itself in three ways. First, condomless sex may confer the perception of trust between primary partners and in turn foster greater intimacy within the relationship. By engaging in condomless sex, transwomen may perceive themselves as expressing trust in and commitment to their primary partners (Nemoto, Operario, Keatley, & Villegas, 2004). Second, give the reported high rates of condom use with commercial partners, engaging in condomless sex with primary partners serves as a way to distinguish between these two different partnerships. As one transwoman sex worker stated, "I allow him [primary partner] to penetrate me because I love the guy. He's the only man I allow to penetrate me without the condom" (Nemoto, Operario, Keatley, & Villegas, 2004, p. 730). By removing the physical barrier between partners, condomless sex confers the perception of a more intimate relationship with primary male partners; in contrast, negotiating and using condoms with paying partners maintains the perception that commercial sex is a business transaction devoid of personal relevance. Finally, the social stigma experienced by transwomen, especially those who engage in sex work, is perceived to be remedied through sexual intimacy with a primary partner. In-depth interviews by Melendez and Pinto (2007) found that exposure to community stigma and social rejection contributed to transwomen's need to feel secure, loved, and desired by romantic partners. Transgender women reported these needs were partially met through intimacy and condomless sex with male primary partners. As one woman stated:

> You just want to be loved, that's it. Being ridiculed so much, called this, called that, being used. . . . It's just like after a certain point in your life you just . . . you get needy, I guess. . . . And a lot of people don't want to admit it, but a lot of people settle. A lot of us settle. . . . I really think that it's so many of us that are getting this [HIV] because we want to be loved and you know . . . and a lot of times you meet somebody and you feel as though this person's going to love you, so you . . . you risk a lot of things that . . . you know what I'm saying? To make this person happy, you know, you feel as though if you don't use it [condom] it's going to be closer, it's going to make him love you even more. (Melendez & Pinto, 2007, p. 241)

Economic Hardship

As other chapters discuss, transwomen are driven to sex work because of difficulties securing formal employment. Although transwomen who engage in sex work report higher rates of condom use with commercial partners compared with primary partners, research still shows significant HIV risk within the context of commercial sex transactions (Operario et al., 2008). Research indicates that transwomen frequently have strict "100% condom rules" for sex with paying partners because they view condom use as an occupational safety measure (Nemoto, Operario, Keatley, & Villegas, 2004). However, under severe economic hardship, transgender women may compromise these rules—especially when offered greater compensation to have condomless sex: "A man like that comes up to me . . . and when the rent is due, or . . . You know it depends on your . . . your desperate level [whether you use a condom or not]. It's . . . it's just weird how, you know, people will pay extra. A male will pay you extra without the condom thing" (Nemoto, Operario, Keatley, & Villegas, 2004, p. 729).

Financial motives also contribute to engaging in substance use with commercial male partners, and this dynamic potentially leads to a cyclical pattern of dependency. Substance use aids in attracting paying partners; it can also mitigate feelings of aversion or personal revulsion when engaging with undesirable paying partners (e.g., "the uglier my trick was, the more dope I had to use" [Nemoto, Operario, Keatley, & Villegas, 2004, p. 731]). Yet the use of substances may evolve from a coping mechanism for sex work and turn into a dependency, in which sex work income is required to support substance use. Moreover, commercial male partners commonly offer drugs to the women, facilitating a potential addiction. Economic hardship serves as motivation for both sexual risk behaviors and substance use behaviors in the context of commercial male partnerships.

Role Strain

As noted previously, transwomen predominantly prefer the receptive role during sex with cisgender male partners, which may affirm a more feminine identity. In a recent study, Satcher and colleagues (2015) explored the contexts in which transwomen perform insertive anal sex despite their receptive role preference. They described the notion of "role strain," or the stress experienced when one engages in, or is pressured to engage in, behaviors that are incompatible with one's identified social role. In this case, pressure to be the insertive partner during sex may lead transwomen to experience role strain. This strain may be due, in part, to the personal discomfort and gender disaffirmation felt by transwomen when using their penises to penetrate cisgender male partners. They found that transwomen experiencing greater role strain (i.e., stress from having insertive anal sex when their preference is for receptive anal sex to affirm their feminine social identity) were more likely to use drugs before engaging in sex. In the context of sex work, some male commercial partners are willing to pay more money to a transgender woman who will perform insertive sex. This act may trigger psychological distress, substance use, and other unhealthy consequences.

IMPLICATIONS FOR INTERVENTION AND TREATMENT

In consideration of the interrelated nature of sexual risk and substance use behaviors between tranwomen involved in sex work and their cisgender male partners, interventions to promote health and mitigate poor outcomes need to be reexamined. Transwomen who engage in sex work have been a primary focus for HIV interventions in many global contexts (Poteat et al., 2015). However, interventions have generally overlooked cisgender men who have sex with transwomen, who also warrant attention given the behavioral risk factors discussed in this chapter. Moreover, the complex relationship dynamics between transwomen and cisgender men—both paying and primary partnerships—must be understood as unique contexts for health behaviors such as HIV risk taking and illicit drug use. In light of this insight, we must consider moving beyond solely targeting transwomen as the point of intervention and broaden our focus to interpersonal dynamics and relationship contexts between transwomen and their cisgender male partners, both paying and primary.

Historically, HIV prevention efforts have been compartmentalized within discrete populations: specific groups are targeted on the basis of a categorized identity factor that confers risk. For example, gay, bisexual, and other men who have sex with men are one group identified by government agencies (e.g., Centers for Disease Control and Prevention), clinical service providers, and public health intervention researchers. Efforts to engage this population have relied on men identifying as a member of the population being targeted. Other HIV prevention efforts have focused on transwomen, especially those engaged in sex work; these efforts also rely on individuals identifying themselves as transgender or sex workers (or both). Cisgender men who have sex with transwomen may elude such public health outreach and intervention strategies, which rely on identity labels to categorize individuals, given the heterogeneity and fluidity in their individual self-identification.

An alternative strategy to reach both transwomen and their male partners is through a stepwise approach. Because transwomen are likely to identify and affiliate themselves with the transgender community, strategies for reaching and engaging this population in health-promotion programs are feasible. Capitalizing on transwomen's group identification and connecting them to HIV and substance use treatments and programs could, through referrals by the women, reach their cisgender male partners. This strategy may also be useful for reaching commercial partners who may feel reluctant to disclose their sexual behaviors to public health outreach workers.

This strategy was recently demonstrated to be feasible and promising for delivering a couples-focused HIV prevention program to transwomen and their cisgender primary male partners (Operario et al., 2016). In this study transwomen who reported being in a primary partnership were recruited from community venues in San Francisco and screened into a couples-focused HIV prevention program. These women then referred their male partners to the program. Couples received HIV prevention counseling together, in which they discussed their risk behaviors, relationship dynamics, and experiences of stigma and stress, and made commitments to practice healthier behaviors. Compared to a control group, participants who received couples HIV counseling reported significantly less condomless sex and fewer casual outside partners at a three-month follow-up. This study joins the small body of scientific literature on effective HIV interventions for transwomen (reviewed in Poteat et al., 2015). No other known HIV interventions for male partners of transwomen have yet been published.

The research described in this chapter also highlights the need for treatment interventions to address any substance use by both trans women and their cisgender male partners. Recently, our lab conducted a systematic review of the literature to identify effective substance use interventions for transwomen (Glynn & van den Berg, 2017). After searching five digital databases and screening 9,994 manuscripts, we were able to identify only one empirical intervention, which showed preliminary but promising effects of a community-based program for substance use reduction with transwomen who engage in sex work (Nemoto et al., 2005). However, this study had important methodological limitations, and future research is urgently needed to address the high rates of substance use among transwomen. No known substance use intervention studies have been conducted with male partners of transwomen.

CONCLUSION

In summary, this chapter has demonstrated high risk and complex psychosocial and relationship dynamics for HIV, substance use, and other health problems among transwomen and their cisgender male partners. Partnership dynamics—both paying and primary partnerships—contribute in unique ways to the observed health problems in these populations. The partnership dynamics reviewed here include the tenuous relevance of sexual identity categories for these men, the diverse patterns of sexual attraction among cisgender men to transwomen, and the influence of gender affirmation, intimacy motives, economic hardship, and role strain on the sexual and substance use behaviors of transwomen with both paying and primary partners. This is a nascent scientific literature that warrants additional scientific attention and methodological and conceptual innovation to meet the high demonstrated need in these populations.

REFERENCES

Bockting, W. O., Robinson, B. E., & Rosser, B. R. S. (1998). Transgender HIV prevention: A qualitative needs assessment. *AIDS Care, 1* (4), 505–525.

Gamarel, K. E., Reisner, S. L., Laurenceau, J.-P., Nemoto, T., & Operario, D. (2014). Gender minority stress, mental health, and relationship quality: A dyadic investigation of transgender women and their cisgender male partners. *Journal of Family Psychology, 28* (4), 437–447.

Glynn, T. R., Gamarel, K. E., Kahler, C. W., Iwamoto, M., Operario, D., & Nemoto, T. (2016). The role of gender affirmation in psychological well-being among transgender women. *Psychology of Sexual Orientation and Gender Diversity, 3* (3), 336–344.

Glynn, T. R., & van den Berg, J. J. (2017). A systematic review of interventions to reduce problematic substance use among transgender individuals: A call to action. *Transgender Health, 2* (1), 45–59.

Hendricks, M. L., & Testa, R. J. (2012). A conceptual framework for clinical work with transgender and gender nonconforming clients: An adaptation of the Minority Stress Model. *Professional Psychology: Research and Practice, 43* (5), 460–467.

Melendez, R. M., & Pinto, R. (2007). "It's really a hard life": Love, gender, and HIV risk among male-to-female transgender persons. *Culture, Health & Sexuality, 9* (3), 233–245.

Meyer, I. H. (2003). Prejudice, social stress, and mental health in lesbian, gay, and bisexual populations: Conceptual issues and research evidence. *Psychological Bulletin, 129* (5), 674–697.

Nemoto, T., Operario, D., Keatley, J., Han, L., & Soma, T. (2004). HIV risk behaviors among male-to-female transgender persons of color in San Francisco. *American Journal of Public Health, 94* (7), 1193–1199.

Nemoto, T., Operario, D., Keatley, J., Nguyen, H., & Sugano, E. (2005). Promoting health for transgender women: Transgender Resources and Neighborhood Space (TRANS) program in San Francisco. *American Journal of Public Health, 95* (3), 382–384.

Nemoto, T., Operario, D., Keatley, J., & Villegas, D. (2004). Social context of HIV risk behaviours among male-to-female transgenders of colour. *AIDS Care, 16* (6), 724–735.

Operario, D., Burton, J., Underhill, K., & Sevelius, J. (2008). Men who have sex with transgender women: Challenges to category-based HIV prevention. *AIDS and Behavior, 12* (1), 18–26.

Operario, D., Gamarel, K. E., Iwamoto, M., Suzuki, S., Suico, S., Darbes, L., & Nemoto, T. (2016). Couples-focused prevention program to reduce HIV risk among transgender women and their primary male partners: Feasibility and promise of the Couples HIV Intervention Program. *AIDS and Behavior,* 1–12. doi: 10.1007/s10461-016-1462-2.

Operario, D., Nemoto, T., Iwamoto, M., & Moore, T. (2011). Risk for HIV and unprotected sexual behavior in male primary partners of transgender women. *Archives of Sexual Behavior, 40* (6), 1255–1261.

Operario, D., Soma, T., & Underhill, K. (2008). Sex work and HIV status among transgender women: Systematic review and meta-analysis. *Journal of Acquired Immune Deficiency Syndrome, 48* (1), 97–103.

Operario, D., Yang, M.-F., Reisner, S. L., Iwamoto, M., & Nemoto, T. (2014). Stigma and the syndemic of HIV-related health risk behaviors in a diverse sample of transgender women. *Journal of Community Psychology, 42* (5), 544–557.

Poteat, T., Wirtz, A. L., Radix, A., Borquez, A., Silva-Santisteban, A., Deutsch, M. B., Khan, S. I., Winter, S., & Operario, D. (2015). HIV risk and preventive interventions in transgender women sex workers. *Lancet, 385* (9964), 274–286.

Reisner, S. L., Gamarel, K. E., Nemoto, T., & Operario, D. (2014). Dyadic effects of gender minority stressors in substance use behaviors among transgender women and their non-transgender male partners. *Psychology of Sexual Orientation and Gender Diversity, 1* (1), 63–71.

Rodríguez-Madera, S., & Toro-Alfonso, J. (2005). Gender as an obstacle in HIV/AIDS prevention: Considerations for the development of HIV/AIDS prevention efforts for male-to-female transgenders. *International Journal of Transgenderism, 8* (2–3), 113–122.

Satcher, M., Segura, E., Silva-Santisteban, A., Reisner, S., Sanchez, J., Lama, J., & Clark, J. (2015). Exploring contextual differences for receptive and insertive role strain among transgender women and men who have sex with men in Lima, Peru. *Sexually Transmitted Infections, 91* (Suppl. 2), A106.

Sausa, L. A., Keatley, J., & Operario, D. (2007). Perceived risks and benefits of sex work among transgender women of color in San Francisco. *Archives of Sexual Behavior, 36* (6), 768–777.

Sevelius, J. M. (2013). Gender affirmation: A framework for conceptualizing risk behavior among transgender women of color. *Sex Roles, 68* (11), 675–689.

Sevelius, J. M., Reznick, O. G., Hart, S. L., & Schwarcz, S. (2009). Informing interventions: The importance of contextual factors in the prediction of sexual risk behaviors among transgender women. *AIDS Education and Prevention, 21* (2), 113–127.

SECTION IV

MENTAL HEALTH AND SUBSTANCE USE ISSUES AMONG TRANSWOMEN IN THE SEX TRADE

Whether or not they are involved in the sex trade, transwomen have been described as suffering from certain mental health issues, depressed affect in particular, and substance use. Depression is thought to be extremely prevalent among transwomen sex workers, but empirical studies of this issue are rare. First, Operario and colleagues describe reports of depression, and their correlates, among transwomen with a history of sex work in San Francisco. Then Nuttbrock describes the association between sex work and depressive symptoms and shows that this association is mediated by both gender abuse and substance use. A current review of substance use among transwomen by Hoffman follows.

CHAPTER 6

Mental Health and Transphobia among Transwomen Sex Workers

Application and Extension of Minority Stress Models

Don Operario[1]
Tiffany R. Glynn[2]
Tooru Nemoto[3]

1 Professor of public health in the Department of Behavior and Social Sciences at Brown University.
2 PhD student in clinical health psychology at Miami University.
3 Research program director at the Public Health Institute.

SUMMARY

The aims of this chapter are to (1) describe the literature on mental health problems and their social determinants among transwomen sex workers, including findings from a study of 573 transgender women from San Francisco with a history of sex work, and (2) examine the Gender Minority Stress Model and its applicability to transgender female sex workers. On the basis of this analysis, we suggest implications for research and for social and health service providers working with transgender female sex workers.

KEY TERMS

depressive symptoms; exposure to violence; gender minority stress; minority stress; transphobia

Nuttbrock, Larry, *Transgender Sex Work and Society*
dx.doi.org/10.17312/harringtonparkpress/2017.11.tsws.006
© 2018 by Harrington Park Press

Over the past two decades, there has been increasing research addressing the mental health problems facing individuals in the transgender community. Many of the research studies contributing to this body of knowledge have exclusively included or have high proportions of transwomen involved in sex work, and collectively these research studies point to the alarmingly high prevalence of mental health vulnerability and psychological disorders among these women. During this time, a large body of research has also more generally examined mental health disparities affecting sexual minority populations (i.e., cisgender lesbian, gay, bisexual [LGB] men and women); many studies interpret their findings in terms of the Minority Stress Model (Graham et al., 2011).

The Minority Stress Model posits that repeated exposure to stigma, discrimination, and mistreatment owing to one's stigmatized sexual identity leads to mental health problems (Meyer, 2003). Thus, mental health disparities among LGB people are attributed to the experience of LGB-related stigma and discrimination. Likewise, transphobia—defined as exclusion of and stigma attached to transgender-identified people—can explain the high occurrence of mental health problems among transgender populations (Bockting et al., 2013). Researchers have recently adapted the principles of the Minority Stress Model to explain the social causation of mental health problems among transgender populations, referring to this adapted framework as the Gender Minority Stress Model (Hendricks & Testa, 2012). However, the types of stressors that transgender sex workers uniquely experience, and their potential effects on mental health, have not been directly examined.

SOCIAL CONTEXT OF MENTAL HEALTH PROBLEMS AMONG TRANSWOMEN IN SEX WORK

Mental health issues among transwomen have been well documented in the research literature; findings indicate the high prevalence of suicidal ideation and suicide attempts, depression, anxiety, and low self-esteem (Clements-Nolle, Marx, & Katz, 2006). A systematic review of published reports involving transwomen found that 54% reported having suicidal thoughts and 31% had attempted suicide (Herbst et al., 2008). Another review of the literature on suicidality among sexual and gender minority populations estimated the incidence of completed suicides at 800 for every 100,000 postsurgery transgender persons, which is strikingly high compared with estimates drawn from the general US population of 11.5 suicides per 100,000 persons (Haas et al., 2010).

Because of societal stigma and transphobia, transgender individuals face multiple life stressors, which contribute to their risk of having poor psychological well-being. Some of the more commonly identified stressors experienced by transgender individuals include experiences of violence (Clements-Nolle et al., 2006; Testa et al., 2012), difficulties being employed (Garofalo et al., 2006), risk of being homeless (Wilson et al., 2009), and a lack of social support (Glynn et al., 2016).

Previously, Nemoto, Bödeker, and Iwamoto (2011) examined the prevalence and associations among depression, transphobia, social support, and exposure to violence among transgender women in San Francisco and Oakland, California, with a history of sex work. This cross-sectional study used purposive and snowball sampling techniques to recruit 573 adults who identified as transgender or transsexual, had a history of sex work, and identified as African American, Asian or Asian American, Latina, or white. Participants completed a onetime survey that included validated measures of depression and transphobia (adapted from a measure of homophobic stigma; Díaz et al., 2001) and items that assessed history of violence (physical assault, rape, or sexual assault) and social support. Overall, 51% of the sample met criteria for current depressive symptomatology, and 35% had a history of attempted suicide. Notably, transwomen who were recently involved in sex work (i,e., during the preceding 30 days) reported significantly higher depressive symptoms compared with those who had not recently been involved in sex work (M = 19.48 versus 15.27, respectively, $p < .01$). The overall sample evinced alarming levels of physical and sexual assault: 50% had been physically assaulted, 37% had been raped before the age of 18, and 30% had been raped as an adult (age 18 or older). Physical assault and abuse were reported in the context of sex work: 19% of the sample reported being physically assaulted by a sex work customer, and 16% reported being raped as an adult by a customer. Indicators of transphobia reported in the sample included harassment by the police (66%), having to move away from family or friends because of one's transgender identity (54%), losing a job or career owing to one's transgender identity (43%), being told that transgender people are not normal (74%), and being the object of jokes or ridicule (73%). In a multivariable regression model, levels of depression were significantly greater among participants reporting higher levels of transphobia; conversely, depression was significantly lower among participants who had high levels of social support as well as high levels of education and income. This study provided compelling evidence of the deleterious mental health consequences of transphobia and the protective effects of social support and socioeconomic resources.

As findings from the Nemoto and colleagues (2011) study suggest, engagement in sex work can lead to increased risk for mental health problems because of exposures to physical abuse, violence, and victimization, which are frequently embedded in the context of sex work. Moreover, transwomen sex workers who experience abuse or violence may lack access to security and protections provided by law enforcement—and may even be victimized by police—which can contribute to overall feelings of vulnerability, threat, and powerlessness.

Having access to supportive communities and social networks within sex work populations may provide transwomen sex workers a source of resilience and empowerment, as the findings described earlier noted. Our team's previous experience conducting interventions with transgender sex workers provided insight into the empowering role of group cohesion and collective support in promoting the sense of self-esteem and self-efficacy among these women (Nemoto et al., 2005). For example, transwomen sex workers who have supportive peer networks can share basic survival tips and strategies for navigating sex work environments—such as skills to maximize safety through self-defense and self-advocacy, ways to identify dangerous situations or challenging encounters with customers or law enforcement, information about gender-affirmation or transition procedures, as well as alternative means for financial support, employment, housing, and social services (Sausa et al., 2007). Indeed, HIV prevention and health promotion programs designed for transwomen of color have emphasized the role of building social support within the transgender community as a key strategy to improve wellness (Collier et al., 2015; Taylor et al., 2011). These interventions are especially noteworthy in their emphasis on empowerment within and derived from the transgender community, rather than solely noting psychological and other vulnerabilities that are due to environmental hazards such as sex work and transphobia.

MINORITY STRESS AND GENDER MINORITY STRESS

Since its initial publication in 2003, Minority Stress Theory (Meyer, 2003) has become one of the most frequently cited frameworks to analyze the social causation of mental health disparities among sexual minority people. The basic premise of Minority Stress Theory is that identification as a sexual minority is associated with social stress, which becomes manifest in the form of lived experiences, anticipated experiences, or internalized beliefs about stigma and inferiority because of one's LGB status. Minority stressors can be both distal (i.e., external to the individual, such as instances of interpersonal or structural antigay prejudice and discrimination) or proximal (i.e., internal to the individual, such as the fear of being discriminated against or sensitivity toward LGB-related microaggressions) (Meyer, 2003). Another premise of Minority Stress Theory is that these stressors are chronic and persistent, so that sexual minority individuals experience repeated exposure to LGB-related stressors over the life course. Consequently, the cumulative experience of chronic exposure to minority stressors can lead to compromised coping resources, resulting in emotional dysregulation and maladaptive behaviors that give rise to mental health problems or psychological disorders (Hatzenbuehler, 2009).

The Minority Stress Theory has received abundant support in the empirical literature, and it offers a conceptual framework to explain health disparities that negatively affect LGB populations, including disparities related to substance use, smoking, and physical health (Blosnich et al., 2013; Goldbach et al., 2014; Lick et al., 2013). Although there have been some attempts to use the Minority Stress Theory to examine mental health outcomes among transgender people (e.g., Kelleher, 2009), the original formulation of this theory focused primarily on the experiences of sexual minority populations. The experiences of LGB-related stigma and discrimination might not be relevant to and might overlook important dimensions of transgender-related stigma and discrimination, such as the basic challenges that preclude many transgender people from obtaining employment, legal documents, housing, and healthcare.

There is now emerging a nascent literature on Gender Minority Stress in which researchers examine some of the chronic distal and proximal stressors faced by transgender individuals that lead to mental health problems (Hendricks and Testa, 2012). Unlike the original Minority

Stress Theory, which posits that homophobia and heterosexism impose stress on LGB people, the Gender Minority Stress framework begins with the assumption that violation of the gender binary leads to exclusion and marginality for transgender people. Gender minority stressors can be both distal (such as interpersonal harassment or systematic bias against transgender people) or proximal (such as fear of being "discovered" as transgender). Other examinations of gender minority stressors have been described previously in this chapter and are further elaborated on elsewhere (Gamarel et al., 2014; Hughto et al., 2015; Reisner et al., 2015). A measure of Gender Minority Stress and Resilience (GMSR) has been developed and psychometrically validated (Testa et al., 2015); it includes nine subdimensions of stress: gender-related discrimination, rejection, victimization, identity nonaffirmation, internalized transphobia, anticipatory transphobia, nondisclosure, community connectedness, and pride.

Gender minority stress can be conceptualized as both a determinant of sex work and a consequence of sex work among transwomen. Each of the dimensions assessed in the GMSR measure can explain why many transwomen enter sex work—for example, discrimination and rejection that prevent their ability to obtain formal labor, victimization that compromises their basic sense of self-efficacy and social functioning, identity nonaffirmation and nondisclosure that impel them to remain hidden from general society, and so on. In turn, engagement in sex work can exacerbate preexisting experiences of victimization, internalized and anticipatory transphobia, identity nonaffirmation, and so forth.

Notably, the final two dimensions of the GMSR measure reflect important assets that can be facilitated in transgender sex work networks—community connectedness and pride. These two dimensions reflect sources of resilience that transwomen sex workers can harness to empower themselves and promote their wellness. Indeed, some researchers on sex work have called for conceptual and empirical frameworks that counteract the unidimensional view that sex workers are disempowered victims, and instead have advocated for more nuanced perspectives of sex workers as having a strong capacity for community empowerment and mobilization (Weitzer, 2009).

TRANSGENDER SEX WORK MINORITY STRESS AND MENTAL HEALTH

As this chapter and others in this volume describe, the context of sex work for transwomen can often be characterized in terms of extreme levels of socioeconomic disadvantage, daily harassment, social isolation and alienation, risk for physical and sexual abuse and violence, and risk for substance use and HIV (Nadal et al., 2014). The severity of these sex work–related factors arguably extends beyond the levels of everyday stressors frequently considered in models of minority stress. Although Weitzer (2009) and others (Harcourt & Donovan, 2005; Kerrigan et al., 2015; Vanwesenbeeck, 2001) have argued for more complex views of sex workers that neither pathologize nor belittle the agency of sex workers, many studies of transwomen sex workers have highlighted the substantial and severe hardships that these women frequently face (Operario et al., 2008; Poteat et al., 2015; Weinberg et al., 1999). Consequently, the mental health challenges of transwomen sex workers can be especially acute and difficult to treat.

For example, levels of physical and sexual violence and victimization experienced by transwomen sex workers can have human-rights implications (Decker et al., 2015; Mizock & Lewis, 2008), which possibly suggests a reconsideration of health and legal policies to better promote the social inclusion and basic rights of transwomen. Confronted with repeated exposure to violence and victimization, many transwomen might have serious levels of trauma or addiction disorders that require highly sensitive intervention and treatment services (Hoffman, 2014; Nadal et al., 2014; Singh & McKleroy, 2011). Thus, the Gender Minority Stress Model and transgender-focused psychological interventions will require additional complexity because of the multilevel cumulative factors that shape the mental health of transwomen sex workers. Trauma-informed and gender-affirmative interventions can build on the Gender Minority Stress Model to address mental health problems and co-occurring health issues in this population.

CONCLUSIONS

In this chapter we have described some of the research indicating the high burden of mental health and psychological problems among transwomen, including depression and suicidality, and we have argued that these problems arise in large part because of the social context of transphobia that marginalizes these women. The Gender Minority Stress Model (Hendricks and Testa, 2012) is an emerging conceptual framework for understanding the social causation of mental health disparities among transgender people. We have also argued that transwomen sex workers face multiple levels of risk that are due to the cumulative structural, social, and interpersonal challenges that these women often confront. The basic premises of the Gender Minority Stress Model may need to be reconceptualized in order for us to understand and accommodate some of the extreme social and health vulnerabilities of transwomen sex workers.

Future research and interventions to address the mental health problems of transwomen sex workers must therefore take a multilevel approach in accordance with the multiple and complex layers of causality that impel these women to engage in sex work and that shape their psychological functioning. Intervention strategies must target individual-level, community-level, and structural-level determinants of both sex work risk factors and mental health problems. Efforts to address the likely co-occurrence of mental health issues, trauma, substance use, HIV, and socioeconomic problems are warranted by the literature. Mental health research and interventions for this population must refrain from pathologizing and further stigmatizing it. Community-participatory research and community-empowerment interventions may be particularly useful for engaging transwomen sex workers in research and interventions that acknowledge their agency, complexity, and humanity.

REFERENCES

Blosnich, J., Lee, J. G., & Horn, K. (2013). A systematic review of the aetiology of tobacco disparities for sexual minorities. *Tobacco Control, 22* (2), 66–73.

Bockting, W. O., Miner, M. H., Swinburne Romine, R. E., Hamilton, A., & Coleman, E. (2013). Stigma, mental health, and resilience in an online sample of the US transgender population. *American Journal of Public Health, 103* (5), 943–951.

Clements-Nolle, K., Marx, R., & Katz, M. (2006). Attempted suicide among transgender persons: The influence of gender-based discrimination and victimization. *Journal of Homosexuality, 51,* 53–69.

Collier, K. L., Colarossi, L. G., Hazel, D. S., Watson, K., & Wyatt, G. E. (2015). Healing Our Women for transgender women: Adaptation, acceptability, and pilot testing. *AIDS Education and Prevention, 27* (5), 418–431.

Decker, M. R., Crago, A. L., Chu, S. K., Sherman, S. G., Seshu, M. S., Buthelezi, K., . . . & Beyrer, C. (2015). Human rights violations against sex workers: Burden and effect on HIV. *Lancet, 385* (9963), 186–199.

Díaz, R. M., Ayala, G., Bein, E., Henne, J., & Marin, B. V. (2001). The impact of homophobia, poverty, and racism on the mental health of gay and bisexual Latino men: Findings from 3 US cities. *American Journal of Public Health, 91* (6), 927–932.

Gamarel, K. E., Reisner, S. L., Laurenceau, J. P., Nemoto, T., & Operario, D. (2014). Gender minority stress, mental health, and relationship quality: A dyadic investigation of transgender women and their cisgender male partners. *Journal of Family Psychology, 28* (4), 437.

Garofalo, R., Deleon, J., Osmer, E., Doll, M., & Harper, G. W. (2006). Overlooked, misunderstood and at-risk: Exploring the lives and HIV risk of ethnic minority male-to-female transgender youth. *Journal of Adolescent Health, 38* (3), 230–236.

Glynn, T. R., Gamarel, K. E., Kahler, C. W., Iwamoto, M., Operario, D., & Nemoto, T. (2016). The role of gender affirmation in psychological well-being among transgender women. *Psychology of Sexual Orientation and Gender Diversity, 3* (3), 336.

Goldbach, J. T., Tanner-Smith, E. E., Bagwell, M., & Dunlap, S. (2014). Minority stress and substance use in sexual minority adolescents: A meta-analysis. *Prevention Science, 15* (3), 350–363.

Graham, R., Berkowitz, B., Blum, R., Bockting, W., Bradford, J., de Vries, B., . . . & Makadon, H. (2011). *The health of lesbian, gay, bisexual, and transgender people: Building a foundation for better understanding.* Washington, DC: Institute of Medicine.

Haas, A. P., Eliason, M., Mays, V. M., Mathy, R. M., Cochran, S. D., D'Augelli, A. R., . . . & Russell, S. T. (2010). Suicide and suicide risk in lesbian, gay, bisexual, and transgender populations: Review and recommendations. *Journal of Homosexuality, 58* (1), 10–51.

Harcourt, C., & Donovan, B. (2005). The many faces of sex work. *Sexually Transmitted Infections, 81* (3), 201–206.

Hatzenbuehler, M. L. (2009). How does sexual minority stigma "get under the skin"? A psychological mediation framework. *Psychological Bulletin, 135* (5), 707.

Hendricks, M. L., & Testa, R. J. (2012). A conceptual framework for clinical work with transgender and gender nonconforming clients: An adaptation of the Minority Stress Model. *Professional Psychology—Research and Practice, 43* (5), 460.

Herbst, J. H., Jacobs, E. D., Finlayson, T. J., McKleroy, V. S., Neumann, M. S., Crepaz, N., & HIV/AIDS Prevention Research Synthesis Team. (2008). Estimating HIV prevalence and risk behaviors of transgender persons in the United States: A systematic review. *AIDS and Behavior, 12* (1), 1–17.

Hoffman, B. R. (2014). The interaction of drug use, sex work, and HIV among transgender women. *Substance Use & Misuse, 49* (8), 1049–1053.

Hughto, J. M. W., Reisner, S. L., & Pachankis, J. E. (2015). Transgender stigma and health: A critical review of stigma determinants, mechanisms, and interventions. *Social Science & Medicine, 147,* 222–231.

Kelleher, C. (2009). Minority stress and health: Implications for lesbian, gay, bisexual, transgender, and questioning (LGBTQ) young people. *Counselling Psychology Quarterly, 22* (4), 373–379.

Kerrigan, D., Kennedy, C. E., Morgan-Thomas, R., Reza-Paul, S., Mwangi, P., Win, K. T., . . . & Butler, J. (2015). A community empowerment approach to the HIV response among sex workers: Effectiveness, challenges, and considerations for implementation and scale-up. *Lancet, 385* (9963), 172–185.

Lick, D. J., Durso, L. E., & Johnson, K. L. (2013). Minority stress and physical health among sexual minorities. *Perspectives on Psychological Science, 8* (5), 521–548.

Meyer, I. H. (2003). Prejudice, social stress, and mental health in lesbian, gay, and bisexual populations: Conceptual issues and research evidence. *Psychological Bulletin, 129* (5), 674.

Mizock, L., & Lewis, T. K. (2008). Trauma in transgender populations: Risk, resilience, and clinical care. *Journal of Emotional Abuse, 8* (3), 335–354.

Nadal, K. L., Davidoff, K. C., & Fujii-Doe, W. (2014). Transgender women and the sex work industry: Roots in systemic, institutional, and interpersonal discrimination. *Journal of Trauma & Dissociation, 15* (2), 169–183.

Nemoto, T., Bödeker, B., & Iwamoto, M. (2011). Social support, exposure to violence and transphobia, and correlates of depression among male-to-female transgender women with a history of sex work. *American Journal of Public Health, 101* (10), 1980–1988.

Nemoto, T., Operario, D., Keatley, J., Nguyen, H., & Sugano, E. (2005). Promoting health for transgender women: Transgender Resources and Neighborhood Space (TRANS) program in San Francisco. *American Journal of Public Health, 95* (3), 382–384.

Operario, D., Soma, T., & Underhill, K. (2008). Sex work and HIV status among transgender women: Systematic review and meta-analysis. *Journal of Acquired Immune Deficiency Syndrome, 48* (1), 97–103.

Poteat, T., Wirtz, A. L., Radix, A., Borquez, A., Silva-Santisteban, A., Deutsch, M. B., . . . & Operario, D. (2015). HIV risk and preventive interventions in transgender women sex workers. *Lancet, 385* (9964), 274–286.

Reisner, S. L., Greytak, E. A., Parsons, J. T., & Ybarra, M. L. (2015). Gender minority social stress in adolescence: Disparities in adolescent bullying and substance use by gender identity. *Journal of Sex Research, 52* (3), 243–256.

Sausa, L. A., Keatley, J., & Operario, D. (2007). Perceived risks and benefits of sex work among transgender women of color in San Francisco. *Archives of Sexual Behavior, 36* (6), 768–777.

Singh, A. A., & McKleroy, V. S. (2011). "Just getting out of bed is a revolutionary act": The resilience of transgender people of color who have survived traumatic life events. *Traumatology, 17* (2), 34–44.

Taylor, R. D., Bimbi, D. S., Joseph, H. A., Margolis, A. D., & Parsons, J. T. (2011). Girlfriends: Evaluation of an HIV-risk reduction intervention for adult transgender women. *AIDS Education and Prevention, 23* (5), 469–478.

Testa, R. J., Habarth, J., Peta, J., Balsam, K., & Bockting, W. (2015). Development of the Gender Minority Stress and Resilience Measure. *Psychology of Sexual Orientation and Gender Diversity, 2* (1), 65.

Testa, R. J., Sciacca, L. M., Wang, F., Hendricks, M. L., Goldblum, P., Bradford, J., & Bongar, B. (2012). Effects of violence on transgender people. *Professional Psychology: Research and Practice, 43* (5), 452–459.

Vanwesenbeeck, I. (2001). Another decade of social scientific work on sex work: A review of research, 1990–2000. *Annual Review of Sex Research, 12* (1), 242–289.

Weinberg, M. S., Shaver, F. M., & Williams, C. J. (1999). Gendered sex work in the San Francisco Tenderloin. *Archives of Sexual Behavior, 28* (6), 503–521.

Weitzer, R. (2009). Sociology of sex work. *Annual Review of Sociology, 35,* 213–234.

Wilson, E. C., Garofalo, R., Harris, R. D., Herrick, A., Martinez, M., Martinez, J., . . . & Adolescent Medicine Trials Network for HIV/AIDS Interventions. (2009). Transgender female youth and sex work: HIV risk and a comparison of life factors related to engagement in sex work. *AIDS and Behavior, 13* (5), 902–913.

CHAPTER 7

Sex Work and Major Depression among Transwomen in New York City

Mediating Effects of Gender Abuse and Substance Use

Larry A. Nuttbrock[1]

1 Previously affiliated with the National Development and Research Institutes (NDRI) and now a private consultant living in New York City.

SUMMARY

This chapter provides rare longitudinal data about the association between sex work among transwomen and serious depressive symptomatology in the form of DSM major depression. After the strength of this association was evaluated, the extent to which it is mediated by gender-related abuse and substance use was systematically examined. The results suggest that sex work among transwomen is strongly associated with clinical depression in large part because of increased levels of gender abuse and substance use.

KEY TERMS

gender abuse; major depression; sex work; statistical mediation; substance use

Earlier studies have observed extremely high levels of depressive symptoms among transgender women (Bockting et al., 2013; Hoffman, 2014; Rotandi et al., 2011). Studies using an established CES-D (Center for Epidemiologic Studies Depression Scale) (Radloff, 1977) cut score

Nuttbrock, Larry, *Transgender Sex Work and Society*
dx.doi.org/10.17312/harringtonparkpress/2017.11.tsws.007
© 2018 by Harrington Park Press

have suggested that more than half of these women may be classified as clinically depressed (Clements-Nolle et al., 2001; Nemoto, Bödeker, & Iwamoto, 2011). Using diagnostic criteria for assessing *DSM-IV*-TR major depression (American Psychiatric Association, 2000), a prospective study of transwomen by me and my colleagues found that 17.8% of them met the criteria for major depression at baseline; the yearly incidence was 15.9% (Nuttbrock et al., 2014a).

In our longitudinal study, new experiences of psychological or physical abuse stemming from gender nonconformity were associated with new cases of major depression, suggesting a causal association (Nuttbrock et al., 2014a). Experiences of gender abuse were also found to trigger substance use (Nuttbrock et al., 2014b), and substance use may, in turn, lead to increased depressive symptomatology (Nemoto et al., 2011).

The current study further examined this set of findings in conjunction with sex work as an antecedent variable. An overall association of sex work with major depression was hypothesized; additional predictions that this association would be mediated by increases in gender abuse and substance use ensued. Following the four steps for evaluating mediation (Baron & Kenny, 1986), four hypotheses were posed: (1) sex work is associated with major depression; (2) sex work is associated with gender abuse and substance use (the presumed mediators); (3) gender abuse and substance use are associated with major depression (showing that the presumed mediators affect depression); and (4) the association between sex work and major depression is reduced when gender abuse and substance use are controlled (suggesting a mediation effect). These hypotheses were tested in conjunction with background variables (age, ethnicity, employment, nativity, sexual orientation, and hormone therapy) that were evaluated as potential confounders and controlled, as appropriate.

METHOD

Transgender or gender-variant individuals were actively involved in all aspects and phases of this project, including design of the instrument, recruitment, interviewing, data collection, and some of the data analysis. The Institutional Review Board (IRB) of the National Development and Research Institutes (NDRI) approved all the research protocols.

Selection of Study Participants

A total of 571 transwomen from the New York metropolitan area between the ages of 19 and 59 were initially recruited to participate in the New York Transgender Project. All these individuals were assigned as male at birth but subsequently did not regard themselves as "completely male" in all situations or roles (reflecting an MTF/transgender spectrum). Study participants who were biologically assayed as HIV-negative (60.4%, or 345/571) were then randomly assigned to participate in a three-year prospective study designed to evaluate risk factors for new cases of HIV/STI (prospective study N = 230). To improve efficiency of the research design, the randomization incorporated an overweighting for high-risk sexual behavior for HIV and younger age.

The study participants were initially recruited through transgender organizations in the New York metropolitan area, the Internet, newspaper advertisements, the streets, clubs, client referrals of other clients, and paid assistants from transgender communities who worked on a day-to-day basis with the field staff. Because of time constraints associated with this project, there was variation in the duration of time the study participants could potentially be followed. The recruitment phase, which began in December 2004, was extended to September 2007 so that all participants in the prospective study could potentially be followed for at least twelve months (135 and 74 could potentially be followed for 24 and 36 months, respectively).

The percentages of potentially available study participants who were actually interviewed were 149/230 (64.8%), 171/230 (74.3%), 92/135 (68.1%), and 56/74 (75.7%) at 6, 12, 24, and 36 months, respectively. Longitudinal modeling for this report used five assessment points: baseline and the four follow-ups (6, 12, 24, and 36 months).

Measurements

Study participants completed face-to-face interviews in conjunction with the Life Review of Transgender Experiences (LRTE). Gender abuse, major depression, and other factors were assessed at baseline, and changes in these variables were assessed during follow-ups. The English version of the LRTE was fully translated to Spanish, and 19% (44/230) were interviewed in Spanish with a fluent interviewer. Study participants were compensated $40 for completing all the protocols associated with a given assessment period.

BACKGROUND VARIABLES *Age* was included as a continuous variable from 19 through 59. *Education* was scaled as less than high school, high school graduate, some college, and college graduate or higher. Ethnicity was coded using preestablished census categories and classified for this report as non-Hispanic white versus all other categories (nonwhite ethnicity). *Employment* was defined as working full- or part-time at any regular job (on or off the books) during the previous six months. Self-reports of being born in the United States, compared to being born outside the United States (coded high), were labeled as *nativity*. *Sexual orientation* was based on reports of sexual attraction to men only, women only, men and women, and neither men nor women. This variable was grouped in this report as sexual attraction to men only (androphilic) versus all other categories. *Hormone therapy* was assessed at all points and defined as using any type of female hormone supplements or anti-androgen products during the preceding six months.

SEX WORK Study participants were queried at all assessment points about having received any money, drugs, or gifts in exchange for sex during the previous six months (sex work).

GENDER ABUSE At all assessment points, study participants were queried about whether they had been "verbally abused or harassed" (psychological gender abuse) and thought it was because of their gender identity or presentation. A parallel item asked about being "physically abused or beaten" (physical gender abuse).

SUBSTANCE USE Respondents were asked at all assessment times about their use of alcohol (five or more drinks on a given occasion); cannabis (marijuana or hashish); cocaine (crack or powder); heroin; amphetamines or methamphetamines; downers or tranquilizers; phencyclidine or PCP; LSD or other hallucinogens; ecstasy or XTC; poppers, nitrates, or other inhalants; misused prescription drugs; or any other drug during the preceding month. Substance use was quantified for this report by the number of different substances used (capped at five to reduce skewing and outliers) and an overall summary of days of using a particular drug added across all drugs that were used (capped at 15).

MAJOR DEPRESSION This variable was codified and assessed using the Mini International Neuropsychiatric Interview (M.I.N.I. Plus) (English version 5.0.0), which was designed as a brief, structured interview for the major Axis I psychiatric disorders in *DSM-IV* (Sheehan et al., 1998). Validation and reliability studies comparing the M.I.N.I. to the other diagnostic instruments (Structured Clinical Interview for DSM and the Comprehensive International Diagnostic Interview) show that the M.I.N.I. has acceptably high validation and reliability scores, but it can be administered in a much shorter time. In the current study, interviewers were trained to complete the M.I.N.I. by the principal investigator (LN), a psychiatric epidemiologist with experience in the assessment of psychopathology in high-risk populations.

Assessment of major depression proceeded in four steps:

1. *Diagnostic Screening.* Respondents were asked: "Were you consistently depressed or down, most of the day, every day for at least two weeks?" or "Were you less interested in most things or less able to enjoy the things you used to enjoy most of the time for at least two weeks?"

2. *Diagnostic Symptomatology.* If either of these screens was positive, the presence of seven diagnostic symptoms was determined — appetite increase or decrease; trouble sleeping; fidgeting or restlessness; tiredness or lack of energy; feeling worthless or guilty; difficulty concentrating or making decisions; or suicidal ideation.

3. *Diagnostic Criteria.* If three or more of these diagnostic symptoms were present, the interviewer inquired whether the symptoms overlapped and occurred during the same time frame (DSM symptom overlap criteria) and whether the symptoms of depression caused "significant distress or impaired the ability to function at work, socially, or in some other important way" (DSM impairment criteria).

4. *Diagnostic Rule-Outs.* If the diagnostic criteria were met, further inquiries were made as to whether the indicated symptoms were due to the loss of a loved one (bereavement rule-out); whether there was a medical illness just before the symptoms began (medical rule-out); and whether drugs were taken just before the symptoms began (substance use rule-out). Time-varying assessments

of major depression, across all the assessment times, reflected whether depression occurred during the previous six months.

Statistical Techniques

Generalized estimating equations (GEE) with a binomial link were used for dichotomous outcomes, and the effects were expressed as odds ratios (OR) (Hardin & Hilbe, 2012). GEE with an identity link was used for continuous outcomes, and the effects were expressed as unstandardized betas (betas). For both effects, 95% confidence intervals were calculated; statistical significance was indicated by exclusion of the null effects: 1.00 for odds ratios and .00 for betas. Clustering within individuals across time was modeled with an exchangeable working correlation structure. All the data were analyzed using version 9 of Stata. Effects of the background variables (except hormone therapy) were evaluated using baseline measurements only. Hormone therapy and all the other variables were analyzed across follow-ups and included in the analysis as time-varying covariates or end points.

Mediation was assessed using the four steps noted above, which were originally proposed by Baron and Kenny (1986).[1] Mediation was claimed if an initial effect was reduced by 10% or more with controls for hypothesized mediators (Selvin, 2004). Estimates of mediation may be biased if the initial association is confounded by other variables (MacKinnon et al., 2002). To reduce potential confounding, background variables associated with outcome variables were controlled in the analysis, as appropriate.

RESULTS

Study Attrition

Attrition included those who were not followed at a given point because of study time constraints (administrative attrition) and the potentially available participants at given points who were not located and interviewed (client-related attrition). The subsets of the 230 study participants followed at years one, two, and three were compared to those not so followed with regard to baseline measurements of background variables, gender abuse, depressive symptoms, and other variables (combined administrative and client-related attrition). Only older age with study completion at years one ($r = .15$; $p < .05$) and three ($r = .16$; $p < .05$) was significant. Because study attrition was, for the most part, not predicted from variables included in the analysis, the analysis may not be significantly biased by missing data.

Study Participants

Study participants were by design between 19 to 59 years of age (mean = 34.0; SD = 12.4). Less than half (42.2%) did not graduate from high school; 6.1% were college graduates or higher. More than half (53.0%) were employed part- or full-time in a regular job. Ethnicity was 35.7% Hispanic; 35.2% non-Hispanic white; 17.4% non-Hispanic black; and 11.7% any other identification. Less than one-fourth (22.4%) were foreign-born. Most (58.9%) were attracted to men only (androphilic), 25.4% to women only, 13.8% to men and women, and 1.8% to neither men nor women. At baseline, 52.2% reported hormone therapy during the previous six months.

At baseline, 53.0% indicated psychological gender abuse during the preceding six months; a yearly incidence was reported during follow-up of 40.8% (126 episodes/309 person years). During this time frame, 10.0% indicated physical gender abuse during the previous six months, and a yearly incidence during follow-up of 9.7% (30 episodes/309 person years). The prevalence of any substance use exceeded 70.0% across assessment points. Poly-substance use (two or more drugs) exceeded 30.0% at all points. At baseline, 17.8% reported major depression during the preceding six months, and a yearly incidence during follow-up of 15.9% (49 episodes/309 person years).

Background Variables with Major Depression

In separate bivariate analyses, two of the background variables—nativity (OR = .53) and hormone therapy (OR = 2.96)—were associated with major depression. In a multivariate analysis, with these variables simultaneously included, both nativity (OR = .57) and hormone therapy (OR = 2.96) remained statistically significant. These variables were therefore controlled in some of the analysis below.

Sex Work with Major Depression

Sex work was associated with major depression (OR = 3.35) and remained statistically significant (OR = 2.90) when background variables (nativity and hormone therapy) were controlled (Table 7.1).

TABLE 7.1

Sex Work with Major Depression

	MAJOR DEPRESSION	
	OR	(95% CI)
Sex work		
Uncontrolled	3.35	(2.28, 4.93)
Background controlled[a]	2.90	(1.90, 4.41)

NOTE: Odds ratios based on GEE with a binomial link.
[a] Hormone therapy and nativity controlled.

Sex Work with Gender Abuse and Substance Use

Sex work was associated with psychological gender abuse (OR = 5.30), and this effect was reduced but still statistically significant (OR = 3.76) with background variables controlled. Sex work was strongly associated with physical gender abuse (OR = 10.37); this effect was reduced but still statistically significant and strong with background variables controlled (OR = 7.52) (Table 7.2).

Sex work was also associated with the number of substances used (beta = 1.90), this effect being reduced but still significant with background variables controlled (beta = .87). Sex work was also associated with number of days using substances (beta = 1.57), and this effect was

TABLE 7.2

Sex Work with Gender Abuse

	GENDER ABUSE			
	PSYCHOLOGICAL		PHYSICAL	
	OR	(95% CI)	OR	(95% CI)
Sex work				
Uncontrolled	5.30	(3.67, 7.69)	10.37	(5.47, 19.67)
Background controlled[a]	3.76	(2.45, 5.77)	7.52	(3.76, 15.06)

NOTE: Odds ratios based on GEE with a binomial link.
[a] Hormone therapy and nativity controlled.

TABLE 7.3

Sex Work with Substance Use

	DRUG USE			
	NUMBER OF SUBSTANCES[a]		DAYS USING SUBSTANCES[b]	
	beta	(95% CI)	beta	(95% CI)
Sex work				
Uncontrolled	1.90	(.91, 1.27)	1.57	(1.25, 1.88)
Background controlled[c]	.87	(.70, 1.08)	1.35	(1.01, 1.69)

NOTE: Unstandardized betas based on GEE with an identity link.
[a] Number of substances used during the previous month with a range of 0 through 5.
[b] Cumulative measure of number of substances and number of days each was used during the previous month with a range of 0 through 15.
[c] Hormone therapy and nativity controlled.

reduced but still statistically significant with background variables controlled (beta = 1.35) (Table 7.3).

Gender Abuse and Substance Use with Major Depression

Psychological (OR = 5.02) and physical (OR = 3.54) gender abuse was associated with major depression, and these effects were reduced (ORs of 4.21 and 2.62) but still statistically significant with background variables controlled. Number of substances (beta = 1.77) and days using substances (beta = 1.30) were also associated with major depression; these effects were reduced (betas of 1.63 and 1.23) but still statistically significant with background variables controlled (Table 7.4).

Sex Work with Major Depression Controlling for Gender Abuse and Substance Use

The basic background-controlled effect of sex work on major depression (OR = 2.90) (see Table 7.1) was reduced by approximately 25% with gender abuse (OR = 2.16) and substance use (OR = 2.16) separately controlled. The basic effect was reduced by approximately 30% with both gender abuse and substance use controlled (OR = 1.89) (Table 7.5). These data suggest that the association of sex work with major depression is significantly mediated by gender abuse and substance use.

TABLE 7.4

Gender Abuse and Substance Use with Major Depression

	MAJOR DEPRESSION	
	OR	(95% CI)
GENDER ABUSE		
UNCONTROLLED		
Psychological	5.02	(3.29, 7.66)
Physical	3.54	(2.05, 5.99)
BACKGROUND CONTROLLED[a]		
Psychological	4.21	(2.59, 6.84)
Physical	2.62	(1.42, 4.84)
SUBSTANCE USE		
UNCONTROLLED		
Number of substances[b]	1.77	(1.50, 2.08)
Days using substances[c]	1.30	(1.18, 1.43)
BACKGROUND CONTROLLED[a]		
Number of substances[b]	1.63	(1.36, 1.96)
Days using substances[c]	1.23	(1.10, 1.37)

NOTE. Unstandardized betas based on GEE with an identity link.
[a] Hormone therapy and nativity controlled.
[b] Number of substances used during the previous month with a range of 0 through 5.
[c] Cumulative measure of number of substances and number of days each was used during the previous month with a range of 0 through 15.

DISCUSSION

Using *DSM-IV-TR* criteria for assessing major depression, I found that that 17.8% of the transwomen in the prospective component of the New York Transgender Project were suffering from major depression at baseline, an estimate that is approximately four times higher than the prevalence of major depression in the general population (Eaton et

TABLE 7.5

Sex Work with Major Depression with Controls for Gender Abuse and Drug Use

	MAJOR DEPRESSION	
	OR	(95% CI)
SEX WORK		
CONTROLS		
Gender abuse[a]	2.16	(1.27, 3.67)
Drug use[b]	2.16	(1.25, 3.71)
Gender abuse and drug use[c]	1.89	(1.08, 3.29)

NOTE: Odds ratios based on GEE with a binomial link. Background variables hormone therapy and nativity controlled throughout.
[a] Psychological and physical gender abuse controlled.
[b] Number of drugs and number of days using drugs controlled.
[c] Psychological and physical gender abuse, number of drugs, and number of days using drugs controlled.

al., 1997). The estimated prevalence of major depression among transwomen, while extremely high, is significantly lower than earlier estimates that were based on a CES-D cut score.[2]

The data suggest that sex work is associated with a twofold increase in *DSM-IV*-TR major depression among transwomen in New York City. Sex work was also associated with a fourfold increase in psychological abuse and an eightfold increase in physical abuse stemming from gender nonconformity, and this abuse was in turn associated with three- to fourfold increases in major depression. On the basis of effect sizes typically observed in the behavioral sciences, and substantive considerations, these associations may be characterized as moderately strong to strong in magnitude (Valentine & Cooper, 2003). A mediation analysis suggested that the association of sex work with major depression (noted above) significantly reflects increased gender-related abuse association with sex work.

Sex work was associated with using one additional substance during the preceding month and using these substances an additional one and one-half days. Increased substance use was, in turn, associated with major depression. A mediation analysis suggested that the association between sex work and major depression significantly reflects increased substance use associated with sex work.

These data suggest that sex work, gender abuse, and substance use are intertwined major risk factors for serious psychiatric symptomatology in the form of major depression among transwomen. These individuals are in need of holistic transgender-friendly services through which these intertwined and complex issues are observed and properly understood in the context of transwomen's lives.

NOTES

This research was supported by a grant from the National Institute on Drug Abuse (NIDA) (1 R01 DA018080) (Larry Nuttbrock, principal investigator).

1. Since Baron and Kenny's seminal publication in 1986, new approaches have been developed for mediation analysis (MacKinnon, 2008). My colleagues and I have used some of these techniques (Nuttbrock et al., 2014b), but they are less well developed and more statistically cumbersome when the outcome variable is dichotomous. Mediation analyses with dichotomous outcomes, using these new techniques, have seldom been published in the applied literature. In the interest of accessibility and economy, the four-step approach of Baron and Kenny are used in this and other reports in this volume.

2. Surveys of transwomen in the San Francisco area, using a cut score of 16 on the CES-D, estimated major depression in this population at 48.7% (Nemoto et al., 2011) and 63.0% (Clements-Nolle et al., 2001). This discrepancy may be largely explained by the low positive predicted value of the CES-D with diagnosed major depression; only about 50% of those above established cut points on the CES-D are depressed on the basis of diagnostic protocols (Thomas et al., 2001).

REFERENCES

American Psychiatric Association. (2000). *Diagnostic and statistical manual of mental disorders* (4th ed., rev.). Washington, DC: American Psychological Association.

Baron, R. M., & Kenny, D. A. (1986). The moderator-mediator variable distinction in social psychological research: Conceptual, strategic, and statistical considerations. *Journal of Personality and Social Psychology, 51,* 1173–1182.

Bockting, W. O., Miner, M., Swinburne Romine, R. E., & Coleman, E. (2013). Stigma, mental health, and resilience in an online sample of the U.S. transgender population. *American Journal of Public Health, 103,* 943–951.

Clements-Nolle, K., Marx, R., Guzman, R., & Katz, M. (2001). The prevalence, risk behaviors, health care use, and mental health status of transgender persons: Implications for public health intervention. *American Journal of Public Health, 91,* 915–921.

Eaton, W. W., Anthony, J. C., Gallo, J., Cai, G., Tien, A., Romanoski, A., . . . & Chen, L. S. (1997). Natural history of Diagnostic Interview Schedule/DSM-IV major depression: The Baltimore Epidemiologic Catchment Area follow-up. *Archives of General Psychiatry, 54,* 993–999.

Hardin, J. R., & Hilbe, J. R. (2012). *Generalized estimating equations* (2nd ed.). New York: CRC Press.

Hoffman, B. (2014). An overview of depression among transgender women. *Depression Research and Treatment.* Article ID 394283, 9 pages.

MacKinnon, D. P. (2008). *An introduction to statistical mediation analysis.* New York: Lawrence Erlbaum.

MacKinnon, D. P., Lockwood, C. M., Hoffman, J. M., West, S. G., & Sheets, V. (2002). A comparison of methods to test mediation and other intervening variable effects. *Psychological Methods, 7,* 83–104.

Nemoto, T., Bödeker, B., & Iwamoto, M. (2011). Social support, exposure to violence, and transphobia, and correlates of depression among male-to-female transgender women with a history of sex work. *American Journal of Public Health, 101,* 1980–1988.

Nuttbrock, L., Bockting, W. O., Rosenblum, A., Hwahng, S., Mason, M., Marci, M., & Becker, J. (2014). Gender abuse and major depression among male-to-female transgender persons: A prospective study of vulnerability and resilience. *American Journal of Public Health, 104,* 2191–2198.

———. (2013). Gender abuse, depressive symptoms, and substance use among transgender women: A three-year prospective study. *American Journal of Public Health, 103,* 300–307.

Radloff, L. S. (1977). The CES-D scale: A self-report depression scale for research in the general population. *Applied Psychological Measurement, 1,* 385–401.

Rotandi, G., Bauer, R., Travers, A., & Travers, R. (2011). Depression in male-to-female Ontarians: Results from the trans PULSE project. *Canadian Journal of Community Mental Health, 30,* 113–133.

Selvin, S. (2004). *Statistical analysis of epidemiologic data* (3rd ed.). New York: Oxford University Press.

Sheehan, D. V., Lecrubier, Y., Sheehan, K. H., Amorim, P., Janavs, J., Weiller, E., . . . & Baker, R. (1998). Mini-International Neuropsychiatric Interview (M.I.N.I.): The development and validation of a structured diagnostic psychiatric interview for DSM-IV and ICD–10. *Journal of Clinical Psychiatry, 59* (Suppl. 20), 22–33.

Thomas, J. L., Jones, G. N., Scarinci, I. C., Mehan, D. J., & Brantley, P. J. (2001). The utility of the CES-D as a depression screening measure among low-income women attending primary care clinics. *International Journal of Psychiatry in Medicine, 31,* 25–40.

Valentine, J. C., & Cooper, H. (2003). *Effect size substantive interpretation guidelines: Issues in the interpretation of effect sizes.* Washington, DC: What Works Clearinghouse.

CHAPTER 8

Substance Use among Transgender Sex Workers

Beth R. Hoffman[1]

1 Associate professor in the Public Health Department at California State University, Los Angeles.

SUMMARY

The last chapter showed that sex work among transwomen is strongly associated with measurements of substance use; however, systematic reviews of these associations have not been provided in the literature. This chapter presents a review of this literature.

KEY TERMS

depression; sex work; stigma; substance use; transwomen; violence

Rates of substance use are higher in transgender females than in the general population. Though the prevalence of substance use in transwomen is unclear, a meta-analysis by Herbst and colleagues (2008) indicated that transwomen used alcohol at lower rates than females in the general population and were approximately equivalent in marijuana use, but they had significantly higher use rates of cocaine or crack, heroin, and other injection drugs (SAMHSA, 2014). The accuracy of these numbers is unknown and may be skewed high because of oversampling of certain subgroups of transwomen. Because studies have tended to recruit from venues frequented by transwomen in urban areas (e.g., bars and HIV service centers; Hughes & Eliason, 2002), samples are skewed in favor of young transwomen of color engaging in high-risk behaviors such as drug use and sex work (Rosser et al., 2007).

Nuttbrock, Larry, *Transgender Sex Work and Society*
dx.doi.org/10.17312/harringtonparkpress/2017.11.tsws.008

Though few studies examine rates of substance use in transgender female sex workers, there is evidence that sex work results in increased rates of substance use among this population (Operario & Nemoto, 2005). In the United States, participating in black-market economies (sex work or drug sales) results in twice the rate of substance use as a coping mechanism compared to those who don't participate in these economies (Grant et al., 2011). A study of transgender female (*kathoey*) sex workers in Bangkok, Thailand, found that nearly all participants had used alcohol in the past year, approximately 33% had used marijuana, 36% had used ecstasy, 20% had used ketamine, and 10% had used non-injecting methamphetamine (Nemoto et al., 2012).

Sex work and drug use are inexorably linked. Sex work yields money quickly, which can be used to pay for drugs (Bith-Melender et al., 2010). Sex work can also be physically, emotionally, and spiritually taxing, leading some sex workers to use drugs to escape from their daily reality (Bith-Melender et al., 2010; Sausa, Keatley & Operario, 2007). Qualitative analyses indicate that both sex work and drug use are seen as "rites of passage" by certain transwomen (Nemoto, Operario, Keatley, & Villegas, 2004). A quantitative study found that transgender females who engaged in sex work in the previous 30 days were 600% more likely to engage in illicit drug use than transgender females not engaging in sex work (Operario & Nemoto, 2005).

FACTORS AFFECTING SUBSTANCE USE

Violence and Stigma

Violence is a constant threat to transwomen (Chestnut, Dixon, & Jindasurat, 2013), and the low status and taboo nature of sex work further marginalize transwomen in this occupation. Sex workers have reported incidents of rape, robbery, physical attacks, and murder by clients (Sausa, Keatley, & Operario, 2007). Police are frequently unsympathetic, often participating in violent behavior themselves by harassing transgender females, pulling their wigs off, or demanding forced sex (Sausa, Keatley, & Operario, 2007). Preliminary evidence indicates that exposure to acute or ongoing violence has been associated with substance use in transwomen (Testa et al., 2012).

Violence can be classified in at least three types: physical violence (attacks), sexual violence (forced sexual activity), and verbal violence (threats, intimidation, discrimination). Though there is limited research regarding type of violence and effects on transwomen (and even less research on this topic with transgender female sex workers), there is evidence that type of violence may have varying effects on the drug use of victims. For example, a study of predominantly white transwomen in Virginia indicated that substance use was associated not with a history of experiencing physical violence but with a history of sexual violence (Testa et al., 2012). Other studies have found that verbal violence is linked to depression, but sexual and physical violence are not (Bockting et al., 2013; Nemoto, Bödeker, & Iwamoto, 2011).

Depression

The relationship between depression and drug use has not been adequately explored among transgender females, let alone among transgender female sex workers. To date there has not been a quantitative study of depression and drug use among transwomen (Hoffman, 2014). While several studies have found no link between sex work and depression in transwomen (Bazargan & Galvan, 2012; Nuttbrock et al., 2013; Nemoto, Bödeker, & Iwamoto, 2011), other studies have indicated that transgender sex workers engage in substance use to alleviate mental distress (Bith-Melender et al., 2010; Nemoto, Operario, Keatley, & Villegas, 2004).

Clients' Drug Use

Drug use by transwomen with their sex work clients is a common occurrence. Clients provide sex workers with drugs (Nemoto, Operario, Keatley, & Villegas, 2004) and may even prefer sex workers who are intoxicated (Sausa, Keatley, & Operario, 2007). Study respondents have reported that some clients will pay more if the sex worker engages in drug use with them (Nemoto et al., 1999; Sausa, Keatley, & Operario, 2007; Bith-Melender et al., 2010). Thus, it is not surprising that engagement in sex work while intoxicated is common; one study indicates that over half of transgender women respondents with commercial sex partners had engaged in sex while intoxicated in the previous 30 days (Nemoto, Operario, Keatley, Han, & Soma, 2004). Further, those engaging in sex work are more likely to have sex while intoxicated (Operario & Nemoto, 2005).

Hormone Use

Many transwomen use hormones (estrogen as well as androgen blockers) to create and maintain the appearance and feelings of femininity. Hormones obtained medically are in the form of an oral preparation or a transdermal patch; however, some transwomen obtain these hormones in the black market in injectable form because of the ease of access or a perception that these hormones are more effective (Nemoto et al., 1999). Because sex workers probably have less access to medical care and more access to black-market contacts than those in licit occupations, transgender female sex workers are more likely to use injectable hormones. Though injecting hormones is not equivalent to substance use, some studies of substance use may conflate the two if the act of injecting substances is measured (as opposed to measures of the use of injectable drugs: Reback & Fletcher, 2014).

CONSEQUENCES OF SUBSTANCE USE

Riskier Sexual Behavior

Though results are mixed, transgender female sex workers have demonstrated safer sex behavior with commercial partners than with other types of partners. A study of transwomen of color (Latina, Asian/Pacific Islander, and African American) indicated that using drugs or alcohol during sex was associated with increased rates of receptive anal sex regardless of partner type (primary, casual, and commercial). When it came to unprotected receptive anal sex, however, substance use during sex was not associated with this behavior for commercial partners, but it was for primary and casual partners (Nemoto, Operario, Keatley, Han, & Soma, 2004). In contrast, a study of kathoey in Thailand found that substance use predicted less likelihood of condom use with commercial partners (Nemoto et al., 2012). Taken together, these findings may mean that sex workers in the United States are aware of the dangers of unprotected sex with clients and protect themselves accordingly, but they do not see the danger inherent in unprotected sex with their primary and casual partners.

HIV and Other STDs

The association among sex work, intravenous drug use (IDU), and high-risk sexual behavior may vary across countries. For example, studies of transgender sex workers in Pakistan are yielding results that vary from those typically seen in Western countries. *Hijra* (transgender) sex workers (HSWs) from Larkana, Pakistan, where HIV rates were 27.6% (compared to a national prevalence rate for HSWs of 6.4%) were more likely than HSWs from other towns in Pakistan to use alcohol during intercourse with clients (Altaf, Zahidie, & Agha, 2012). Another study of male and transgender sex workers (MTSW) in Pakistan found that over one-fifth of MTSW reported clients who were IDUs, and approximately one-eighth of their sexual networks injected drugs (Collumbien et al., 2008). Though few MTSW were using injection drugs, those with IDU partners were more likely to smoke hash and drink alcohol, which, in theory, should lead to riskier sexual behavior. However, MTSWs with IDU clients were more likely than other MTSWs to use condoms, despite lower knowledge of HIV/AIDS and HIV transmission (Collumbien et al., 2008).

In the United States, study results are mixed. Drug use is higher in transwomen in San Francisco who are HIV-positive compared to those who are HIV-negative (Clements-Nolle et al., 2001), though the causative agent in this association is unclear. This study also indicated that HIV-positive transwomen are more likely to have receptive anal intercourse (RAI) with their main partner, but there was no difference in engagement in RAI, whether protected or unprotected, with sex work clients by HIV status (Clements-Nolle et al., 2001). However, a qualitative study in San Francisco indicated that some transgender sex workers may neglect to use condoms with commercial partners while intoxicated (Sausa, Keatley, & Operario, 2007).

MODELS EXPLAINING SUBSTANCE USE

Minority Stress Model

The Minority Stress Model was created by Meyer (2003) to explain high rates of mental disorders in LGB populations and was based on constructs of social psychology. The model is based on the concept that alienation, stigma, and discrimination from mainstream society result in feelings of isolation and stress, leading to high rates of mental disorders and coping mechanisms, some of which may be maladaptive (such as substance use). Hendricks and Testa (2012) adapted this model for transgender and gender-variant individuals to explain the prevalence of stress disorders and the effects of this stress on these populations.

According to Bradford and colleagues (2013), factors associated with being a victim of discrimination are living in a suburban area, being female-to-male, being a member of a racial or ethnic minority group, having a low level of education, earning a low income, and lacking health insurance. The last four of these characteristics can be used to describe most transgender female sex workers, which suggests that this group may experience discrimination at high levels, even apart from the discrimination and violence experienced because of their occupation. Studies of transgender participants have indicated a connection between mental distress and drug use (Clements-Nolle, Marx, & Katz, 2006) and between sexual violence and substance use (Testa et al., 2012). In addition, samples of transgender women that included sex workers indicated that they engaged in substance use to cope with stress and discrimination (Nemoto, Operario, Keatley, & Villegas, 2004; Van Devanter et al., 2011), which further supports the Minority Stress Model.

Stress Process Model

The Stress Process Model proposes that stress from various sources results in increased levels of maladaptive coping, leading to illness (Pearlin et al., 1981). This model is older than the Minority Stress Model, and, unlike that model, it focuses more on internal coping mechanisms to stress. However, much of the evidence discussed above indicating substance use as a response to stress would support this model as well as the Minority Stress Model (Clements-Nolle, Marx, & Katz, 2006; Nemoto, Operario, Keatley, & Villegas, 2004; Testa et al., 2012; Van Devanter et al., 2011). One study (Hotton et al., 2013) directly tested this model in a sample of transwomen, about half of whom had participated in high-risk sexual behaviors that included sex work. Results indicated that substance use mediated the relationship between stressful life events and sexually risky behavior. This result not only is in line with studies indicating the relationship between substance use and sex work but also provides support for rehabilitation models that address substance use when aiding transgender sex workers in finding less risky forms of employment.

TREATMENT RECOMMENDATIONS

This evidence certainly supports the need for substance-use treatment programs for transwomen and for transgender sex workers as a subset of that group. Relatively few papers have been published regarding treatment programs for transwomen, let alone transgender sex workers. The few that have been (Craft & Mulvey, 2001; Kammerer, Mason, & Conners, 1999; Lombardi & van Servellin, 2000; Nemoto et al., 2005; Oggins & Eichenbaum, 2002; Senreich, 2011) do provide valuable recommendations for practitioners and others working on substance use treatment for this group.

Recruitment

The biggest challenge in providing drug treatment for transwomen sex workers may lie in recruiting clients. Potential clients may not consider themselves in need of drug treatment if they are not using needles or may consider their primary problem to be one of gender, not drug abuse (Kammerer, Mason, & Connors, 1999). Oggins and Eichenbaum (2002) report that outreach to prospective clients is most effective to those who are in jail, are homeless, or are suffering from acute addiction; outreach to sex workers on the street or in bars is particularly ineffective, as it is distracting and potentially offensive. In other words, treatment is likely to be more effective with transgender females who are interested in leaving sex work or have already faced negative effects from either drug use or sex work, while those who are making a living through sex work are not likely to be interested in drug treatment if they are not finding that their drug use is negatively affecting their lives.

Population Served

Programs must be specifically targeted intersectionally for transgender sex workers (in other words, targeted for both transgender females and for sex workers) in order to adequately serve that group. Programs for cisgender sex workers will not suffice to provide support from either staff or clients for those in treatment (Kammerer, Mason, & Connors, 1999). Though transgender sex workers share some of the struggles of cisgender sex workers, there are additional challenges caused by the added stigma they face owing to others' reactions to their transgender status that require the support of those who understand these issues. Additionally, programs that cater to LGB populations may not be particularly appealing to transgender clients; past and current tensions between these groups and transgender populations may result in transwomen feeling unwelcome in both feminist and LGB spaces (Kammerer, Mason, & Connors, 1999). Further, a transgender female sex worker who is attracted to men may not consider herself to fall under the umbrella of LGB, as her sexual orientation is that of women attracted to men, and therefore heterosexual (Lombardi & van Servellin, 2000; Oggins & Eichenbaum, 2002; Senreich, 2011).

Challenges Faced in Treatment

As mentioned earlier, the challenges transgender clients face in treatment go further than addressing the dynamics related to substance use. Transwomen may be struggling with issues related to gender identity, acceptance of this identity by friends and family, violence of various types, and potentially comorbid depression or other mental illnesses in addition to substance use problems. Transgender sex workers may additionally be coping with a loss of income or consequences of incarceration or other legal problems relating to sex work. All transgender clients may require assistance in finding and maintaining employment or in transitioning at work; sex worker treatment clients must also face the challenge of a gap in their résumés or of having no legal work experience to speak of (Lombardi & van Servellin, 2000; Oggins & Eichenbaum, 2002).

Cultural Sensitivity Training

Staff of programs must receive ongoing training to treat transgender sex worker clients with respect and understanding. Therapists and counselors must be educated in the areas of gender identity, internalized transphobia, adaptive coping with stressors, self-esteem and self-acceptance issues, and challenges of living with HIV, among other areas related to substance use (Craft & Mulvey, 2001; Lombardi & van Servellin, 2000). If facilities or programs also serve cisgender clients, these clients should participate in regular training as well to orient them to the basics of transgender identity and in how to treat transgender clients appropriately (Oggins & Eichenbaum, 2002).

Ultimately, as Nemoto and colleagues (2005) suggest, transgender females, especially those who are former sex workers, may be the best choice to staff substance use treatment programs for transgender female sex workers. In addition to personally understanding the challenges that transgender sex worker clients face, transgender staff may be most knowledgeable of the effects of hormone use on mental health and may be best able to monitor clients starting or continuing hormones (Oggins & Eichenbaum, 2002). Finally, transgender professionals who were formerly clients are excellent role models for current clients, providing a picture of what life can be after achieving sobriety and leaving sex work (Oggins & Eichenbaum, 2002).

Facilities and Procedures

Physical spaces and policies should allow for gender expression of transgender clients. Clients should be able to participate in programs on the basis of the gender with which they most identify, including restrooms, lodging, and gender-based support-group sessions (Lombardi & van Servellin, 2000; Oggins & Eichenbaum, 2002). Though many substance use treatment programs encourage plain dress and minimal makeup so that the focus can be on recovery rather than on attraction, such policies may be alienating to transwomen who use clothing and cosmetics to express their gender identity. Therefore, clients should be encouraged to wear clothing and cosmetics in which they feel comfortable, even as efforts are taken to educate clients that revealing clothing is not appropriate for this setting (Lombardi & van Servellin, 2000; Oggins & Eichenbaum, 2002).

Legal Use of Hormones

As mentioned earlier, clients may have used hormones in the past. However, the hormones used may have been acquired through the black market. Further, some clients may need to restart hormone use after cessation of use during a period of incarceration. Other transgender clients may have never used hormones but have an interest in doing so. It is recommended that clients be given access to medical-grade hormones and counseled on their use, as well as provided counseling regarding feminization surgeries, if requested (Oggins & Eichenbaum, 2002).

Supplemental Services

Treatment programs must also include vocational training if the client is to avoid sex work upon reentry into the community. The drug treatment program for transgender females at Walden House in San Francisco provides clients with listings of employers friendly to hiring transgender employees, provides interviewing tips through focus groups, and directly invites clients to use the site's vocational program, which provides courses and workshops on English language, computer applications, and résumé development, among other topics (Oggins & Eichenbaum, 2002). Clients should also be connected with health insurance and transgender-friendly medical providers to ensure continuity of health services (including access to hormones) upon leaving treatment programs (Craft & Mulvey, 2001).

In summary, there are several components that must be put in place to provide substance treatment programs that will meet the needs of transgender female sex workers. While recommendations exist, few programs have reported on their efficacy for this group. In light of the clear needs of this group for interventions to reduce substance use, sex work, and ultimately HIV, creation of culturally sensitive drug treatment programs should be a priority for pro-transgender practitioners.

REFERENCES

Altaf, A., Zahidie, A., & Agha, A. (2012). Comparing risk factors of HIV among *hijra* sex workers in Larkana and other cities of Pakistan: An analytical cross sectional study. *BMC Public Health, 12*, 1–9.

Bazargan, M., & Galvan, F. (2012). Perceived discrimination and depression among low-income Latina male-to-female transgender women. *BMC Public Health, 12*, 1–8.

Bith-Melender, P., Sheoran, B., Sheth, L., Bermudez, C., Drone, J., Wood, W., & Schroeder, K. (2010). Understanding sociocultural and psychological factors affecting transgender people of color in San Francisco. *Journal of the Association of Nurses in AIDS Care, 21* (3), 207–220.

Bockting, W. O., Miner, M. H., Swinburne Romine, R. E., Hamilton, A., & Coleman E. (2013). Stigma, mental health, and resilience in an online sample of the US transgender population. *American Journal of Public Health, 103* (5), 943–951.

Bradford, J., Reisner, S. L., Honnold, J. A., & Xavier, J. (2013). Experiences of transgender-related discrimination and implications for health: Results from the Virginia Transgender Health Initiative Study. *American Journal of Public Health, 103*, 1820–1829.

Chestnut, S., Dixon, E., & Jindasurat, E. (2013). *Lesbian, gay, bisexual, transgender, queer, and HIV-affected hate violence in 2012.* New York: NCAVP.

Clements-Nolle, K., Marx, R., Guzman, R., & Katz, M. (2001). HIV prevalence, risk behaviors, health care use, and mental health status of transgender persons: Implications for public health intervention. *American Journal of Public Health, 91,* 915–921.

Clements-Nolle, K., Marx, R., & Katz, M. (2006). Attempted suicide among transgender persons. *Journal of Homosexuality, 51* (3), 53–69.

Collumbien, M., Chow, J., Qureshi, A. A., Rabbani, A., & Hawkes, S. (2008). Multiple risks among male and transgender sex workers in Pakistan. *Journal of LGBT Health Research, 4* (2–3), 71–79.

Craft, E. M., & Mulvey, K. P. (2001). Addressing lesbian, gay, bisexual, and transgender issues from the inside: One federal agency's approach. *American Journal of Public Health, 91,* 889–891.

Grant, J. M., Mottet, L. A., Tanis, J., Harrison, J., Herman, J. L., & Keisling, M. (2011). *Injustice at every turn: A report of the National Transgender Discrimination Survey.* Washington, DC: National Center for Transgender Equality and National Gay and Lesbian Task Force.

Hendricks, M. L. & Testa, R. J. (2012). A conceptual framework for clinical work with transgender and gender nonconforming clients: An adaptation of the Minority Stress Model. *Professional Psychology: Research and Practice, 43* (5), 460–467.

Herbst, J. H., Jacobs, E. D., Finlayson, T. J., McKleroy, V. S., Neumann, M. S., Crepaz, N., & HIV/AIDS Prevention Research Synthesis Team. (2008). Estimating the HIV prevalence and risk behaviors of transgender persons in the United States: A systematic review. *AIDS and Behavior, 12,* 1–17.

Hoffman, B. (2014). An overview of depression among transgender women. *Depression Research and Treatment,* Article ID 394283, 1–9.

Hotton, A. L., Garofalo, R., Kuhns, L. M., & Johnson, A. K. (2013). Substance use as a mediator of the relationship between life stress and sexual risk among young transgender women. *AIDS Education and Prevention, 25* (1), 62–71.

Hughes, T. L., & Eliason, M. (2002). Substance use and abuse in lesbian, gay, bisexual, and transgender populations. *Journal of Primary Prevention, 22* (3), 263–298.

Kammerer, N., Mason, T., & Connors, M. (1999). Transgender health and social service needs in the context of HIV risk. *International Journal of Transgenderism, 3,* 1–2.

Lombardi, E. L., & van Servellin, G. (2000). Building culturally sensitive substance use prevention and treatment programs for transgendered populations. *Journal of Substance Abuse Treatment, 19,* 291–296.

Meyer, I. H. (2003). Prejudice, social stress, and mental health in lesbian, gay, and bisexual populations: Conceptual issues and research evidence. *Psychological Bulletin, 129* (5), 674–697.

Nemoto, T., Bödeker, B., & Iwamoto, M. (2011). Social support, exposure to violence and transphobia, and correlates of depression among male-to-female transgender women with a history of sex work. *American Journal of Public Health, 101* (10), 1980–1988.

Nemoto, T., Iwamoto, M., Perngparn, U., Areesantichai, C., Kamitani, E., & Sakata, M.

(2012). HIV-related risk behaviors among kathoey (male-to-female transgender) sex workers in Bangkok, Thailand. *AIDS Care, 24* (2), 210–219.

Nemoto, T., Luke, D., Mamo, L., Ching, A., & Patria, J. (1999). HIV risk behaviours among male-to-female transgenders in comparison with homosexual or bisexual males and heterosexual females. *AIDS Care, 11* (3), 297–312.

Nemoto, T., Operario, D., Keatley, J., Han, L., & Soma, T. (2004). HIV risk behaviors among male-to-female transgender persons of color in San Francisco. *American Journal of Public Health, 94* (7), 1193–1199.

Nemoto, T., Operario, D., Keatley, J., Nguyen, H., & Sugano, E. (2005). Promoting health for transgender women: Transgender Resources and Neighborhood Space (TRANS) program in San Francisco. *American Journal of Public Health, 95,* 382–384.

Nemoto, T., Operario, D., Keatley, J., & Villegas, D. (2004). Social context of HIV risk behaviors among male-to-female transgenders of color. *AIDS Care, 16* (6), 724–735.

Nuttbrock, L., Bockting, W., Rosenblum, A., Hwahng, S., Mason, M., Macri, M., & Becker, J. (2013). Gender abuse, depressive symptoms, and HIV and other sexually transmitted infections among male-to-female transgender persons: A three-year prospective study. *American Journal of Public Health, 103* (2), 300–307.

Oggins, J., & Eichenbaum, J. (2002). Engaging transgender substance users in substance use treatment. *International Journal of Transgenderism, 6* (2), 1–16.

Operario, D., & Nemoto, T. (2005). Sexual risk behavior and substance use among a sample of Asian-Pacific Islander transgendered women. *AIDS Education & Prevention, 17* (5), 430–443.

Pearlin, L. I., Menaghan, E. G., Lieberman, M. A., & Mullan, J. T. (1981). The stress process. *Journal of Health and Social Behavior, 22* (4), 337–356.

Reback, C. J., & Fletcher, J. B. (2014). HIV prevalence, substance use, and sexual risk behaviors among transgender women recruited through outreach. *AIDS and Behavior, 18,* 1359–1367.

Rosser, B. R. S., Oakes, J. M., Bockting, W. O., & Miner, M. (2007). Capturing the social demographics of hidden sexual minorities: An Internet study of the transgender population in the United States. *Sexuality Research & Social Policy, 4* (2), 50–64.

Sausa, L. A., Keatley, J., & Operario, D. (2007). Perceived risks and benefits of sex work among transgender women of color in San Francisco. *Archives of Sex Behavior, 36,* 768–777.

Senreich, E. (2011). The substance abuse treatment experiences of a small sample of transgender clients. *Journal of Social Work Practice in the Addictions, 11,* 295–299.

Substance Abuse and Mental Health Services Administration (SAMHSA). (2014). *Results from the 2013 National Survey on Drug Use and Health: Summary of national findings.* NSDUH Series H-48, HHS Publication No. (SMA) 14-4863. Rockville, MD: Substance Abuse and Mental Health Services Administration.

Testa, R. J., Sciacca, L. M., Wang, F., Hendricks, M. L., Goldblum, P., & Bradford, J. (2012). Effects of violence on transgender people. *Professional Psychology: Research and Practice, 43* (5), 452–459.

Van Devanter, N., Duncan, A., Raveis, V. H., Birnbaum, J., Burrell-Piggott, T., & Siegel, K. (2011). Continued sexual risk behaviour in African American and Latino male-to-female transgender adolescents living with HIV/AIDS: A case study. *Journal of AIDS & Clinical Research, S1,* 1–2.

Since the 1990s, extremely high levels of HIV have been observed among transwomen; reviews of this literature suggest that the prevalence of HIV may be even higher among those in the sex trade. This section begins with a review by Scheim and colleagues of the current literature on the prevalence of HIV among transwomen sex workers. This is followed by a look at the association between HIV and substance use by Glynn and colleagues. Then Nuttbrock examines the association between sex work and incidence of HIV/STI among transwomen in the New York Transgender Project, showing here that this association reflects increased levels of abuse, depressive symptoms, and substance use. The final chapter in this section addresses the little-studied issue of access to medical care among transwomen sex workers. Among HIV-positive transwomen included in the baseline component of the New York Transgender Project, Nuttbrock found that sex work was associated with self-reports of not receiving HIV medications (antiviral therapies).

CHAPTER 9

The Prevalence of HIV among Transwomen Sex Workers

A Review of Current Literature

Ayden I. Scheim[1]
Laura Winters[2]
Zack Marshall[3]
Daze Jefferies[4]
Stefan D. Baral[5]

1 Pierre Elliott Trudeau Foundation Scholar in Epidemiology and Biostatistics at Western University in London, Canada.
2 Graduate student in sociology at the University of New Brunswick.
3 Assistant professor at Renison University College, University of Waterloo.
4 Graduate student in gender studies at Memorial University of Newfoundland, Canada.
5 Physician epidemiologist and associate professor in the Department of Epidemiology at the Johns Hopkins Bloomberg School of Public Health.

SUMMARY

Transgender (trans) women and women who engage in sex work are groups that face a higher burden of HIV relative to other populations. Women at the intersection of these identities and occupations experience compounded vulnerabilities to the acquisition and transmission of HIV. In this chapter we provide an overview of recent research on HIV prevalence and incidence among transwomen who engage in sex work globally, and the multiple factors contributing to their HIV-related risk and resilience.

KEY TERMS

HIV incidence; HIV prevalence; HIV risk; sex work; transwomen

Nuttbrock, Larry, *Transgender Sex Work and Society*
dx.doi.org/10.17312/harringtonparkpress/2017.11.tsws.009
© 2018 by Harrington Park Press

Transwomen who engage in sex work are a heterogeneous group: the term *transwoman* encompasses great variability in identities, embodiments, and lived experiences. Similarly, there is a wide spectrum of sex work involvement. Sex work takes place in many contexts and forms, and the people who do it have varying levels of control over their work and the conditions in which this work occurs. Individuals who were assigned the male sex at birth but who identify as female or feminine, and who engage in sex work, do not necessarily identify as "transwomen sex workers," a term we use in this chapter for economy.

HIV BURDEN AMONG TRANS SEX WORKERS

In a 2008 systematic review, Operario and colleagues meta-analyzed HIV prevalence data for trans sex workers and comparison groups published between 1988 and 2006, including 3,159 transwomen (2,139 of whom were sex workers) across 14 countries (Operario, Soma, & Underhill, 2008). They found pooled prevalence of 27% among trans sex workers, which was significantly higher than among female sex workers (relative risk = 4.02, 95% CI 1.60–10.11) but not significantly different from prevalence among non–sex working transwomen in the included studies.

Baral, Poteat, and colleagues (2013) conducted a systematic review of laboratory-confirmed HIV prevalence data for transwomen globally, including publications from 2000 through 2011. Combining data for 11,066 transwomen in ten low- and middle-income and five high-income countries (all with concentrated epidemics), they found pooled global prevalence of 19% (95% CI 17–21). Compared to all reproductive-age adults, the odds of HIV infection among transwomen were 48.8 times as high (95% CI 31.2–76.3), and this number did not differ significantly by country income (low and middle versus high). Many studies did not report the proportion of respondents with a history of sex work, which precluded subgroup analyses.

To provide an updated picture of the HIV burden among trans sex workers, we reviewed data on HIV prevalence and incidence published from 2008 to 2015, drawing on publications identified in two recent systematic reviews (Reisner et al., 2016; Poteat et al., 2016). Tables 9.1, 9.2, and 9.3 summarize results for Latin America, Asia, and Europe and North America, respectively. No disaggregated data for trans sex workers were located for other regions. Prevalence estimates are based on laboratory-confirmed HIV infection, unless otherwise specified.

In three studies from Argentina that predominantly sampled sex workers, seroprevalence ranged from 27% to 34%. Elsewhere in Latin America, one study each reported seroprevalence among predominantly sex-working transwomen in Ecuador, El Salvador, Mexico, Paraguay, and Peru, with estimates between 17% and 32%. Of three studies from

TABLE 9.1

HIV Prevalence and Incidence among Transgender Women Sex Workers in Latin America, 2008–2015

Citation	Location	N	Sampling	% Sex Workers (Definition)	HIV (CI)	Method for Ascertaining HIV Status
Dos Ramos Farías et al., 2011	Argentina	273	Convenience; community organizations	100% (regular or occasional transactional sex + identification as sex worker)	Prevalence: 34% (29–40) Estimated incidence: 10.7 per 100 PY (3.8–17.7)	Laboratory
Socías et al., 2014	Argentina	452	Convenience	85% (lifetime); 61% (current)	27%	Self-report
Toibaro et al., 2009	Argentina (Buenos Aires)	105	STI clinic	100% (not specified)	28%	Laboratory
Fernandes et al., 2015	Brazil (Campo Grande)	152	Venue-based (bar, massage parlor, street)	76% (ever exchanged sex for money or goods)	24%	Laboratory
Martins et al., 2013	Brazil (Fortaleza)	304	Respondent-driven sampling	87% (received money for sex, lifetime, unweighted) 66% (past month, unweighted)	12% (unweighted)	Self-report
Costa et al., 2014	Brazil (Rio Grande do Sul)	284	Gender-identity clinic patients	29% (lifetime)	History of sex work: 39% No sex work: 19% ($p = .003$)	Laboratory
Solomon et al., 2015	Ecuador (Guayaquil)	131	Clinical trial screening	74% (ever received money for sex)	17%	Laboratory
Barrington et al., 2012	El Salvador (San Salvador)	67	Respondent-driven sampling	54% (CI 34–76; sold sex in past year)	19% (5–39)	Laboratory

Citation	Location	N	Sampling	% Sex Workers (Definition)	HIV (CI)	Method for Ascertaining HIV Status
Colchero et al., 2015	Mexico (Mexico City)	585	Convenience; meeting places, HIV clinic, detention centers	39% (transactional sex as consistent or primary income source)	47% overall, 19–32% for participants not sampled from HIV clinic. HIV infection not associated with current sex work.	Laboratory
Aguayo Munoz, & Aguilar, 2013	Paraguay	237	Not specified	89% (unspecified)	27% (21–32)	Laboratory
Silva-Santisteban et al., 2012	Peru (Lima)	450	Respondent-driven sampling	64% (CI 56–74; currently works as sex worker)	30% (23–39) HIV infection not associated with current sex work.	Laboratory

Brazil, one that included laboratory-confirmed prevalence data and disaggregation by lifetime sex work status found that 39% of trans sex workers were HIV-positive, significantly higher than the 19% prevalence among other transwomen ($p = .003$) (Costa et al., 2014). However, two other studies from the region found that HIV prevalence was not significantly higher among sex workers (Colchero et al., 2015; Silva-Santisteban et al., 2012).

Published studies in Asia and the Pacific came from India (N = 3), Pakistan (N = 4), and Thailand (N = 3). One Indian study reported laboratory-confirmed seroprevalence from a majority-sex-worker sample, finding 18% prevalence among transwomen (described as *hijra*), with an 87% lifetime prevalence of sex work (Brahmam et al., 2008). In Pakistan, transwomen (described as *hijra, jogta,* and *khusra*) included in studies were almost universally sex workers. HIV prevalence was relatively low (1–7%), but the burden of active STIs was very high where measured (49–59%). In a study comparing trans sex workers across cities in Pakistan, HIV seroprevalence was markedly higher in the city with the highest level of economic reliance on sex work as a sole source of income, and where average number of clients was highest (28% versus 6% overall; Altaf, Zahidie, & Agha, 2012). In Thailand, seroprevalence

TABLE 9.2

HIV Prevalence and Incidence among Transgender Women Sex Workers in Asia, 2008–2015

Citation	Location	N	Sampling	% Sex Workers (Definition)	HIV (CI)	Method for Ascertaining HIV Status
Brahmam et al., 2008	India	575	Time-location	87% (lifetime); 64% (main income source)	18%	Laboratory
Subramani-an et al., 2013	India (Tamil Nadu)	404 (2006) 403 (2009)	Multistage & time-location cluster sampling	20% (sex work as main source of income, 2006); 41% (2009)	12% (2006) 10% (2009)	Laboratory
Chakrapani et al., 2015	India (multisite, urban and rural)	300	Convenience	71% (paid for sex in past 3 months); 26% (reported employment as sex worker)	9%	Self-report
Emmanuel et al., 2013	Pakistan	3,714	Convenience; peer referral	100% (home- or dera-based [communal home overseen by guru])	7.2% (6.8–7.5%)	Laboratory
Altaf, Zahidie, & Agha, 2012	Pakistan (multi-city)	619	Network-based sampling	100% (inclusion criteria = "undertakes sexual activity with a man in return for money or other financial benefits")	6% overall; range from 0 to 28% by city	Laboratory
Khan et al., 2008	Pakistan (Lahore and Karachi)	409	Cluster sampling	84% (sold sex in the past month); 99% (sold sex in the past year)	1% (58% had any STI)	Laboratory
Hawkes et al., 2009	Pakistan (Rawalpindi)	253	Respondent-driven sampling (not weighted)	100% (sold sex in past 30 days)	2.4% (0.4–4.3%); 49% with active syphilis	Laboratory

Citation	Location	N	Sampling	% Sex Workers (Definition)	HIV (CI)	Method for Ascertaining HIV Status
Nemoto et al., 2012	Thailand	112	Venue-based (bars, street)	100% (current sex worker)	0%, 53% ever tested	Self-report
Chemnasiri et al., 2010	Thailand (Bangkok)	241	Time-location	Not specified, at least 51% recruited from sex work venues	10%	Laboratory
Guadamuz et al., 2011	Thailand (multicity)	474	Venue-day-time sampling	61% (ever received money, gifts, or valuables for sex)	17% among those with a history of sex work; 9% among those without ($p < .05$)	Laboratory

among transwomen with a history of sex work was higher than among other transwomen (17% versus 9%, $p < .05$; Guadamuz et al., 2011).

Only small studies of trans sex workers were available in the European literature. In Portugal (two studies), 80% of 20 trans sex workers had laboratory-confirmed HIV infection, and 17% of 81 trans sex workers self-reported being HIV-positive. In one study from the United Kingdom, 38% of 24 trans sex workers (23 transwomen) were seropositive. All six studies from the United States drew on samples in San Francisco or Los Angeles. In four samples with mixed-sex work histories, self-reported HIV prevalence ranged from 14% to 24%. Among sex workers only, a 30% overall self-reported prevalence was found (Nemoto et al., 2014). In a San Francisco study with relatively low sex work engagement (11% in the previous six months), 40% had laboratory-confirmed HIV, and seroprevalence was not associated with sex work (Rapues et al., 2013).

In summary, we found a heavy burden of HIV among trans sex workers, which is consistent with previous reviews (Baral, Poteat, et al., 2013; Operario et al., 2008), but limited data that allow for direct comparison of burden between transwomen with and without sex work involvement. Where comparative data were available, such as in Operario and colleagues

TABLE 9.3

HIV Prevalence and Incidence among Transgender Women Sex Workers in Europe and North America, 2008–2015

Citation	Location	N	Sampling	% Sex Workers (Definition)	HIV (CI)	Method for Ascertaining HIV Status
Almeida et al., 2014	Portugal (Lisbon)	20*	Clinic for sex workers	100% (unspecified)	80%	Laboratory
Dias et al., 2015	Portugal (multi-city)	81	Convenience, venue-based	100% (sex work in past 12 months)	17% (8–27%)	Self-report (among those ever tested)
Hill et al., 2011	United Kingdom (London)	24 (incl. 1 trans-man)	STI clinic	100% (unspecified)	38%	Laboratory
Brennan & Kuhns, 2012	United States (Chicago and Los Angeles)	151 (ages 15–24)	Convenience, multiple sources	67% (lifetime transactional sex)	16%	Self-report
Fletcher, Kisler, & Reback, 2014	United States (Los Angeles)	517	Convenience; HIV prevention program participants	49% (past-month transactional sex)	24%	Self-report
Reback & Fletcher, 2013	United States (Los Angeles)	2,136	Convenience; HIV prevention outreach	73% (sex for money or drugs in past month)	14%	Self-report
Nemoto et al., 2014	United States (San Francisco)	573	Convenience	100% ("self-report-ed history of sex work")	Total: 30% White: 18% API: 13% Latina: 25% Black: 47% $p < 0.01$	Self-report
Rapues et al., 2013	United States (San Francisco)	314	Respon-dent-driven sampling	11% (commercial sex work in past 6 months)	40% (32–48%) HIV infection not associated with current sex work.	Laboratory

Citation	Location	N	Sampling	% Sex Workers (Definition)	HIV (CI)	Method for Ascertaining HIV Status
Sevelius et al., 2009	United States (San Francisco)	153	Convenience	34% (transactional sex in past year)	22%	Self-report

*Gender spectrum/natal sex not specified.

(2008), we found that the HIV burden was not consistently higher among transwomen with a history of sex work, as compared to other transwomen. In large part, this may be due to the high burden of HIV among transwomen overall and shared contexts of social marginalization irrespective of sex work involvement, particularly among the higher-risk transwomen whom convenience sampling methods tend to select for. In addition, sex work involvement is the norm for transwomen in some settings, rendering it a ubiquitous determinant that is not detectable in within-group analyses of transwomen.

This seeming inconsistency may also be an artifact of how sex work involvement is operationalized. Among those studies reporting HIV prevalence stratified by sex work history, a pattern emerges: lifetime sex work is associated with prevalent HIV infection (Costa et al., 2014; Guadamuz et al., 2011; Lombardi & Friedman, 2012; Nuttbrock et al., 2009), but current sex work is not (Colchero et al., 2015; Rapues et al., 2013; Silva-Santisteban et al., 2012). This pattern suggests a particularly high HIV burden among former trans sex workers, who will be older on average and may have left sex work because of HIV diagnosis or disease progression.

RACE, ETHNICITY, IMMIGRATION, AND HIV PREVALENCE AMONG TRANS SEX WORKERS

In the United States, transwomen of color, particularly African Americans and Latinas, experience far higher rates of HIV than their white peers (Grant et al., 2011; Herbst et al., 2008). These numbers mirror well-documented broader racial disparities in HIV incidence and prevalence in the United States (White House Office of National AIDS Policy, 2015).

Among transwomen sex workers specifically, available data from the United States indicate profound racial and ethnic disparities in both sex work participation and HIV burden. In each of the studies from the United States included in Table 9.3, more than half of the sample was African American or Latina. Nemoto and colleagues (2014) found significant variation ($p < .01$) in self-reported HIV prevalence among trans sex workers in San Francisco, the highest prevalence (47%) being among African Americans and the lowest among Asians and Pacific Islanders (13%). Differences in self-reported prevalence, however, may reflect variation in uptake of HIV testing as well as true differences in seroprevalence. Similarly, being African American was independently associated with HIV infection among Los Angeles trans sex workers (Reback & Fletcher, 2013). In a report from the largest US trans survey to date, 3% of non-Hispanic white trans sex workers (including transmen and transwomen) reported being HIV-positive, versus 26% of trans sex workers of color and 41% of African American trans sex workers (Fitzgerald et al., 2015).

Globally, evidence of racial and ethnic disparities in HIV among transwomen is limited but can be expected in settings where broader disparities exist. For instance, in Canada, where aboriginal people are disproportionately affected by HIV, prevalence appeared elevated in aboriginal trans people (Bauer et al., 2012). In European data, the majority of both trans sex workers and HIV-infected trans sex workers are migrant workers, most often from Latin America (Almeida et al., 2014; Dias et al., 2015; Fernández-Balbuena et al., 2014; Patrascioiu et al., 2013). Less is known about HIV prevalence among nonimmigrant and racial and ethnic majority trans sex workers in Europe.

FACTORS CONTRIBUTING TO HIV RISK AMONG TRANS WOMEN WHO ENGAGE IN SEX WORK

In this section, we summarize recent research on factors associated with HIV-related risk and HIV infection among transwomen sex workers (Table 9.4), and situate these findings in the context of the extant literature on trans and sex worker health. A multitude of structural, interpersonal, and individual factors related to what it means to be trans, as well as what it means to do sex work, in a stigmatizing social context contribute to trans sex workers' vulnerability to HIV infection. The situation is complex, as these factors not only contribute to risk inde-

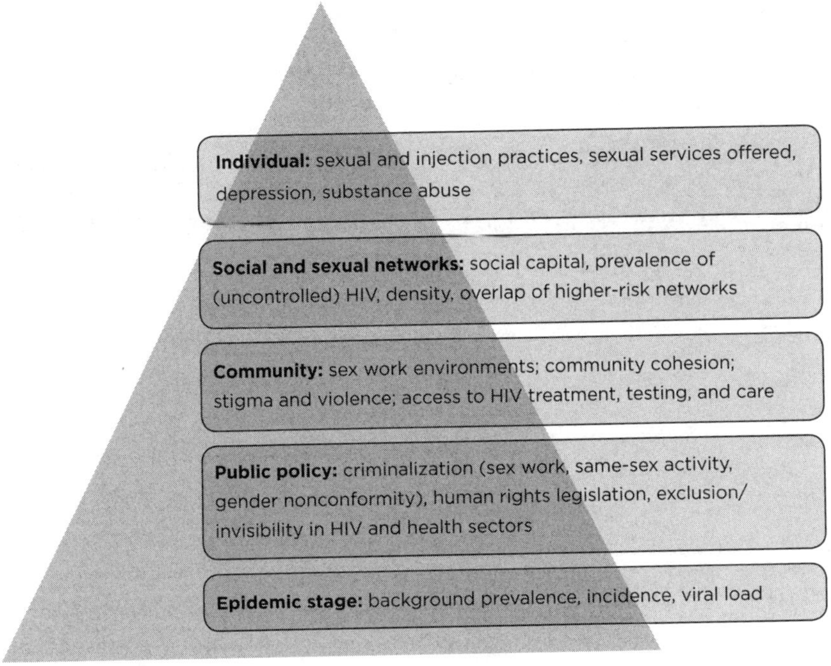

FIGURE 9.1

Modified Social Ecological Model for HIV Risks among Transwomen Sex Workers.
Source: Adapted from Baral, Logie, et al. (2013).

pendently, but also interact to heighten risk. Simply being trans and engaging in any sex work does not necessitate increased HIV risk, but being trans and doing sex work for certain individuals, under certain conditions, does. We adapt Baral and colleagues' Modified Social Ecological Model (Baral, Logie, et al., 2013) (MSEM) to begin to tease apart the relationships between intersecting levels of HIV risk for transwomen who engage in sex work. In this model (Figure 9.1), risks are contextualized in relation to the individual, her social and sexual networks, her community, and public policy; we extend the model to consider factors related to sex work at each level.

The MSEM emphasizes the role of supra-individual factors in the production of HIV acquisition and transmission risk in vulnerable populations, with the premise that interventions targeting these factors have greater potential to reduce HIV risk at the population level than interventions addressing more proximal sexual and injection risk behaviors.

TABLE 9.4

Risk and Protective Factors among Transgender Women Sex Workers, 2008–2015

Citation	Location	N	% Sex Workers	Risk/Protective Factor	Masure of Association (CI)
Chakrapani et al., 2015	India (multisite, urban and rural)	300	71% (past 3 months)	Number of psychosocial health conditions (depression, victimization, frequent alcohol use)	Adjusted odds ratio (AOR) for inconsistent condom use with male partners;
				1 condition	1.42 (0.53, 3.80)
				2 conditions	4.12 (1.54, 11.00)
				3 conditions	15.77 (4.71, 52.84)
Hawkes et al., 2009	Pakistan (Rawalpindi)	253	100% (past month)		AOR for current STI
				Any non–sex work income	1.97 (1.05, 3.68)
				Condom use during last anal sex	0.33 (0.17, 0.65)
				First sex with a man was forced	2.96 (1.44, 6.09)
Silva-San-tisteban et al., 2012	Peru (Lima)	450	64% (current)		AOR for HIV infection:
				Over 35 years old	4.7 (1.3, 17.4)
				Recent syphilis	8.2 (1.7, 39.4)
				Herpes simplex 2–positive	6.3 (1.1, 36.2)
Dias et al., 2015	Portugal (multicity)	81	100% (current)	Higher number of clients in last working day, vs. cisgender sex workers	$p = .013$
				trans vs. male sex workers	AOR for HIV-positive, self-report: 6.4 (1.7, 24.3)

Citation	Location	N	% Sex Workers	Risk/Protective Factor	Masure of Association (CI)
Nemoto et al., 2012	Thailand	112	100%		Multiple linear regression for frequency of condom use for anal sex with exchange partners, past 6 months:
				Completed sex reassignment surgery	$\hat{a} = -.32, p < .001$
				Ever abused by brother or father	$\hat{a} = -.27, p < .05$
				Past-year illicit drug use	$\hat{a} = -.34, p <. 001$
Brennan & Kuhns, 2012	United States (Chicago and Los Angeles)	151 (ages 15–24)	67% lifetime	3 or 4 syndemic index factors (low self-esteem, polydrug use, victimization, intimate partner violence) vs. 0	AOR for HIV infection = 6.61 (1.25, 34.85)
				Sex work	B for association with syndemic index = 0.70, SE = 0.20, $p < 0.01$
Nemoto et al., 2014	United States (San Francisco)	573 (history of sex work)	100% lifetime		AOR for unprotected receptive anal intercourse:
				Depression	Primary partner = 2.58 (1.24, 5.38)
				Safe sex self-efficacy	Primary partner = 0.48 (0.25, 0.91); sex work partner = 0.27 (0.10, 0.76)
				Transphobia	Sex work partner = 2.56 (1.12, 5.87)
Nuttbrock et al., 2009	United States (New York)	367 (of color)	not specified	Lifetime number of sex work partners	AOR for HIV infection = 1.02, $p < 0.05$

(continued)

(Table 9.4 cont.)

Citation	Location	N	% Sex Workers	Risk/Protective Factor	Masure of Association (CI)
Nuttbrock et al., 2013 and 2015	United States (New York)	230 (HIV-nega-tive at base-line)	39% in past 6 mo.		Hazard ratio (HR) for unprotected receptive anal intercourse with commercial partners:
				Gender abuse	3.72 (2.27, 6.09)
				Depressive symptoms	1.07 (1.05, 1.10)
				Sex work	Adjusted HR for incident HIV/STI: 3.46 (1.63, 7.34)
Reback & Fletcher, 2013	United States (Los Angeles)	2,136	73% in past month		AOR for self-re-ported HIV-posi-tive:
				African American/ black	2.97 (1.65, 5.83)
				Methamphetamine use	2.09 (1.52, 2.88)
				Crack use	2.19 (1.21, 3.97)
				Lifetime injection drug or hormone use	1.65 (1.21, 2.25)
				Anal sex with exchange partner	0.51 (0.31, 0.84)
				Unprotected anal sex with exchange partner	2.24 (1.09, 4.60)
Lombardi & Friedman, 2012	United States	3,577	Not specified		AOR for self-re-ported HIV-posi-tive status:
				Lifetime sex work, overall	6.08 (3.5, 10.58)
				Lifetime sex worker in high HIV prevalence city (versus non–sex worker)	0.34 (0.14, 0.88)

Citation	Location	N	% Sex Workers	Risk/Protective Factor	Masure of Association (CI)
Clements-Nolle, Guzman, & Harris, 2008	United States (San Francisco)	190	100% (current)		AOR for inconsistent condom use for anal sex with exchange partners, past six months:
				Low self-esteem	3.09 (1.28, 7.47)
				History of sexual assault	2.91 (1.06, 8.01)
				Crack cocaine use	2.59 (1.09, 6.13)
Wilson et al., 2010	United States (Los Angeles and Chicago)	120 (ages 16–24)	40% (commercial partner in past 3 months)	Commercial versus main partner	AOR for consistent condom use for anal intercourse: 4.3 (1.4, 13.3)
Wilson et al., 2014	United States (San Francisco)	235	18% of sexual relationships were with commercial partners	Commercial vs. primary partner	AOR for condomless anal intercourse: 0.20 (0.10, 0.43)

Public Policy

The negative effects of the criminalization of sex work (including the criminalization of clients) on the lives of women who do sex work, including their health, is well documented (Krüsi et al., 2014). Criminalization has enabled widespread human rights violations against sex workers. Among cisgender sex workers, these violations have been demonstrated to potentiate HIV acquisition and transmission risk (Decker et al., 2015), while legal protections have been associated with reduced HIV prevalence (Oldenburg et al., 2016). Within the criminal justice system, abuses against sex workers include physical and sexual violence at the hands of police; arbitrary arrest and imprisonment; seizure of condoms or syringes and their use as evidence; theft and extortion; and impunity for perpetrators of violence against sex workers. Moreover, even in the absence of direct mistreatment by state actors, criminalization of sex work—including criminalization of clients—and attendant policing practices limit sex workers' control over the work environment. This lack of control restricts their capacity to screen clients and negotiate the terms of sexual interaction (Shannon & Csete, 2010). For instance, police crackdowns on street-based sex work often displace workers to industrial, dark, or deserted urban areas in which they are particularly vulnerable (Krüsi et al., 2014; Shannon et al., 2008).

Same-sex sexual activity and cross-sex gender expression continue to be criminalized in approximately 75 countries (Carroll & Itaborahy, 2015), and human-rights violations against transwomen are commonplace even in settings without anti-transgender legal sanctions. Consequently, as compared to other sex workers, transwomen are disproportionately affected by violence from state actors (Cohan et al., 2006). In fact, transwomen—regardless of sex work status—commonly report mistreatment by police. In Canada, a relatively progressive policy environment for trans people, one-quarter of transwomen reported being harassed by police because of being trans (Marcellin, Bauer, & Scheim, 2013). In Los Angeles, in a sample of Latina transwomen (53% undocumented immigrants; 80% lifetime sex work), verbal, physical, and sexual assault by police were reported by 67%, 21%, and 22% of participants, respectively (Woods et al., 2013). Abuse by law enforcement was independently associated with a sex work history (adjusted OR = 5.43, 95% CI 2.55, 11.54).

In settings where anal intercourse between natal males and gender-nonconforming persons is criminalized, trans sex workers are multiply criminalized and highly vulnerable to police violence and extortion. For example, in Sri Lanka, trans sex workers described ubiquitous and highly gendered forms of violence. In addition to verbal, physical, and sexual abuse, extortion, and failure to protect, they reported being forced to engage in stereotypically feminine behavior, such as dancing or cleaning for police who were detaining them (Nichols, 2010).

As is discussed elsewhere in this volume, exclusion from the formal labor market and concomitant poverty contribute to the high levels of sex work involvement in trans communities, particularly for members of racial and ethnic minority groups and those with precarious migration status. Socioeconomic exclusion can also increase vulnerability to HIV for trans sex workers by leading them to focus on earnings over safer sex practices. Clients frequently offer more money in exchange for condomless intercourse, and sex workers with greater economic need or with less negotiating power (or both) owing to social stigma are more likely to accept such offers (Deering et al., 2013).

Indeed, trans sex workers report increased earning potential as a cause of condom nonuse with clients (Nemoto et al., 2012; Reisner et al., 2009), and sexual and gender minority sex workers in Canada (including trans sex workers) were more likely than heterosexual female sex workers to accept higher pay in exchange for condomless sex (Deering et al., 2013).

Health systems, including the HIV sector, have the potential to reduce or exacerbate HIV risk. Unfortunately, the illegality of sex work in most countries hampers the development of accessible and acceptable healthcare services for sex workers, whose experiences with healthcare providers are often characterized by judgment and ridicule, hostility, and denial of treatment (Baral et al., 2015; Scorgie et al., 2013). Trans people face similar manifestations of stigma in healthcare (Safer et al., 2016) and are often made invisible in healthcare education, policy, and practice (Bauer et al., 2009).

Community

Along with exposure to state violence under criminalization, transwomen sex workers frequently experience stigma, harassment, and violence in the communities where they live and work. Gender-related stigma and abuse have been associated with condomless receptive anal intercourse with commercial partners in the United States (Nemoto et al., 2014; Nuttbrock et al., 2013) and Thailand (Nemoto et al., 2012). A history of sexual assault predicted inconsistent condom use with commercial partners in the United States (Clements-Nolle, Guzman, & Harris, 2008) and current STI in Pakistan (Hawkes et al., 2009).

As was described earlier, the interaction of stigmas related to sex work, trans identity, sex between members of the same natal sex, and HIV profoundly limits the availability and accessibility of healthcare for trans sex workers, including HIV testing, treatment, and care (Logie et al., 2011; Roche & Keith, 2014). Healthcare services sensitive to the needs and identities of trans sex workers are scarce; even services specifically supporting sex workers may alienate trans sex workers by failing to affirm their gender identities. Transwomen living with HIV experience unique barriers to engagement and retention in HIV care, including stigma in healthcare settings, lack of integration with transition-related care, competing priorities (e.g., basic needs), and concerns about interactions between antiretroviral medications and hormones for gender affirmation (Poteat, Reisner, & Radix, 2014). These same factors may limit their access to and interest in pre-exposure prophylaxis and other HIV prevention technologies that require interaction with the healthcare system (Wilson et al., 2015). Trans sex workers also face financial barriers to care, extending to settings with public healthcare systems where they may receive nonstigmatizing treatment only in private clinics (Scorgie et al., 2013) or need to pay for non-insured procedures related to gender transition (Rotondi et al., 2013). As a result of these barriers, transwomen often engage in medically unsupervised feminizing body modification, including illicit hormone use and injection of soft-tissue fillers (e.g., industrial silicone; Rotondi et al., 2013; Silva-Santisteban et al., 2012). In addition to posing a range of health risks, these practices may increase risk of HIV related to shared injection equipment. However, these procedures may be important for trans sex workers' income generation.

Also at the community level, sex work environments play a critical role in enabling or hindering HIV prevention practices (Harcourt, 2005). For instance, ethnographic research in New York City suggests that racial disparities in HIV prevalence among transwomen are tied to the racially stratified transgender sex work market in which African American and Latina trans sex workers predominate in street-level high-risk survival work, Asian trans sex workers are more commonly found in moderate-risk indoor survival sex work, and white trans sex workers more often engage in occasional, indoor work (Hwahng & Nuttbrock, 2007).

Social and Sexual Networks

It appears that structurally determined network characteristics, rather than individual sexual and drug use behaviors, account for the racial disparities in HIV infection among transwomen in the United States. For example, among African American cisgender men who have sex with men (MSM), high levels of undiagnosed or untreated HIV and STIs within sexual networks contribute to elevated HIV incidence (Millett et al., 2007), in a context of high racial assortativity in African American MSM sexual networks because of racial stratification in MSM communities (Matthews et al., 2016). Research on this topic is lacking for transwomen, but one study did identify higher racial assortativity among African American and Latina transwomen in San Francisco (Wilson et al., 2014).

Little is known about the primary, casual, or commercial partners of trans sex workers, although some evidence indicates that cisgender men who have sex with transwomen (paid and unpaid) are themselves at elevated risk of HIV because of sexual and drug use behaviors (Coan, Schrager, & Packer, 2005; Operario et al., 2011; Reisner et al., 2012). As is the case for sex workers in general, trans sex workers are most likely to consistently use condoms with commercial partners, and least likely with primary partners (Wilson et al., 2014; Wilson et al., 2010). However, even infrequent condomless sex can contribute to substantial HIV risk in the context of anal intercourse with a high volume of clients. In a Portuguese study, trans sex workers had a higher volume of clients than cisgender sex workers (Dias et al., 2015), and among trans sex workers in New York, an increasing number of sex workers was predictive of HIV infection (Nuttbrock et al., 2009).

Individual Level

Trans sex workers are at elevated risk for substance use and poor mental health that are related to the stigma, social exclusion, criminalization, and violence they face both as sex workers and as transwomen (Hoffman, 2014; Nadal, Davidoff, & Fujii-Doe, 2014). In turn, substance use and mental health issues are associated with HIV-related sexual risk behavior and HIV infection. Among trans sex workers, use of illicit drugs (particularly stimulants such as crack cocaine and methamphetamines) have been associated with self-reported HIV-positivity (Reback & Fletcher, 2013) and inconsistent condom use for anal intercourse with commercial partners (Clements-Nolle et al., 2008; Nemoto et al., 2012). Depression has also been related to condomless anal intercourse with commercial (Clements-Nolle et al., 2008) and primary (Nemoto et al., 2014) partners.

These individual-level risk factors may interact to potentiate HIV risk and poor health outcomes for those living with HIV. Syndemic approaches to HIV posit that mutually reinforcing psychosocial health problems resulting from social marginalization interact to increase HIV risk (Singer, 1996; Stall et al., 2003). Sex work engagement and HIV infection among young transwomen in the United States have been associated with a syndemic of polydrug use, victimization, and intimate partner violence (Brennan & Kuhns, 2012). In India, syndemic depression, frequent alcohol use, and victimization were associated with inconsistent condom use among trans sex workers (Chakrapani et al., 2015).

Although research in this area has tended to focus on the production of risk, the MSEM accounts for the possibility of protective factors at each level. For example, at the individual level, those with a better relationship to sex work (i.e., feeling empowered rather than disempowered by participation in sex work) may be at decreased risk for HIV through consistent condom use, in both private and professional encounters (Almeida, 2011).

ENHANCING DATA COLLECTION ON HIV AMONG TRANS SEX WORKERS

Our review reinforces the assertion that the HIV burden among trans sex workers remains unacceptably high, and that multilevel interventions targeting biological, behavioral, and social-structural determinants of HIV vulnerability are urgently needed (Poteat et al., 2015). At the same time, though the volume of trans health data has increased exponentially in recent years, much remains to be investigated concerning HIV among trans sex workers. Basic epidemiologic data on HIV prevalence in trans sex workers are largely absent for most countries and for regions in which the HIV burden is greatest, specifically in sub-Saharan Africa (International Reference Group on Transgender People and HIV, 2016). Lack of data collection and lack of data disaggregation jointly contribute to this absence. Collection and disaggregation of data on trans sex workers are challenged by political will, but also by cultural variations in the degree to which gender and sexual orientation are considered distinct phenomena that define mutually exclusive groups of MSM and transwomen.

Disaggregated data for transwomen sex workers are necessary, but not sufficient, for developing appropriately specific and evidence-based interventions. Studies among transwomen should collect more granular data on sex work, assessing timing, duration, extent, and type of sex work involvement. There is a wide spectrum of sex work, ranging from occasional or opportunistic exchange of sex for goods to full-time employment as a self-identified sex worker. Thus, the level of economic reliance on sex work varies. For some, sex work is a sole source of income or goods for survival, whereas for others it provides supplementary income for discretionary purchases (Harcourt, 2005). Sex work can be further differentiated by the multitude of social contexts in which it occurs, which vary in the level of occupational health and safety they provide (Harcourt, 2005). In general, sampling methods in sex work research overrepresent sex workers in higher-risk (i.e., street-based) segments of the sex industry (Bungay, Oliffe, & Atchison, 2015). However, trans sex workers may in fact be disproportionately represented in street-based sex work because of employment discrimination and stratification within the sex industry, and their relatively limited ability to rely on family, peers, or the state to meet basic needs for shelter, food, and healthcare. Finally, assessment of HIV burden by current sex work status may underestimate the relationship between sex work involvement and HIV risk among transwomen.

HIV RISK AND RESILIENCE OF TRANS SEX WORKERS UNDER CRIMINALIZATION

The heavy burden of HIV borne by transwomen sex workers necessitates a focus on risk factors amenable to intervention at the individual, network, community, and policy levels. Nevertheless, a risk orientation has the potential to reinforce stereotypes about the connections among transwomen, sex work, and HIV risk. In her work on LGBT youths and policing, Dwyer (2014) notes the "tension between the need for recognition of LGBT youthful riskiness and how categories of LGBT youth riskiness . . . then become taken for granted" (p. 66).

Recent work drawing attention to the structural production of HIV risk for sex workers (Shannon et al., 2015) challenges taken-for-granted assumptions about the relationship between sex work and HIV risk, underscoring the potential of public policy interventions to alter the "risk environment" (Rhodes, 2002) for sex workers. Where sex work is decriminalized and community responses to HIV prevention are commonplace, sex work even has the potential to be protective; for example, in New South Wales, Australia, sex workers have lower rates of HIV than the general population (Jeffreys, Fawkes, & Stardust, 2012). Given the greater biological transmission risks faced by transgender versus cisgender women sex workers (i.e., because of the higher per-act transmission probability associated with anal intercourse), upstream interventions to improve the environments in which trans sex workers live and work are critical.

Despite these observations, we found that factors examined in studies of HIV risk among transwomen sex workers between 2008 and 2015 (see Table 9.4) were most often at the individual level. As Lyons and colleagues discuss in Chapter 24, we take the view that criminalization of sex work is a key contributor to the risks faced by transwomen who engage in it. Greater emphasis is required on the role of public policy in creating risky environments for transwomen sex workers—risks including, but not limited to, HIV. Legal and policy changes, such as removal of criminal sanctions and introduction of protective laws, have the potential to create safer work environments for transwomen who wish to engage in sex work (which can contribute to economic stability, community support, and validation of gender identity for transwomen), and to expand the range of labor options available to transwomen.

ACKNOWLEDGMENTS

We wish to thank the transwomen who participated in the included studies, and Sari Reisner for generously sharing data. A.I. Scheim is supported by the Pierre Elliott Trudeau Foundation and Vanier Canada Graduate Scholarships.

REFERENCES

Aguayo, N., Munoz, S. R., & Aguilar, G. (2013). HIV and syphilis prevalence and behavior, practices and attitudes of the TRANS population in Paraguay, 2011. *Sexually Transmitted Infections, 89* (Suppl. 1), A254.

Almeida, A., Brasileiro, A., Costa, J., Eusébio, M., & Fernandes, R. (2014). Prevalence of and factors mediating HIV infection among sex workers in Lisbon, Portugal: The 5-year experience of a community organisation. *Sexually Transmitted Infections, 90,* 497.

Almeida, M. (2011). Sex work and pleasure: An exploratory study on sexual response and sex work. *Sexologies, 20,* 229–232.

Altaf, A., Zahidie, A., & Agha, A. (2012). Comparing risk factors of HIV among hijra sex workers in Larkana and other cities of Pakistan: An analytical cross sectional study. *BMC Public Health, 12,* 279.

Baral, S. D., Friedman, M. R., Geibel, S., Rebe, K., & Bozhinov, B. (2015). Male sex workers: Practices, contexts, and vulnerabilities for HIV acquisition and transmission. *Lancet, 385* (9964), 260–273.

Baral, S. D., Logie, C. H., Grosso, A., Wirtz, A. L., & Beyrer, C. (2013). Modified social ecological model: A tool to guide the assessment of the risks and risk contexts of HIV epidemics. *BMC Public Health*, 13, 482.

Baral, S. D., Poteat, T., Strömdahl, S., Wirtz, A. L., Guadamuz, T. T., & Beyrer, C. (2013). Worldwide burden of HIV in transgender women: A systematic review and meta-analysis. *Lancet Infectious Diseases*, 13, 214–222.

Barrington, C., Wejnert, C., Guardado, M. E., Nieto, A. I., & Bailey, G. P. (2012). Social network characteristics and HIV vulnerability among transgender persons in San Salvador: Identifying opportunities for HIV prevention strategies. *AIDS and Behavior*, 16, 214–224.

Bauer, G. R., Hammond, R., Travers, R., Kaay, M., Hohenadel, K. M., & Boyce, M. (2009). "I don't think this is theoretical; this is our lives": How erasure impacts health care for transgender people. *Journal of the Association of Nurses in AIDS Care*, 20, 348–361.

Bauer, G. R., Travers, R., Scanlon, K., & Coleman, T. (2012). High heterogeneity of HIV-related sexual risk among transgender people in Ontario, Canada: A province-wide respondent-driven sampling survey. *BMC Public Health*, 12, 292.

Brahmam, G. N. V., Kodavalla, V., Rajkumar, H., Rachakulla, H. K., Kallam, S., Myakala, S. P., et al. (2008). Sexual practices, HIV and sexually transmitted infections among self-identified men who have sex with men in four high HIV prevalence states of India. *AIDS*, 22 (Suppl. 5), S45–57.

Brennan, J., & Kuhns, L. (2012). Syndemic theory and HIV-related risk among young transgender women: The role of multiple, co-occurring health problems and social marginalization. *American Journal of Public Health*, 102, 1751–1757.

Bungay, V., Oliffe, J., & Atchison, C. (2015, November 20). Addressing underrepresentation in sex work research: Reflections on designing a purposeful sampling strategy. *Qualitative Health Research*, e-pub ahead of print. doi:10.1177/104973 2315613042.

Carroll, A., & Itaborahy, L. P. (2015). *State sponsored homophobia 2015: A world survey of laws: Criminalisation, protection and recognition of same-sex love*. Geneva: ILGA.

Chakrapani, V., Newman, P. A., Shunmugam, M., Logie, C. H., & Samuel, M. (2015, October 12). Syndemics of depression, alcohol use, and victimisation, and their association with HIV-related sexual risk among men who have sex with men and transgender women in India. *Global Public Health*, e-pub ahead of print. doi:10.1080/17441692.2015.1091024.

Chemnasiri, T., Netwong, T., Visarutratana, S., Varangrat, A., Li, A., Phanuphak, P., et al. (2010). Inconsistent condom use among young men who have sex with men, male sex workers, and transgenders in Thailand. *AIDS Education and Prevention*, 22, 100–109.

Clements-Nolle, K., Guzman, R., & Harris, S. G. (2008). Sex trade in a male-to-female transgender population: Psychosocial correlates of inconsistent condom use. *Sexual Health*, 5, 49–54.

Coan, D. L., Schrager, W., & Packer, T. (2005). The role of male sexual partners in HIV infection among male-to-female transgendered individuals. *International Journal of Transgenderism, 8* (2–3), 21–30.

Cohan, D., Lutnick, A., Davidson, P., Cloniger, C., Herlyn, A., Breyer, J., et al. (2006). Sex worker health: San Francisco style. *Sexually Transmitted Infections, 82*, 418–422.

Colchero, M. A., Cortés-Ortiz, M. A., Romero-Martínez, M., Vega, H., González, A., Román, R., et al. (2015). HIV prevalence, sociodemographic characteristics, and sexual behaviors among transwomen in Mexico City. *Salud Pública de México, 57* (Suppl. 2), s99–s106.

Costa, A. B., Fontanari, A. M. V., Jacinto, M. M., da Silva, D. C., Lorencetti, E. K., da Rosa Filho, H. T., et al. (2014). Population-based HIV prevalence and associated factors in male-to-female transsexuals from southern Brazil. *Archives of Sexual Behavior, 44*, 521–524.

Decker, M. R., Crago, A. L., Chu, S., & Sherman, S. G. (2015). Human rights violations against sex workers: Burden and effect on HIV. *Lancet, 385* (9963), 186–199.

Deering, K. N., Lyons, T., Feng, C. X., Nosyk, B., Strathdee, S. A., Montaner, J. S. G., & Shannon, K. (2013). Client demands for unsafe sex: The socioeconomic risk environment for HIV among street and off-street sex workers. *Journal of Acquired Immune Deficiency Syndrome, 63*, 522–531.

Dias, S., Gama, A., Fuertes, R., Mendão, L., & Barros, H. (2015). Risk-taking behaviours and HIV infection among sex workers in Portugal: Results from a cross-sectional survey. *Sexually Transmitted Infections, 91*, 346–352.

Dos Ramos Farías, M. S., Garcia, M. N., Reynaga, E., Romero, M., Vaulet, M. L. G., Fermepín, M. R., et al. (2011). First report on sexually transmitted infections among trans (male to female transvestites, transsexuals, or transgender) and male sex workers in Argentina: High HIV, HPV, HBV, and syphilis prevalence. *International Journal of Infectious Diseases, 15* (9), e635–640.

Dwyer, A. (2014). "We're not like these weird feather boa–covered AIDS-spreading monsters": How LGBT young people and service providers think riskiness informs LGBT youth–police interactions. *Critical Criminology, 22*, 65–79.

Emmanuel, F., Salim, M., Akhtar, N., Arshad, S., & Reza, T. E. (2013). Second-generation surveillance for HIV/AIDS in Pakistan: Results from the 4th round of Integrated Behavior and Biological Survey, 2011–2012. *Sexually Transmitted Infections, 89* (Suppl. 3), iii23–iii28.

Fernandes, F. R. P., Zanini, P. B., Rezende, G. R., Castro, L. S., Bandeira, L. M., Puga, M. A., et al. (2015). Syphilis infection, sexual practices and bisexual behaviour among men who have sex with men and transgender women: A cross-sectional study. *Sexually Transmitted Infections, 91*, 142–149.

Fernández-Balbuena, S., Belza, M. J., Urdaneta, E., Esteso, R., Rosales-Statkus, M. E., & de la Fuente, L. (2014). Serving the underserved: An HIV testing program for populations reluctant to attend conventional settings. *International Journal of Public Health, 60*, 121–126.

Fitzgerald, E., Patterson, S. E., Hickey, D., Biko, C., & Tobin, H. J. (2015). *Meaningful work: Transgender experiences in the sex trade.* Best Practices Policy Project, Red Umbrella Project, National Center for Trans Equality. Retrieved from www .bestpracticespolicy.org/wp-content/uploads/2015/12/Meaningful-Work-Full-Report.pdf.

Fletcher, J. B., Kisler, K. A., & Reback, C. (2014). Housing status and HIV risk behaviors among transgender women in Los Angeles. *Archives of Sexual Behavior, 43,* 1651–1661.

Grant, J. M., Mottet, L. A., Tanis, J., Harrison, J., Herman, J. L., & Keisling, M. (2011). *Injustice at every turn: A report of the National Transgender Discrimination Survey.* Washington, DC: National Center for Transgender Equality and National Gay and Lesbian Task Force.

Guadamuz, T. T., Wimonsate, W., Varangrat, A., Phanuphak, P., Jommaroeng, R., McNicholl, J. M., et al. (2011). HIV prevalence, risk behavior, hormone use, and surgical history among transgender persons in Thailand. *AIDS and Behavior, 15,* 650–658.

Harcourt, C. (2005). The many faces of sex work. *Sexually Transmitted Infections, 81,* 201–206.

Hawkes, S., Collumbien, M., Platt, L., Lalji, N., Rizvi, N., Andreasen, A., et al. (2009). HIV and other sexually transmitted infections among men, transgenders, and women selling sex in two cities in Pakistan: A cross-sectional prevalence survey. *Sexually Transmitted Infections, 85* (Suppl. 2), ii8–ii16.

Herbst, J. H., Jacobs, E. D., Finlayson, T. J., McKleroy, V. S., Neumann, M. S., Crepaz, N., & HIV/AIDS Prevention Research Synthesis Team. (2008). Estimating HIV prevalence and risk behaviors of transgender persons in the United States: A systematic review. *AIDS and Behavior, 12,* 1–17.

Hill, S. C., Daniel, J., Benzie, A., Ayres, J., King, G., & Smith, A. (2011). Sexual health of transgender sex workers attending an inner-city genitourinary medicine clinic. *International Journal of STD & AIDS, 22,* 686–687.

Hoffman, B. R. (2014). The interaction of drug use, sex work, and HIV among transgender women. *Substance Use & Misuse, 49,* 1049–1053.

Hwahng, S. J., & Nuttbrock, L. (2007). Sex workers, fem queens, and cross-dressers: Differential marginalizations and HIV vulnerabilities among three ethnocultural male-to-female transgender communities in New York City. *Sexuality Research and Social Policy, 4* (4), 36–59.

International Reference Group on Transgender People and HIV. (2016). *Counting trans people in: Advancing global data collection on trans people and HIV.* Oakland, CA: Global Forum on MSM and HIV.

Jeffreys, E., Fawkes, J., & Stardust, Z. (2012). Mandatory testing for HIV and sexually transmissible infections among sex workers in Australia: A barrier to HIV and STI prevention. *World Journal of AIDS, 2,* 203–211.

Khan, A. A., Rehan, N., Qayyum, K., & Khan, A. (2008). Correlates and prevalence of

HIV and sexually transmitted infections among hijras (male transgenders) in Pakistan. *International Journal of STD & AIDS, 19*, 817–820.

Krüsi, A., Pacey, K., Bird, L., Taylor, C., Chettiar, J., & Allan, J., et al. (2014). Criminalisation of clients: Reproducing vulnerabilities for violence and poor health among street-based sex workers in Canada—A qualitative study. *BMJ Open, 4*, e005191.

Logie, C. H., James, L., Tharao, W., & Loutfy, M. R. (2011). HIV, gender, race, sexual orientation, and sex work: A qualitative study of intersectional stigma experienced by HIV-positive women in Ontario, Canada. *PLoS Medicine, 8*, e1001124.

Lombardi, E. L., & Friedman, M. (2012, July 23). Influence of structural factors on the HIV status and sex work activity of trans women. Poster presented at the XIX International AIDS Conference. Washington, DC.

Marcellin, R. L., Bauer, G. R., & Scheim, A. I. (2013). Intersecting impacts of transphobia and racism on HIV risk among trans persons of colour in Ontario, Canada. *Ethnicity and Inequalities in Health and Social Care, 6* (4), 97–107. Retrieved from http://doi.org/10.1108/EIHSC-09-2013-0017.

Martins, T. A., Kerr, L., Macena, R., Mota, R. S., & Kendall, C. (2013). Travestis, an unexplored population at risk of HIV in a large metropolis of northeast Brazil: A respondent-driven sampling survey. *AIDS Care, 25*, 606–612.

Matthews, D. D., Smith, J. C., Brown, A. L., & Malebranche, D. J. (2016). Reconciling epidemiology and social justice in the public health discourse around the sexual networks of black men who have sex with men. *American Journal of Public Health, 106*, 808–816.

Millett, G. A., Flores, S. A., Peterson, J. L., & Bakeman, R. (2007). Explaining disparities in HIV infection among black and white men who have sex with men: A meta-analysis of HIV risk behaviors. *AIDS, 21*, 2083–2091.

Nadal, K. L., Davidoff, K. C., & Fujii-Doe, W. (2014). Transgender women and the sex work industry: Roots in systemic, institutional, and interpersonal discrimination. *Journal of Trauma & Dissociation, 15*, 169–183.

Nemoto, T., Bödeker, B., Iwamoto, M., & Sakata, M. (2014). Practices of receptive and insertive anal sex among transgender women in relation to partner types, sociocultural factors, and background variables. *AIDS Care, 26*, 434–440.

Nemoto, T., Iwamoto, M., Perngparn, U., Areesantichai, C., Kamitani, E., & Sakata, M. (2012). HIV-related risk behaviors among kathoey (male-to-female transgender) sex workers in Bangkok, Thailand. *AIDS Care, 24*, 210–219.

Nichols, A. (2010). Dance Ponnaya, dance! Police abuses against transgender sex workers in Sri Lanka. *Feminist Criminology, 5*, 195–222.

Nuttbrock, L., Bockting, W. O., Rosenblum, A., Hwahng, S. J., Mason, M., Macri, M., & Becker, J. (2015). Gender abuse and incident HIV/STI among transgender women in New York City: Buffering effect of involvement in a transgender community. *AIDS and Behavior, 19*, 1446–1453.

———. (2013). Gender abuse, depressive symptoms, and HIV and other sexually transmitted infections among male-to-female transgender persons: A three-year prospective study. *American Journal of Public Health, 103,* 300–307.

Nuttbrock, L., Hwahng, S. J., Bockting, W. O., Rosenblum, A., Mason, M., Macri, M., & Becker, J. (2009). Lifetime risk factors for HIV/sexually transmitted infections among male-to-female transgender persons. *Journal of Acquired Immune Deficiency Syndrome, 52* (3), 417–421.

Oldenburg, C. E., Perez-Brumer, A. G., Reisner, S. L., Mayer, K. H., Mimiaga, M. J., Hatzenbuehler, M. L., & Bärnighausen, T. (2016, March 16). Human rights protections and HIV prevalence among MSM who sell sex: Cross-country comparisons from a systematic review and meta-analysis. *Global Public Health,* e-pub ahead of print. doi:10.1080/17441692.2016.1149598.

Operario, D., Nemoto, T., Iwamoto, M., & Moore, T. (2011). Risk for HIV and unprotected sexual behavior in male primary partners of transgender women. *Archives of Sexual Behavior, 40,* 1255–1261.

Operario, D., Soma, T., & Underhill, K. (2008). Sex work and HIV status among transgender women: Systematic review and meta-analysis. *Journal of Acquired Immune Deficiency Syndrome, 48,* 97–103.

Patrascioiu, I., Lopez, C. Q., Porta, M. M., Velazquez, G. B. A., Hanzu, F. A., Gómez-Gil, E., et al. (2013). Characteristics of the HIV positive transgender population of Catalonia. Paper presented at the 15th European Congress of Endocrinology, Copenhagen. *Endocrine Abstracts, 32,* 341.

Poteat, T., Reisner, S. L., & Radix, A. (2014). HIV epidemics among transgender women. *Current Opinion in HIV and AIDS, 9,* 168–173.

Poteat, T., Scheim, A., Xavier, J., Reisner, S. L., & Baral, S. (2016). Global epidemiology of HIV infection and related syndemics affecting transgender people. *Journal of Acquired Immune Deficiency Syndrome, 72* (Suppl. 3), S210–219.

Poteat, T., Wirtz, A. L., Radix, A., Borquez, A., Silva-Santisteban, A., Deutsch, M. B., et al. (2015). HIV risk and preventive interventions in transgender women sex workers. *Lancet, 385* (9964), 274–286.

Rapues, J., Wilson, E. C., Packer, T., Colfax, G. N., & Raymond, H. F. (2013). Correlates of HIV infection among transfemales, San Francisco, 2010: Results from a respondent-driven sampling study. *American Journal of Public Health, 103,* 1485–1492.

Reback, C., & Fletcher, J. B. (2013). HIV prevalence, substance use, and sexual risk behaviors among transgender women recruited through outreach. *AIDS and Behavior, 18,* 1359–1367.

Reisner, S. L., Mimiaga, M. J., Bland, S. E., Driscoll, M. A., Cranston, K., & Mayer, K. H. (2012). Pathways to embodiment of HIV risk: Black men who have sex with transgender partners, Boston, Massachusetts. *AIDS Education and Prevention, 24,* 15–26.

Reisner, S. L., Mimiaga, M. J., Bland, S., Mayer, K. H., Perkovich, B., & Safren, S. A. (2009). HIV risk and social networks among male-to-female transgender sex workers in Boston, Massachusetts. *Journal of the Association of Nurses in AIDS Care, 20,* 373–386.

Reisner, S. L., Poteat, T., Keatley, J., Cabral, M., Mothopeng, T., Dunham, E., Holland, C. E., Max, R., & Baral, S. D. (2016). Global health burden and needs of transgender populations. *Lancet, 388*, 412–436.

Rhodes, T. (2002). The "risk environment": A framework for understanding and reducing drug-related harm. *International Journal of Drug Policy, 13*, 85–94.

Roche, K., & Keith, C. (2014). How stigma affects healthcare access for transgender sex workers. *British Journal of Nursing, 23*, 1147–1152.

Rotondi, N. K., Bauer, G. R., Scanlon, K., Travers, A., Kaay, M., & Travers, R. (2013). Nonprescribed hormone use and self-performed surgeries: "Do-it-yourself" transitions in transgender communities in Ontario, Canada. *American Journal of Public Health, 103*, 1830–1836.

Safer, J. D., Coleman, E., Feldman, J. L., Garofalo, R., Hembree, W., Radix, A., & Sevelius, J. (2016). Barriers to healthcare for transgender individuals. *Current Opinion in Endocrinology & Diabetes and Obesity, 23*, 168–171.

Scorgie, F., Nakato, D., Harper, E., Richter, M., Maseko, S., Nare, P., et al. (2013). "We are despised in the hospitals": Sex workers' experiences of accessing health care in four African countries. *Culture, Health & Sexuality, 15*, 450–465.

Sevelius, J., Reznick Grinstead, O., Hart, S. L., & Schwarcz, S. (2009). Informing interventions: The importance of contextual factors in the prediction of sexual risk behaviors among transgender women. *AIDS Education & Prevention, 21*, 113–127.

Shannon, K., & Csete, J. (2010). Violence, condom negotiation, and HIV/STI risk among sex workers. *JAMA, 304*, 573–574.

Shannon, K., Kerr, T., Allinott, S., Chettiar, J., Shoveller, J., & Tyndall, M. W. (2008). Social and structural violence and power relations in mitigating HIV risk of drug-using women in survival sex work. *Social Science & Medicine, 66*, 911–921.

Shannon, K., Strathdee, S. A., Goldenberg, S. M., Duff, P., Mwangi, P., Rusakova, M., et al. (2015). Global epidemiology of HIV among female sex workers: Influence of structural determinants. *Lancet, 385* (9962), 55–71.

Silva-Santisteban, A., Raymond, H. F., Salazar, X., Villayzan, J., Leon, S., McFarland, W., & Cáceres, C. F. (2012). Understanding the HIV/AIDS epidemic in transgender women of Lima, Peru: Results from a sero-epidemiologic study using respondent driven sampling. *AIDS and Behavior, 16*, 872–881.

Singer, M. (1996). A dose of drugs, a touch of violence, a case of AIDS: Conceptualizing the SAVA syndemic. *Free Inquiry in Creative Sociology, 24*, 99–110.

Socías, M. E., Marshall, B. D. L., Arístegui, I., Romero, M., Cahn, P., Kerr, T., & Sued, O. (2014). Factors associated with healthcare avoidance among transgender women in Argentina. *International Journal for Equity in Health, 13*, 81.

Solomon, M. M., Nurena, C. R., Tanur, J. M., Montoya, O., Grant, R. M., & McConnell, J. (2015). Transactional sex and prevalence of STIs: A cross-sectional study of MSM and transwomen screened for an HIV prevention trial. *International Journal of STD & AIDS, 26*, 879–886.

Stall, R. D., Mills, T. C., Williamson, J., Hart, T., Greenwood, G., Paul, J., et al. (2003). Association of co-occurring psychosocial health problems and increased vulnerability to HIV/AIDS among urban men who have sex with men. *American Journal of Public Health, 93,* 939–942.

Subramanian, T., Ramakrishnan, L., Aridoss, S., Goswami, P., Kanguswami, B., Shajan, M., et al. (2013). Increasing condom use and declining STI prevalence in high-risk MSM and TGs: Evaluation of a large-scale prevention program in Tamil Nadu, India. *BMC Public Health, 13,* 857.

Toibaro, J. J., Ebensrtejin, J. E., Parlante, A., Burgoa, P., Freyre, A., Romero, M., & Losso, M. H. (2009). [Sexually transmitted infections among transgender individuals and other sexual identities]. *Medicina, 69,* 327–330.

White House Office of National AIDS Policy. (2015). *National HIV/AIDS Strategy for the United States: Updated to 2020.* Washington, DC. Retrieved from https://www.aids.gov/federal-resources/national-hiv-aids-strategy/nhas-update.pdf.

Wilson, E. C., Garofalo, R., Harris, D. R., & Belzer, M. (2010). Sexual risk taking among transgender male-to-female youths with different partner types. *American Journal of Public Health, 100,* 1500–1505.

Wilson, E. C., Jin, H., Liu, A., & Raymond, H. F. (2015). Knowledge, indications, and willingness to take pre-exposure prophylaxis among transwomen in San Francisco, 2013. *PLoS One, 10,* e0128971.

Wilson, E. C., Santos, G.-M., & Raymond, H. F. (2014). Sexual mixing and the risk environment of sexually active transgender women: Data from a respondent-driven sampling study of HIV risk among transwomen in San Francisco, 2010. *BMC Infectious Diseases, 14,* 430.

Woods, J. B., Galvan, F. H., Bazargan, M., Herman, J. L., & Chen, Y. T. (2013). Latina transgender women's interactions with law enforcement in Los Angeles County. *Policing, 7,* 379–391.

Chapter 10

HIV and Substance Use among Transwomen Sex Workers

A Vicious Cycle of Socioeconomic Hardship, Unmet Service Needs, and Health Risk

Tiffany R. Glynn[1]
Don Operario[2]
Tooru Nemoto[3]

1 Completed a master's degree at the Brown University School of Public Health and is currently a PhD student in clinical health psychology at the University of Miami.
2 Professor of public health in the Department of Behavioral and Social Sciences at Brown University.
3 Research program director at the Public Health Institute in Oakland, CA.

SUMMARY

In this chapter we focus on two health issues commonly examined in research on transwomen who engage in sex work: HIV risk and substance use. Our goal is to provide a contextualized understanding of the association between sex work and health risks in this population by characterizing the socioeconomic and ecological factors that may motivate transwomen to engage in sex work and that, in turn, determine health challenges among transwomen sex workers.

KEY TERMS

economic hardship; health risk; HIV; substance use

Nuttbrock, Larry, *Transgender Sex Work and Society*
dx.doi.org/10.17312/harringtonparkpress/2017.11.tsws.010
© 2018 by Harrington Park Press

In this chapter we focus on two health issues commonly examined in research on transwomen who engage in sex work: HIV risk and substance use. Our goal is to provide a contextualized understanding of the association between sex work and health risks in this population by characterizing the socioeconomic and ecological factors that may motivate transwomen to engage in sex work and that, in turn, determine health challenges among transwomen sex workers. We argue that a vicious cycle of socioeconomic hardship, social exclusion, and health risks operates synergistically to produce sustained vulnerability among transwomen sex workers. That is, socioeconomic and ecological vulnerabilities can serve as a life-course context that determines sex work as a source of income and other social survival needs, and the health risks that derive from sex work may further contribute to socioeconomic and ecological adversity. Consequently, we will argue that cultural changes and aggressive interventions targeting upstream factors (e.g., socioeconomic inequity, stigma, and exclusion) are needed to disrupt this vicious cycle and reduce the disproportionate concentration of health problems repeatedly documented among transwomen who engage in sex work.

HIV AND SUBSTANCE USE IN TRANSWOMEN

The twin epidemics of HIV and substance use among transwomen sex workers have been well described. Some of the earliest studies on these issues occurred in San Francisco; two surveys estimated between 26% and 35% HIV-positive status in community samples, alongside high levels of illicit drug use and sex while under the influence of drugs (Clements-Nolle et al., 2001; Nemoto, Operario, Keatley, & Villegas, 2004). Several years after these studies were published, a meta-analysis estimated that 28% of transwomen had tested HIV-positive (Herbst et al., 2008), and another meta-analysis estimated HIV-positive rates of 27% among transwomen sex workers compared with 15% in transwomen not engaged in sex work, 15% in cisgender male sex workers, and 5% in cisgender female sex workers (Operario et al., 2008). A review of the global literature by Poteat and colleagues (2015) identified only six evidence-based HIV prevention programs for transwomen, none of which specifically targeted the needs of transwomen sex workers.

Studies across multiple international contexts have also reported high prevalence of drug use among transwomen, including polydrug and injection drug use (Reisner et al., 2016). Recently, an exhaustive review of the published literature by Glynn and van den Berg (2017) was able to identify only one quantitatively evaluated substance use intervention for transwomen (by Nemoto et al., 2005). While these data document high risk among transwomen, especially those involved in sex work, Poteat and colleagues remind us of the need to contextualize HIV and drug use in order to identify the upstream social causes of health risk and to avoid victim blaming.

SOCIOECONOMIC HARDSHIP, UNMET SERVICE NEEDS, AND RISK

As Chapter 3 discussed, social- and structural-level discrimination are consistently experienced by transwomen, and these factors contribute to a cultural context of socioeconomic hardship for many members of this population—characterized by housing instability, exclusion from the formal labor sector, and difficulties in obtaining health and social services, among other problems (Bradford et al., 2013; Kattari et al., 2016). Antidiscrimination legislation has been passed in the United States to protect members of historically marginalized groups. However, transwomen have not yet reaped much benefit from policy changes (Grant et al., 2011). A study examining economic well-being among transgender individuals in California after the passage of antidiscrimination laws still found high rates of unemployment, poverty, and homelessness (Davis & Wertz, 2009). For policies and interventions to affect the wellness of this population, a reconsideration of the more deeply rooted and unique factors contributing to inequity among transwomen is needed.

A life course characterized by transphobic discrimination, institutionalized stigma, and socioeconomic adversity contributes to the need for sex work as a source of income for many transwomen. However, the benefits derived from sex work are not solely economic in nature. Indeed, previous qualitative research by Sausa and colleagues (2007) described how social exclusion—often beginning in the family context and extending to the community, peer networks, labor sector, and health services—can obstruct many transwomen from meeting their basic economic as well as social survival needs. Sex work can offer these women key sources of income as well as a perceived community of support from other transwomen sex workers facing similar socioeconomic and employment circumstances. For example, an interesting finding described in qualitative research by Sausa and colleagues was that many transwomen perceived that entrance into sex work was a "rite of passage" that allowed them to identify peers and mentors who could provide guidance on gender transition processes, hormones, and survival strategies. Quantitative findings from a two-city survey of transwomen (Wilson et al., 2009) corroborated the narrative data in Sausa and colleagues by demonstrating significant associations between having a history of sex work and low educational attainment and homelessness—i.e., transwomen sex workers were more economically vulnerable and marginalized compared with transwomen who did not engage in sex work. Like those of Sausa and colleagues, results from Wilson and colleagues showed that transwomen with a history of sex work reported a nearly twofold greater level of social support compared with transwomen who did not engage in sex work—suggesting that sex work can serve social functions such as providing a community of peers. However, having a supportive peer network is not equivalent to having support from health, social, and legal institutions, and transwomen sex workers may continue to experience barriers to professional social services and clinical care settings (Nemoto, Operario, Keatley, Han, & Soma, 2004).

Other researchers have reviewed the ways by which some cisgender female and male sex workers may subjectively perceive social, personal, and economic benefits from selling sex (Vanwesenbeeck, 2001; Weitzer, 2009), indicating that deriving social or personal value from sex work is not a phenomenon unique to transwomen. However, what might be unique to transwomen sex workers is the role that sex work plays in providing the economic and social capital necessary for gender transitioning and transgender-sensitive healthcare. Poteat and colleagues (2015) reinforced this argument in a recent review paper, stating that "sex work provides funds for livelihood and to pay for gender-affirming hormones, injections, and surgeries; and a more feminine appearance was reported to increase sex work earning power" (p. 276). Because many transwomen lack access to employer-provided insurance or other means to pay for prescription hormones, these women commonly report using nonprescription, off-market hormones or performing silicone self-injections, both of which might have limited effectiveness or unmonitored side effects (de Haan et al., 2015). More generally, exclusion from the formal labor market contributes to limited access to providers in the healthcare system (Sineath et al., 2016), an issue compounded by the lack of providers who are sufficiently competent and sensitive to serve transgender patients (Bauer et al., 2009; Lombardi, 2001).

RESEARCH FINDINGS: BAY AREA TRANSWOMEN SEX WORKER SURVEY

To explore this pattern of relationships—the higher burden of HIV and substance problems, unmet needs, and use of nonprescription hormones among transwomen sex workers—we analyzed data from a large cross-sectional survey of transwomen. All women in the sample had a lifetime history of sex work, but only a subset were engaged in sex work at that time (i.e., during the preceding 30 days). The analytic aims were twofold. First, we compared transwomen currently engaged in sex work with transwomen with a history of past sex work that was characterized by socioeconomic and health issues (HIV, substance use, prescription versus nonprescription hormones, silicone injections) in order to identify differences between these two groups. Second, we examined the presence of unmet health and social service needs between transwomen currently engaged in sex work versus those with a past history of sex work. Here we present relevant survey findings alongside interpretations supported by the published literature. We note, however, that cross-sectional data provide only a single snapshot of group differences and cannot reveal the temporal or cyclical relationships among variables. After reporting on the methods, relevant findings, and interpretation of results from this research survey, we will reconsider the cyclical pattern among economic hardship, unmet needs, and health in order to propose directions for future research and describe implications for intervention and policy.

The sample for this analysis comprised 573 transwomen with a history of sex work living in the San Francisco Bay Area (235 were African American or black, 110 were Asian or Pacific Islander, 110 were Latina, and 118 were white). Participants were recruited using targeted venue-based sampling and individually interviewed using a structured survey questionnaire containing validated measures of HIV, substance use, and health risk factors (see Nemoto, Bödeker, & Iwamoto, 2011, for more details).

For purposes of analysis, the sample was divided into two groups: those who had engaged in sex work in the previous 30 days (current sex workers, N = 250), and those who had not (noncurrent sex workers, N = 313) in order to examine disparities. Bivariate logistic regressions were run between sex work status and sociodemographics, substance use behaviors, health outcomes, medical gender-affirmation behaviors, and status of receiving services needed. Results of regression models are reported as odds ratios (ORs) with 95% confidence intervals (CIs). The level for significance was set to .05 (two-tailed) for each analysis.

Transwomen currently involved in sex work had greater socioeconomic adversity. As Table 10.1 shows, current sex workers were significantly more likely to have less than a high school education (OR = 2.12, 95% CI 1.17, 3.81) and to be living in temporary housing (OR = 2.16, 95% CI 1.5, 3.12) or homeless (OR = 2.16, 95% CI 1.10, 4.21). Additionally, they were less likely to have a full-time job (OR = 0.30, 95% CI 0.19, 0.48). The lack of education, employment, and stable housing among the women currently engaging in sex work highlights the motivation for such work that arises from structural, economic, and social barriers. This result mirrors findings reported by Sausa and colleagues (2007), in which a transwoman described how discrimination in employment instrumentally motivates sex work: "We do not have services for transgender[s]. We are not offered specific job training, and we are discriminated also for our physical appearance. . . . We do not have many option[s], and many of us want to get out of the street, and it is almost impossible" (p. 772). Our quantitative findings reflect this sentiment about the inevitability of turning to sex work because of a lack of employment or education stemming from discrimination.

Table 10.2 presents the comparisons of current versus noncurrent sex workers on substance use in the preceding 30 days. Current sex workers were more likely to be using marijuana (OR = 2.01, 95% CI 1.38, 2.93) or club drugs (OR = 3.4, 95% CI 2.06, 5.63), engaging in noninjection stimulant use (OR = 2.95, 95% CI 2.05, 4.24), and engaging in intravenous drug use (OR = 4.53, 95% CI 2.16, 9.53). These robust findings reflect the large role substance use has among the women engaging in sex work.

The use of substances may evolve as a coping mechanism for dealing with the pressures of sex work and, over time, can turn into a dependency in which sex work income is required to support substance

TABLE 10.1

Sociodemographic Characteristics of the Sample of Transgender Women and Comparisons between Current (Past 30 Days) and Noncurrent Sex Workers (N = 563)

		NOT CURRENTLY SEX WORKERS N = 313	CURRENTLY SEX WORKERS N = 250			
		N (%)	N (%)	OR	95% CI	p
Age		36.98 (9.21)	32.95 (9.22)	0.94	0.94, 0.97	<.001
Race or ethnicity						
	Black	125 (54.1%)	106 (45.9%)	0.86	0.55, 1.35	.522
	Latina	51 (46.4%)	59 (53.6%)	1.18	0.70, 1.99	.542
	API	80 (73.4%)	29 (26.6%)	0.34	0.21, 0.65	.001
	White	57 (50.4%)	56 (49.6%)	REF		
Born in the United States						
	Yes	193 (53%)	171 (47%)	0.74	0.52, 1.06	.097
	No	120 (60.3%)	79 (39.7%)	REF		
Years in the United States						
		29.75 (12.87)	27.54 (12.70)	0.99	0.98, 1.00	.06
Education						
	less than HS	87 (48.6%)	92 (51.4%)	2.12	1.17, 3.81	.013
	HS/GED/ vocational/ technical	99 (55%)	81 (45%)	1.64	0.91, 2.95	.102
	Some college	83 (60.1%)	55 (39.9%)	1.33	0.72, 2.45	.369
	College and above	44 (66.7%)	22 (33.3%)	REF		

		NOT CURRENTLY SEX WORKERS N = 313	CURRENTLY SEX WORKERS N = 250			
Have a full-time job						
	Yes	88 (77.2%)	26 (22.8%)	0.30	0.19, 0.48	<.001
	No	225 (50.1%)	224 (49.9%)	REF		
Living situation past 6 months						
	Permanent housing	170 (64.6%)	93 (35.4%)	REF		
	Temporary housing	97 (44.9%)	119 (55.1%)	2.16	1.5, 3.12	<.001
	Halfway house/ treatment center	18 (78.3%)	5 (21.7%)	0.49	0.18, 1.36	.171
	Homeless (shelter, street)	18 (45%)	22 (55%)	2.16	1.10, 4.21	.025
	Other	9 (56.3%)	7 (43.8%)	1.37	0.50, 3.80	.544

NOTE: Rows may not add up to 100% because of missing data.

use. For example, Nemoto, Operario, Keatley, & Villegas (2004) described a transwoman who explained her reliance on both substance use and sex work: "Eventually, I did not like working [on] the streets, and I didn't like to be touched in a sexual way, and it's like the . . . the uglier my trick was, the more dope I had to use" (p. 731). This cycle is detrimental to women's health in various ways. For instance, drug use lowers inhibitions and impairs the decision-making process with consequences to sexual health (e.g., condom negotiation). Additionally, drug use can disrupt physiological processes and lead to health complications (e.g., cardiovascular failure or seizures). Finally, sharing needles during intravenous drug use increases HIV risk, given that another's HIV-positive blood can stay on the needle or in the drug solution, which leads to direct injection of HIV.

As Table 10.3 shows, analysis of survey data also demonstrated that current sex workers were less likely to be HIV-positive (OR = 0.67, 95% CI 0.46, 0.98) and more likely to have had an STI in the previous year

TABLE 10.2

Comparisons of Past 30 Day Substance Use between Current (Past 30 Days) and Noncurrent Transgender Women Sex Workers (N = 563)

		NOT CURRENTLY SEX WORKERS N = 313	CURRENTLY SEX WORKERS N = 250			
		N (%)	N (%)	OR	95% CI	p
Marijuana						
	Yes	125 (48.1%)	135 (51.9%)	1.77	1.26, 2.47	< .001
	No	188 (62%)	115 (38%)			
Non-injection stimulant use (crack, cocaine, meth)						
	Yes	71 (38%)	116 (62%)	2.95	2.05, 4.24	< .001
	No	242 (64.4%)	134 (35.6%)			
Non-injection opioid use (heroin, non-Rx methadone, opiates)						
	Yes	11 (45.8%)	13 (54.2%)	1.51	0.66, 3.42	.328
	No	302 (56%)	237 (44%)			
Non-injection club drugs (ecstasy, hallucinogens)						
	Yes	25 (30.5%)	57 (69.5%)	3.40	2.06, 5.63	< .001
	No	288 (59.9%)	193 (40.1%)			
Intravenous drug use						
	Yes	18 (37.5%)	30 (62.5%)	2.24	1.21, 4.11	< .001
	No	295 (57.3%)	220 (42.7%)			

NOTES: OR = odds ratio; CI = confidence interval; Rx = prescription; "No" group served as the referent group in all models.

(OR = 1.49, 95% CI 1.02, 2.17). These findings could suggest that when the women find out their positive HIV status, they choose to stop engaging in sex work. Given the potentially higher rates of sexual encounters and multiple partners, women currently engaging in sex work are more likely to acquire STIs. Moreover, in light of economic motivations, many transwomen report engaging in higher-risk (i.e., condomless) sex with clients, which can also contribute to STIs, as a transwoman described in the study by Sausa and colleagues (2007): "Unfortunately, in this business of sexual work, there are days that you do very well; there are days that you don't do well. Then if a client comes and offers more money and you have to pay your hotel room, if not they are going to kick you out, then you don't do it [referring to condom use]" (p. 773).

As Table 10.3 shows, current sex workers had twofold greater odds (OR = 2.09, 95% CI 1.22, 3.60) of having engaged in illicit silicone injection over their lifetime than the noncurrent sex workers. Additionally, current sex workers were less likely to have exclusively used prescription hormones (OR = 0.60, 95% 0.42, 0.85) but more likely to have used only nonprescription hormones (OR = 1.76, 95% CI 1.08, 2.87) over their lifetime. These findings reflect the downstream effect of discrimination by highlighting the health risk behaviors, such as sexual risk and illicit medical gender affirmation, that are influenced by barriers to employment and healthcare and have adverse consequences.

Medical gender affirmation includes any medical procedures or pharmacology (e.g., hormones, surgical body modifications) that validates the women in their felt or expressed gender identity. Not all transwomen want or need medical gender affirmation, but for those who do, it can decrease poor mental health outcomes (Colton Meier et al., 2011; Sevelius, 2013). Because of the discussed systematic discrimination and lack of employment and health insurance, gender-affirmation treatment and surgeries come at a high financial cost to the women. Given the desire to feminize their appearance but their lack of financial means, many women seek out illicit silicone injections. However, not only is the illicit silicone administered by an unlicensed, non–medical professional individual, but it commonly does not contain medical-grade silicone, but rather industrial- or food-grade silicone or some other substance (e.g., cement glue) (Wilson et al., 2014). Thus, serious health complications arise from illicit silicone injections among transwomen. Additionally, multiple barriers to prescription hormone use exist, including a lack of health insurance, access to medical care, and access to a trans-knowledgeable provider (Sanchez et al., 2009). In

TABLE 10.3

Health Outcomes and Medical Gender Affirmation among Current
(Past 30 Days) and Noncurrent Transgender Women Sex Workers
(N = 563)

		NOT CURRENTLY SEX WORKERS N = 313	CURRENTLY SEX WORKERS N = 250			
		N (%)	N (%)	OR	95% CI	p
Last HIV test result[1]						
	Positive	102 (64.2%)	57 (35.8%)	0.67	0.46, 0.98	.040
	Negative	201 (54.5%)	168 (45.5%)	REF		
STI past 12 months						
	Yes	71 (48.3%)	76 (51.7%)	1.49	1.02, 2.17	.039
	No	242 (58.2%)	174 (41.8%)			
Illicit silicone injection, lifetime						
	Yes	24 (39.3%)	37 (60.7%)	2.09	1.22, 3.60	.008
	No	289 (57.6%)	213 (42.4%)	REF		
Exclusively Rx hormone use, lifetime						
	Yes	128 (63.7%)	73 (36.3%)	0.60	0.42, 0.85	.004
	No	185 (51.1%)	177 (48.9%)	REF		
Exclusively non-Rx hormone use, lifetime						
	Yes	33 (43.4%)	43 (56.6%)	1.76	1.08, 2.87	.023
	No	280 (57.5%)	207 (42.5%)	REF		

NOTES: [1] Not all individuals had an HIV testing history; thus N = 528. STI = sexual transmitted infection; OR = odds ratio; CI = confidence interval; Rx = prescription; REF = referent group.

light of these barriers, using hormones acquired from sources other than a physician (e.g., the Internet, the street) is widespread and alarming, given the health problems that can manifest themselves from a lack of monitoring (Rotondi et al., 2013).

The survey asked the women about various types of assistance needed and if they were able to receive such services (see Table 10.4). Current sex workers had significantly higher odds of not getting their needs met on most types of service. Findings showed robust associations ranging from almost twofold to threefold greater odds of having any unmet needs, including basic needs (housing, food, and utility [e.g., electricity] aid), mental health needs (counseling, spiritual support, support groups), substance use treatment, healthcare needs (medical care, urgent care, emergency room care, HIV care), financial needs (Social Security, unemployment, general relief, disability), and sexual health needs (STI screening, prevention, case management). The large gap between services needed and services received among current sex workers promotes a pattern of continued disparity in health and well-being.

This finding is consistent with the literature, as transwomen report high rates of discrimination in assistance services, such as being denied routine medical care, health insurance, housing, and employment (Bradford et al., 2013). Lacking the needed resources, transwomen turn to sex work as a means to support themselves; however, being in sex work facilitates the need for more services they are unable to receive, such as rape crisis support, STI screening, and mental health assistance.

CORROBORATING THE VICIOUS CYCLE, AND THEN DISRUPTING IT

Findings from analysis of these cross-sectional data provide preliminary support to the principles of our argument that socioeconomic adversity and unmet needs—including a need for gender-affirming hormones—provide a contextual motivation for engaging in sex work, and that sex work contributes to a risk for substance use and sexually transmitted infections. Unexpectedly, we found that HIV-positive transwomen were less likely to be currently involved in sex work, which might reveal that these women leave sex work when they learn of their HIV status. As we noted, however, cross-sectional findings cannot allow us to examine the hypothesized temporal ordering or cyclical nature by which health problems that derive from sex work further exacerbate

TABLE 10.4

Unmet Services and Assistance Needed among Current (Past 30 Days) and Noncurrent Transgender Women Sex Workers (N = 563)

		NOT CURRENTLY SEX WORKERS N = 313	CURRENTLY SEX WORKERS N = 250	OR	95% CI	p
		N (%)	N (%)	OR	95% CI	p
Basic assistance						
	Needs unmet	70 (42.4%)	95 (57.6%)	2.13	1.47, 3.08	<.001
	Met or not needed	243 (61.1%)	155 (38.9%)	REF		
Mental health assistance						
	Needs unmet	42 (39.6%)	64 (60.4%)	2.22	1.44, 3.42	<.001
	Met or not needed	271 (59.3%)	186 (40.7%)	REF		
Substance use assistance						
	Needs unmet	16 (38.1%)	26 (61.9%)	2.16	1.13, 4.11	.020
	Met or not needed	297 (57%)	224 (43%)	REF		
Healthcare assistance						
	Needs unmet	27 (43.5%)	35 (56.5%)	1.72	1.01, 2.94	.045
	Met or not needed	286 (57.1%)	215 (42.9%)	REF		
Financial assistance						
	Needs unmet	31 (33.3%)	62 (66.7%)	3.00	1.88, 4.80	<.001
	Met or not needed	282 (60%)	188 (40%)	REF		
Sexual health assistance						
	Needs unmet	20 (40%)	30 (60%)	2.00	1.11, 3.61	.022
	Met or not needed	293 (57.1%)	220 (42.9%)	REF		

		NOT CURRENTLY SEX WORKERS N = 313	CURRENTLY SEX WORKERS N = 250			
Legal assistance						
	Needs unmet	19 (44.2%)	24 (55.8%)	1.64	0.88, 3.07	.120
	Met or not needed	294 (56.5%)	226 (43.5%)	REF		

NOTES: "Met or not needed" served as the referent group for all models; OR = odds ratio; CI = confidence interval.

socioeconomic challenges and unmet needs, and thus potentially reinforce the reliance on sex work.

To truly test the temporal ordering and hypothesized feedback loop described here, a longitudinal study is needed to measure each of these variables over multiple points in time. Ideally, such research can include transwomen currently involved in sex work, those with a past history of sex work, and those who have never engaged in sex work in order to tease out distinctions of immediate and earlier sex work as a determinant of health. In the absence of such resource-intensive research, qualitative research in which transwomen narrate their lived experiences can provide useful insight. Qualitative findings from previous research (which were interspersed with our quantitative results) provide preliminary suggestions that transwomen often cope with the mental and emotional consequences of sex work through substance use; once drug use is initiated, many of these women may feel that continuing in sex work is the only means to support it. Additionally, the synergistic effects of substance use and economic hardship influence condom-use behaviors that can lead to greater HIV and STI risk (Nemoto, Operario, Keatley, & Villegas, 2004). Because of their continuing in sex work, these women may need various forms of assistance (e.g., STI screening, healthcare, crisis services), but again, because of discrimination and other barriers, these needs are often unmet. With the chronic discrimination they face, many transwomen are at a greater need for validation in their female identity and expression; consequently, they seek out gender-affirmation procedures they can afford—such as illicit silicone use and nonprescription hormones—but that carry serious health consequences. The cycle thus returns to the original gender-affirmation motivation for initiating, and now continuing, sex work, and this pattern continues.

In light of preliminary findings reported here and the previous research reviewed, it is evident that transwomen in sex work have elevated risks for sexual health problems and drug use, potentially hazardous gender transition behaviors (injection silicone and nonprescription hormones), and a range of unmet service needs. We have argued that sex work and its associated health problems operate in a context of socioeconomic adversity and exclusion, and thus we conclude that efforts that disrupt upstream factors (stigma, exclusion) must be undertaken to affect midstream (sex work) and downstream (health) outcomes. Owing to upstream factors, such as social and structural discrimination, transwomen's ability to secure employment or education is impeded, which leads to engagement in sex work as one of their only means of financial support. This outcome calls for a cultural shift in society's regard for and validation of transgender people. Although initial strides are being made, especially in Western societies that have evinced recent improvements in transgender visibility (MacCarthy et al., 2015), true change will probably be slow and incremental.

Until such deep cultural shifts are attained and the vicious cycle is disrupted, interventions targeting the context of sex work can potentially have influence. For example, increasing availability of and funding for public health and social services for sex work populations and improving the capacity of health providers to treat transgender sex workers can draw members of this population into networks of care. Supporting transwomen in transition-related services, in addition to providing safe and validated hormones, can potentially minimize the reliance on income derived from sex work. Finally, substance use treatment programs that assist transwomen sex workers in fulfilling their unmet gender-affirmation and socioeconomic needs can provide a multifaceted approach to reducing multiple risks and promoting wellness among these women.

REFERENCES

Bauer, G. R., Hammond, R., Travers, R., Kaay, M., Hohenadel, K. M., & Boyce, M. (2009). "I don't think this is theoretical; this is our lives": How erasure impacts health care for transgender people. *Journal of the Association of Nurses in AIDS Care, 20* (5), 348–361.

Bradford, J., Reisner, S. L., Honnold, J. A., & Xavier, J. (2013). Experiences of transgender-related discrimination and implications for health: Results from the Virginia Transgender Health Initiative Study. *American Journal of Public Health, 103* (10), 1820–1829.

Clements-Nolle, K., Marx, R., Guzman, R., & Katz, M. (2001). HIV prevalence, risk behaviors, health care use, and mental health status of transgender persons: Implications for public health intervention. *American Journal of Public Health, 91* (6), 915.

Colton Meier, S. L., Fitzgerald, K. M., Pardo, S. T., & Babcock, J. (2011). The effects of hormonal gender affirmation treatment on mental health in female-to-male transsexuals. *Journal of Gay & Lesbian Mental Health, 15* (3), 281–299.

Davis, M., & Wertz, K. (2009). When laws are not enough: A study of the economic health of transgender people and the need for a multidisciplinary approach to economic justice. *Seattle Journal for Social Justice, 8,* 467.

de Haan, G., Santos, G. M., Arayasirikul, S., & Raymond, H. F. (2015). Non-prescribed hormone use and barriers to care for transgender women in San Francisco. *LGBT Health, 2* (4), 313–323.

Glynn, T., & van den Berg, J. J. (2017). Interventions to reduce problematic substance use among transgender individuals: A call to action. *Transgender Health, 2* (1), 45–59.

Grant, J. M., Mottet, L., Tanis, J. E., Harrison, J., Herman, J., & Keisling, M. (2011). *Injustice at every turn: A report of the National Transgender Discrimination Survey.* Washington, DC: National Center for Transgender Equality and National Gay and Lesbian Task Force.

Herbst, J. H., Jacobs, E. D., Finlayson, T. J., McKleroy, V. S., Neumann, M. S., Crepaz, N., & HIV/AIDS Prevention Research Synthesis Team. (2008). Estimating HIV prevalence and risk behaviors of transgender persons in the United States: A systematic review. *AIDS and Behavior, 12* (1), 1–17.

Kattari, S. K., Whitfield, D. L., Walls, N. E., Langenderfer-Magruder, L., & Ramos, D. (2016). Policing gender through housing and employment discrimination: Comparison of discrimination experiences of transgender and cisgender LGBQ individuals. *Journal of the Society for Social Work and Research, 7* (3), 427–447.

Lombardi, E. (2001). Enhancing transgender health care. *American Journal of Public Health, 91* (6), 869–872.

MacCarthy, S., Reisner, S. L., Nunn, A., Perez-Brumer, A., & Operario, D. (2015). The time is now: Attention increases to transgender health in the United States but scientific knowledge gaps remain. *LGBT Health, 2* (4), 287–291.

Nemoto, T., Bödeker, B., & Iwamoto, M. (2011). Social support, exposure to violence and transphobia, and correlates of depression among male-to-female transgender women with a history of sex work. *American Journal of Public Health, 101* (10), 1980–1988.

Nemoto, T., Operario, D., Keatley, J., Han, L., & Soma, T. (2004). HIV risk behaviors among male-to-female transgender persons of color in San Francisco. *American Journal of Public Health, 94* (7), 1193–1199.

Nemoto, T., Operario, D., Keatley, J., Nguyen, H., & Sugano, E. (2005). Promoting health for transgender women: Transgender Resources and Neighborhood Space (TRANS) program in San Francisco. *American Journal of Public Health, 95* (3), 382–384.

Nemoto, T., Operario, D., Keatley, J., & Villegas, D. (2004). Social context of HIV risk behaviours among male-to-female transgenders of colour. *AIDS Care, 16* (6), 724–735.

Operario, D., Soma, T., & Underhill, K. (2008). Sex work and HIV status among transgender women: Systematic review and meta-analysis. *Journal of Acquired Immune Deficiency Syndrome, 48* (1), 97–103.

Poteat, T., Wirtz, A. L., Radix, A., Borquez, A., Silva-Santisteban, A., Deutsch, M. B., . . . & Operario, D. (2015). HIV risk and preventive interventions in transgender women sex workers. *Lancet, 385* (9964), 274–286.

Reisner, S. L., Poteat, T., Keatley, J., Cabral, M., Mothopeng, T., Dunham, E., . . . & Baral, S. D. (2016). Global health burden and needs of transgender populations: A review. *Lancet, 388* (10042), 412–436.

Rotondi, N. K., Bauer, G. R., Scanlon, K., Kaay, M., Travers, R., & Travers, A. (2013). Nonprescribed hormone use and self-performed surgeries: "Do-it-yourself" transitions in transgender communities in Ontario, Canada. *American Journal of Public Health, 103* (10), 1830–1836.

Sanchez, N. F., Sanchez, J. P., & Danoff, A. (2009). Health care utilization, barriers to care, and hormone usage among male-to-female transgender persons in New York City. *American Journal of Public Health, 99* (4), 713–719.

Sausa, L. A., Keatley, J., & Operario, D. (2007). Perceived risks and benefits of sex work among transgender women of color in San Francisco. *Archives of Sexual Behavior, 36* (6), 768–777.

Sevelius, J. M. (2013). Gender affirmation: A framework for conceptualizing risk behavior among transgender women of color. *Sex Roles, 68* (11–12), 675–689.

Sineath, R. C., Woodyatt, C., Sanchez, T., Giammattei, S., Gillespie, T., Hunkeler, E., . . . & Sullivan, P. S. (2016). Determinants of and barriers to hormonal and surgical treatment receipt among transgender people. *Transgender Health, 1* (1), 129–136.

Vanwesenbeeck, I. (2001). Another decade of social scientific work on sex work: A review of research, 1990–2000. *Annual Review of Sex Research, 12* (1), 242–289.

Weitzer, R. (2009). Sociology of sex work. *Annual Review of Sociology, 35*, 213–234.

Wilson, E. C., Garofalo, R., Harris, D. R, Herrick, A., Martinez, M., Martinez, J., & Belzer, M. (2009). Transgender Advisory Committee and the Adolescent Medicine Trials Network for HIV/AIDS Interventions Transgender Female Youth and Sex Work: HIV risk and a comparison of life factors related to engagement in sex work. *AIDS and Behavior, 13* (5), 902–913.

Wilson, E., Rapues, J., Jin, H., & Raymond, H. F. (2014). The use and correlates of illicit silicone or "fillers" in a population-based sample of transwomen, San Francisco, 3013. *Journal of Sexual Medicine, 11* (7), 1717–1724.

CHAPTER 11

Sex Work, High-Risk Sexual Behavior, and Incident HIV/STI among Transwomen in New York City

A Study of Mediating Factors

Larry A. Nuttbrock[1]

1 Previously with the National Development and Research Institutes (NDRI) and now a private consultant living in New York City.

SUMMARY

This chapter provides rare longitudinal data on the magnitude of the association between sex work and incident HIV/STI among transwomen in New York City; additional analyses examine the extent to which this association is mediated by gender abuse, depression, and substance use.

KEY TERMS

depression; incident HIV/STI; sex work; substance use; transwomen

As the fourth decade of the HIV pandemic comes to an end, extremely high levels of HIV continue to be observed among transwomen. Surveys of this population in the United States have reported estimates of HIV prevalence of from 22.5% to 48.5%, and yearly incidence rates from 3.5% to 7.8% (Clements-Nolle et al., 2001; Elifson et al., 1993; Herbst et al., 2008; Kellogg et al., 2001; Nuttbrock et al., 2009; Operario, Soma, & Underhill, 2008; Simon, Reback, & Bemis, 2000). The prevalence of HIV among transwomen worldwide has been estimated as 48.8 times higher than the corresponding estimates for men and women of reproductive age in the general population (Baral et al., 2013).

Nuttbrock, Larry, *Transgender Sex Work and Society*
dx.doi.org/10.17312/harringtonparkpress/2017.11.tsws.011
© 2018 by Harrington Park Press

Unprotected receptive anal intercourse (URAI) with committed, casual, or commercial partners is the dominant behavioral mode by which transwomen contract HIV and potentially transmit the virus to others (Clements-Nolle et al., 2001; Herbst et al., 2008; Nuttbrock et al., 2009). Transwomen report frequencies of high-risk sexual behavior (including URAI) with noncommercial and commercial sex partners that are higher than those of other sexual or gender minorities (Nemoto et al., 1999) and much higher than those of the general population (Laumann et al., 1994). Age, education, employment, ethnicity, nativity, sexual orientation, and sex work have been identified as risk factors for HIV in this population (Clements-Nolle et al., 2001; Herbst et al., 2008; Nuttbrock et al., 2009; Nemoto, Operario, Keatley, Han, & Soma, 2004; Reback et al., 2005).

Beyond these demographic, economic, and lifestyle factors, a recent prospective study of transgender women in New York City identified gender-related abuse as an additional risk factor for both URAI and HIV/STI (Nuttbrock et al., 2013). The longitudinal effects of gender abuse on high-risk behavior and new cases of HIV/STI were independent of the risk factors noted above. In conjunction with this analysis, associations of gender abuse with URAI and HIV/STI were mediated by depressive symptoms (Nuttbrock et al., 2013). A further investigation observed associations of gender abuse with substance use (Nuttbrock et al., 2014), which may trigger URAI and ultimately HIV infection (Hotton et al., 2013; Nemoto, Operario, Keatley, & Villegas, 2004).

The current study further investigated this set of findings, focusing on sex work as an antecedent factor that may produce the conditions for gender abuse, depressive symptoms, and substance use, which may then result in URAI and HIV/STI. Stated in statistical terms, associations of sex work with URAI and HIV/STI were hypothesized to be mediated by gender abuse, depressive symptoms, and substance use. Following the four steps for assessing mediation (Baron & Kenny, 1986), four hypotheses were advanced: (1) sex work is associated with URAI and incident HIV/STI; (2) sex work is associated with gender abuse, depressive symptoms, and substance use; (3) gender abuse, depressive symptoms, and substance use are associated with URAI and incident HIV/STI; and (4) the associations of sex work with URAI and incident HIV/STI are reduced when controlled for gender abuse, depressive symptoms, and substance use (final test of mediation).

All these hypotheses are substantively important, and empirically examining them in a prospective study will advance the current literature. A systematic review (Herbst et al., 2008) and meta-analysis (Operario et al., 2008) of this literature concluded that sex work among transwomen is associated with an approximately twofold increase in the prevalence of HIV. The current study estimated the extent to which sex work elevates the risks for URAI and new cases of HIV/STI (Hypothesis 1). Cross-sectional and retrospective studies of this population have highlighted issues of abuse, depression, and substance use, which are thought to be even more prevalent among those who trade sex (Reback et al., 2005). The current study estimated longitudinal associations of sex work with gender abuse, depression, and substance use during three years of follow-up (Hypothesis 2). Lapses in judgment triggered by gender abuse, depression, and substance use are thought, in turn, to increase the odds of URAI and HIV infection (Clements-Nolle, Guzman, & Harris, 2008; Nemoto, Operario, Keatley, & Villegas, 2004; Sausa, Keatley & Operario, 2007). The current study estimated the longitudinal effects of these variables on URAI and incident HIV/STI (Hypothesis 3). Finally, the extent to which all these associations can be understood in terms of a mediation model was evaluated as Hypothesis 4.

Some investigators have suggested that high-risk sexual behavior (URAI) with commercial partners may be associated with elevated odds of URAI with noncommercial partners. Individuals involved in the sex trade may engage in condomless sex with a committed partner in an attempt to define this relationship as intimate and unrelated to work (Jackson et al., 2005). Those in the sex trade may also select high-risk and risk-oriented committed partners (Robertson et al., 2013). Sex work has also been associated with an increased likelihood of URAI with casual sexual partners (Reback & Lombardi, 2001). In light of this literature, measurements of URAI with committed, casual, and all sexual partners were obtained and selectively analyzed.

Levels of sex work were categorized (following Chapter 2) in terms of the number of paying sexual partners (if any). Parallel analyses of the influence of sex work on URAI and incident HIV/STI were conducted. To control for potential confounding, the risk factors for HIV noted above were included as background variables and selectively incorporated in the analysis.

METHOD

Transgender or gender-variant individuals were actively involved in all aspects of this project. They assisted with the design of the instrument, training of the field staff, interviewing, data collection, and some of the data analysis. The Institutional Review Board (IRB) of the National Development and Research Institutes (NDRI) approved all the research protocols.

Selection of Study Participants

A total of 571 study participants were initially recruited for a community-based study of transgender women in the New York metropolitan area. Approached individuals were eligible for the study if they were assigned as male at birth but subsequently did not regard themselves as "completely male" in all situations or roles (reflecting an MTF/transgender spectrum). Eligibility criteria also included age of 19 through 59 and the absence of psychotic ideation. Study participants were broadly recruited through transgender organizations in the New York metropolitan area, the Internet, newspaper advertisements, the streets, clubs, client referrals of other clients, and assistants from transgender communities who worked on a day-to-day basis with the field staff.

From the 571 transgender women initially recruited for the retrospective component of the study, 62% (N = 354) were biologically assayed as HIV-negative. These individuals were then randomly assigned to the prospective component of the study, which was designed to evaluate risk factors for new cases of HIV/STI. To increase the efficiency of the research design, younger respondents and those reporting recent high-risk sexual behavior were oversampled.

Because of time constraints in this five-year study, there was variation in the years that study participants could potentially be followed. The recruitment phase, which began in December 2004, was extended to September 2007 so that all participants could potentially be followed for at least one year. From the randomly selected initial pool of 230 HIV-negatives included in the prospective component, 171/230 (74.3%), 92/230 (40.0%), and 56/230 (24.3%) were followed and interviewed at years one, two, and three, respectively. The percentages of potentially available study participants who were reinterviewed and biologically tested for new HIV/STI were 171/230 (74.3%), 92/135 (68.1%), and 56/74 (75.7%) at years one, two, and three, respectively.

Measurements of Self-Reported Variables

At baseline, and 6, 12, 24, and 36 months thereafter, study participants completed face-to-face interviews in conjunction with the Life Review of Transgender Experiences (LRTE), an instrument designed to collect a broad range of information about transgender experiences, including HIV risks. The English version of the LRTE was translated to Spanish, and 19% (44/230) were interviewed in Spanish with a fluent interviewer. Study participants were compensated $40 for completing all the protocols associated with a given assessment period.

BACKGROUND VARIABLES *Age* was coded as a continuous variable from 19 through 59. *Education* was classified as less than high school, high school graduate, some college, and college graduate or higher. *Employment* was coded as currently working full- or part-time on any job (on or off the books). Preestablished census categories were used to classify *ethnicity*. It was grouped as non-Hispanic white as compared to all other categories (coded high). *Nativity* was defined as a birthplace outside the United States as compared to those born in this country. *Sexual orientation* was based on reports of sexual attraction to men only, women only, men and women, and neither men nor women. This variable was grouped as sexual attraction to men only (androphilic) versus all other categories. *Hormone therapy,* defined as using any type of female hormone supplements during the previous six months, was assessed at all time points.

SEX WORK Respondents were asked at all assessment points if they traded sex for money, drugs, or gifts during the preceding month; if so, they were asked about the number of different sexual partners. As outlined in Chapter 2, the responses were coded as "none" (no paying partner), "low" (1 through 4 partners), "moderate" (5 through 49 partners), and "high" (50 through 400 partners).

GENDER ABUSE Study participants were queried at all assessment points about whether they were "verbally abused or harassed" (verbal abuse) during the previous six months and thought it was because of their gender identity or presentation. A parallel item asked about being "physically abused or beaten" (physical abuse). Gender abuse was categorized as neither verbal nor physical abuse; either verbal or physical abuse; or verbal and physical abuse. Following coping (Lazarus & Folkman, 1984) and microaggression (Sue, 2010) theories, subjective appraisals of abuse, and perceptions that it resulted from one's gender presentation, were deemed integral to the experience (and definition) of gender abuse.

DEPRESSIVE SYMPTOMS This variable was evaluated with the widely used 20-item CES-D (Center for Epidemiologic Studies Depression) scale, which includes experiences of depression during the previous week (Radloff, 1977).

SUBSTANCE USE Respondents were asked at all assessment times about the use of alcohol (five or more drinks on a given occasion); cannabis (marijuana or hashish); cocaine (crack or powder); heroin; amphetamines or methamphetamines; downers or tranquilizers; phencyclidine, or PCP; LSD or other hallucinogens; ecstasy, or XTC; poppers, nitrates, or other inhalants; misused prescription drugs; or any other drug during the preceding month. Substance use was quantified as the total number of different drugs used during this period (capped at "4" to reduce skewing and outliers) and an overall summary of days using a particular drug added across all drugs that were used (capped at "15" to reduce skewing and outliers).

HIGH-RISK SEXUAL BEHAVIOR *(URAI)* Respondents were asked at all assessment points about the number of episodes of receptive anal intercourse with committed, casual, or commercial partners during the previous six months, and whether any of these episodes was unprotected (URAI). Frequencies of URAI with specific partners were too low for a full analysis. Most of the analysis used an overall count of URAI with all sexual partners.

Measurements of HIV/STI
Laboratory tests for HIV/STI, performed by Bendiner Schlesinger (Brooklyn, NY), were conducted at baseline and at yearly intervals thereafter for up to three years. Incident HIV was defined as newly observed HIV antibodies using an enzyme immunoassay (EIA) screen with a Western blot confirmation.

Non-HIV sexually transmitted infections were included as biological markers for HIV infection. Syphilis was determined with a rapid plasma reagin (RPR) screen and a fluorescent treponema antibody (FTA-TP) confirmation. Incident syphilis was defined as a newly observed RPR/FTA-TP, after one, two, or three years of follow-up (suggesting an initial infection) or a doubling of the titer ratio during twelve months of follow-up (suggesting a reinfection). Incident hepatitis B was defined by the presence of newly observed surface antigens (HBsAg). Recent untreated exposures to chlamydia and gonorrhea were detected by DNA amplification using ligase chain reaction (LCR) of urine specimens. Those with no recent treatment or laboratory indication of these bacterial infections who subsequently reported treatment or tested positive were defined as incident cases. Those found to be HIV-positive after 12 or 24 months were removed from further study participation and referred for HIV treatment. Those found to be infected with a non-HIV sexually transmitted infection were referred for treatment but not removed from the study.

Statistical Techniques and Modeling

Generalized estimating equations (GEE) with a binomial link were used for dichotomous outcomes, the effects being expressed as odds ratios (OR) (Hardin & Hilbe, 2012). GEE with an identity link were used for continuous outcomes, the effects being expressed as unstandardized betas. Clustering within individuals across time was modeled with an exchangeable working correlation structure. The longitudinal GEE modeling used five time points (baseline and 6, 12, 24, and 36 months thereafter).

HIV/STI was analyzed with Cox proportional hazards, the effects being expressed as hazard ratios (HR) (Cleves et al., 2008). The Cox analysis is based on time until the occurrence of an identified outcome event, defined here as infection with HIV or an STI. The data analytic modeling used here included the possibility of reoccurring events (e.g., reinfection with syphilis). The Cox analysis used four time points (baseline and 12, 24, and 36 months thereafter). All the data analysis was conducted with version 9 of Stata.

The effects of sex work were analyzed with dummy variable coding. Effects of "low," "moderate," and "high" levels of sex work were estimated using "no sex work" as the reference category. All the background variables (except hormone therapy) were analyzed using only baseline measurements. Hormone therapy and all the other variables were assessed across follow-ups and included in the analysis as time-varying covariates or end points.

Mediation was assessed using the four-step approach originally proposed by Baron and Kenny (1986). Mediation was claimed if an initial effect was reduced by 10% or more with controls for hypothesized mediators (Selvin, 2004). Estimates of mediation may be biased if the initial association is confounded by other variables (MacKinnon et al., 2002). To reduce this problem, background variables associated with a given outcome were controlled. Background variables associated with an outcome in a bivariate analysis were simultaneously included in a multivariate analysis of this outcome. Those variables that remained significant were incorporated, as appropriate, in the analysis. Degree of mediation was gauged as a percentage of reduction in the basic association when controlled for posited mediators (Selvin, 2004).

RESULTS

Study Attrition

Attrition included those who were not followed at a given point because of study time constraints (administrative attrition) and the potentially available participants at given points who were not located and interviewed (client-related attrition). The subsets of the 230 study participants followed at years one, two, and three were compared to those not so followed with regard to baseline measurements of background variables, gender abuse, depressive symptoms, and other variables (combined administrative and client-related attrition). Only older age with study completion at years one ($r = .15; p < .05$) and three ($r = .16; p < .05$) was significant. Because study attrition was, for the most part, not predicted from variables included in the analysis, the analysis may not be significantly biased by missing data.

Study Participants

Study participants were by design between 19 to 59 years of age (mean = 34.0; SD = 12.4). Less than half (42.2%) did not graduate from high school; 6.1% were college graduates or higher. More than half (53.0%) were employed part- or full-time in a regular job. Ethnicity was 35.7% Hispanic, 35.2% non-Hispanic white, 17.4% non-Hispanic black, and 11.7% any other identification. Less than one-fourth (22.4%) were foreign-born. Most (58.9%) were attracted to men only (androphilic), 25.4% to women only, 13.8% to men and women, and 1.8% to neither men nor women. At baseline, 52.2% reported hormone therapy during the preceding six months.

At baseline, 60.0% reported no sex work during the previous six months; 12.4%, 16.7%, and 10.6%, respectively, were classified as engaging in "low," "moderate," or "high" levels of sex work. At baseline, 45.2% reported no gender abuse; 46.5% reported either psychological or physical gender abuse; and 8.3% reported both psychological and physical gender abuse. At this time, 63.0% scored 20 or higher on the CES-D (CES-D mean of 24.0; SD = 12.0). The prevalence of any substance use exceeded 70.0% across assessment points. Polysubstance use (two or more drugs) exceeded 30.0% at all points. At baseline, URAI with committed, casual, and commercial partners was 20.0%, 13.5% and 5.1%, respectively.

HIV/STI Incidence

Forty new cases of HIV/STI were detected during three years of follow-up (40/230 = 17.4%). The yearly incidence of HIV was 2.8% (9 new cases/316 person-years of follow-up). Incidence rates for non-HIV sexually transmitted infections ranged from 2.2% for syphilis to 4.4% for hepatitis B.

Associations among Hypothesized Mediators

At baseline, associations among the gender abuse, depressive symptoms, number of drugs, and substance days (hypothesized mediators) ranged from $r = .34$ for gender abuse with depressive symptoms to .74 for number of drugs with drug days.

Analysis of High-Risk Sexual Behavior (URAI)

BASIC ASSOCIATION OF SEX WORK WITH URAI Compared to no sex work, low (OR = 2.44), moderate (OR = 2.58), and high (OR = 3.13) levels were associated with URAI with all partners (Table 11.1). These effects were reduced by approximately 35% with background variables controlled. Compared to no sex work, low (OR = 1.81), moderate (OR = 2.24), and high (OR = 2.49) levels were associated with URAI with a committed partner. With background variables controlled, a moderate (OR = 1.56) level of sex work remained associated with URAI with a committed partner. Compared to no sex work, low (OR = 2.90), moderate (OR = 2.38), and high (OR = 2.53) levels were associated with URAI with casual partners. These effects were reduced by approximately 35% with background variables controlled. At baseline, URAI with commercial partners was 7.0%, 23.7%, and 20.8%, respectively, for low, moderate, and high levels of sex work. (Note that URAI with commercial partners does not apply to those with no sex work.)

TABLE 11.1

Sex Work with Unprotected Receptive Anal Intercourse (URAI) with All Partners and Committed and Casual Partners

	URAI	
	Uncontrolled	Background Controlled [a]
Sex work[b]	All Partners	
None (reference)	—	—
Low	2.44**	1.77**
Moderate	2.58**	1.71**
High	3.13**	2.21**
	Committed Partner	
None (reference)	—	—
Low	1.81*	1.48
Moderate	2.24**	1.56*
High	2.49**	1.70
	Casual Partners	
None (reference)	—	—
Low	2.90**	2.10*
Moderate	2.38**	1.75*
High	2.53**	1.97**

NOTE: Odds ratios estimated with generalized estimating equations (GEE).
[a] Nativity, sexual orientation, and hormone therapy controlled.
[b] Coded as none (0 partners), low (1–4 partners), moderate (5–49 partners), or high (50–400 partners).
*$p < .05$. **$p < .01$.

SEX WORK WITH HYPOTHESIZED MEDIATORS Compared to no sex work, low ($b = .48$), moderate ($b = .48$), and high ($b = .62$) levels were associated with gender abuse (Table 11.2). These effects were reduced by about 15% with background variables controlled. Compared to no sex work, low ($b = 13.58$), moderate ($b = 14.98$), and high ($b = 16.68$) levels were associated with depressive symptoms. These effects were reduced by about 15% with background variables controlled. Compared to no sex work, low ($b = .93$), moderate ($b = 1.09$), and high ($b = 1.31$) levels were associated with the number of drugs used. These effects were reduced by 20% to 35% with background variables controlled. A similar pattern of effects was observed with total number of drug days as the outcome.

TABLE 11.2

Sex Work with Gender Abuse, Depressive Symptoms, and Substance Use

	OUTCOMES			
	Gender Abuse	Depressive Symptoms	Substance Use	
			Number of Drugs	Drug Days
Uncontrolled Sex work [a]				
None (reference)		—	—	—
Low	.48*	13.58*	.93*	1.14*
Moderate	.48*	14.98*	1.09*	1.60*
High	.62*	16.68	1.31*	2.08*
Background controlled [b] Sex work [a]				
None (reference)	—	—	—	—
Low	.39*	10.41*	.72*	.89*
Moderate	.39*	11.64*	.86*	1.34*
High	.54*	14.02*	1.12*	1.87*

NOTE: Unstandardized betas calculated with generalized estimating equations (GEE).
[a] Coded as none (0 partners), low (1–4 partners), moderate (5–49 partners), or high (50–400 partners).
[b] Education and hormone therapy controlled for gender abuse, depressive symptoms, and drug days. Hormone therapy controlled for number of drugs. *$p < .05$. **$p < .01$.

HYPOTHESIZED MEDIATORS WITH URAI Gender abuse (OR = 2.00), depressive symptoms (OR = 1.04), number of drugs (OR = 1.64), and drug days (OR = 1.31) were associated with URAI with all partners (Table 11.3). These effects were somewhat reduced with controls for background variables.

TABLE 11.3

Gender Abuse, Depressive Symptoms, and Substance Use with Unprotected Receptive Anal Intercourse (URAI) with All Sexual Partners

	URAI WITH ALL SEXUAL PARTNERS	
	Uncontrolled	Background Controlled [a]
Gender abuse	2.00*	1.61*
Depressive symptoms	1.04*	1.03*
Substance use		
Number of drugs	1.64*	1.51*
Drug days	1.31*	1.24*

NOTE: Odds ratios calculated with generalized estimating equations (GEE).
[a] Education, nativity, hormone therapy, and sexual orientation controlled.
*$p < .05$.

CHANGES IN BASIC ASSOCIATIONS WITH POTENTIAL MEDIATORS CONTROLLED Table 11.4 shows the effects of sex work on URAI with all partners with controls for potential mediators. With gender abuse controlled, compared to no sex work, low (OR = 1.90), moderate (OR = 1.98), and high (OR = 2.27) levels remained associated with URAI (all partners). Compared to the basic association shown in Table 11.1, these effects were about 40% lower, which is suggestive of substantial mediation. The effects are somewhat lower with controls for background variables; there are similar percentage differences in the basic and controlled associations.

Compared to the basic associations, controls for depressive symptoms and substance use resulted in similar reductions in effects. With simultaneous controls for gender abuse, depressive symptoms, and substance use, and with controls for background variables, the odds ratios of sex work on URAI approached null values of 1.00 (lower right panel of Table 11.4). These data suggest that the association of sex work with URAI is *almost entirely* explained by the interrelated mediated effects of gender abuse, depressive symptoms, and substance use.

TABLE 11.4

Sex Work with Unprotected Receptive Anal Intercourse (URAI) with All Sexual Partners, Controlling for Gender Abuse, Depressive Symptoms, and Substance Use

| | URAI WITH ALL SEXUAL PARTNERS | |
	Background Uncontrolled	Background Controlled [a]
Sex work [b] Gender abuse controlled		
None (reference)	—	—
Low	1.90*	1.47*
Moderate	1.98*	1.44*
High	2.27*	1.73*
Sex work [b]: Depressive symptoms controlled		
None (reference)	—	—
Low	1.66*	1.35
Moderate	1.62*	1.29
High	1.90*	1.54
Sex work [b]: Substance use controlled		
None (reference)	—	—
Low	1.72*	1.35
Moderate	1.65*	1.17
High	1.86*	1.38
Sex work [b]: All controls		
Low	1.37	1.11
Moderate	1.32	1.00
High	1.44	1.11

NOTE. Odds ratios estimated with generalized estimating equations (GEE).
[a] Nativity, sexual orientation, and hormone therapy controlled.
[b] Coded as none (0 partners); low (1–4 partners), moderate (5–49 partners), or high (50–400 partners).
*$p < .01$.

Analysis of Incident HIV/STI

BASIC ASSOCIATION OF SEX WORK WITH HIV/STI Compared to no sex work, low (HR = 4.85), moderate (HR = 5.53), and high (HR = 7.39) levels were associated with new cases of HIV/STI (Table 11.5). These effects were reduced by 30% to 40% with background variables controlled.

TABLE 11.5

Sex Work with Incident HIV/STI

	INCIDENT HIV/STI	
	Uncontrolled	Background Controlled [a]
Sex work [b]		
None (reference)	—	—
Low	4.85*	3.09*
Moderate	5.53*	2.82*
High	7.39*	4.24*

NOTE: Hazard ratios estimated with Cox proportional hazards analysis.
[a] Sexual orientation and hormone therapy controlled.
[b] Coded as none (0 partners); low (1–4 partners), moderate (5–49 partners), or high (50–400 partners).
*$p < .01$.

HYPOTHESIZED MEDIATORS WITH HIV/STI Gender abuse (HR = 1.89), depressive symptoms (HR = 1.05), number of drugs (HR = 1.51), and drug days (HR = 1.28) were associated with incident HIV/STI (Table 11.6). These effects were somewhat reduced with background variables controlled.

CHANGES IN BASIC ASSOCIATIONS WITH POTENTIAL MEDIATORS CONTROLLED Table 11.7 shows the effects of sex work on incident HIV/STI with controls for potential mediators. With gender abuse controlled, compared to no sex work, low (HR = 4.64), moderate (HR = 5.21), and high (HR = 5.72) levels remained associated with HIV/STI. Compared to the basic association shown in Table 11.5, these effects were 20% to 40% lower. The effects were marginally lower with controls for background variables, and there are similar percentage differences in the basic and controlled associations.

TABLE 11.6

Gender Abuse, Depressive Symptoms, and Substance Use with Incident HIV/STI

| | INCIDENT HIV/STI | |
	Uncontrolled	Background Controlled [a]
Gender abuse	1.89**	1.48*
Depressive symptoms	1.05**	1.03**
Substance use		
Number of drugs	1.51**	1.19*
Drug days	1.28**	1.21*

NOTE: Hazard ratios estimated with Cox proportional hazards analysis.
[a] Sexual orientation and hormone therapy controlled.
*$p < .05$. **$p < .01$.

Compared to the basic associations, controls for depressive symptoms and substance use resulted in similar reductions in effects. With controls for gender abuse, depressive symptoms, and substance use, and with controls for background variables, low (HR = 2.05), moderate (HR = 2.19), and high (HR = 2.53) levels remained moderately strong, albeit significantly reduced (lower right section of Table 11.7). Associations of sex work with incident HIV/STI, according to these data, are *significantly explained* by the interrelated mediated effects of gender abuse, depressive symptoms, and substance use.

TABLE 11.7

Sex Work with Incident HIV/STI Controlling for Gender Abuse, Depressive Symptoms, and Substance Use

| | INCIDENT HIV/STI | |
	Uncontrolled	Background Controlled [a]
Sex work[b]		
Gender abuse controlled		
None (reference)	—	—
Low	4.64**	2.97
Moderate	5.21**	2.72**
High	5.72**	3.01**
Sex work[b]		
Depressive symptoms controlled		
None (reference)	—	—
Low	3.78*	2.92
Moderate	3.84**	2.52*
High	4.25**	3.34**
Sex work[b]		
Substance use controlled		
None (reference)	—	—
Low	4.79*	3.18*
Moderate	4.97**	2.68**
High	6.49**	4.05**
Sex work[b]		
All controls		
None (reference)	—	—
Low	2.01*	2.05
Moderate	3.03**	2.19*
High	3.43**	2.53**

NOTE: Hazards ratios estimated with Cox proportional hazards analysis.
[a] Sexual orientation and hormone therapy controlled.
[b] Coded as none (0 partners), low (1–4 partners), moderate (5–49 partners), or high (50–400 partners).
*$p < .05$. **$p < .01$.

DISCUSSION

This prospective study of transgender women from the New York City area investigated the effects of sex work on high-risk sexual behavior (URAI) and incident HIV/STI, under the general hypothesis that this association is mediated by gender abuse, depressive symptoms, and substance use.

Summary and Interpretation of the Findings

The hypothesized mediators were moderately associated, and they may be understood as interrelated, perhaps synergistic, experiences and psychological states. Gender abuse may trigger depressive symptomatology because it confronts and challenges a psychological central component of identity associated with gender. Depression may then prompt substance use, which may feed back and cause a further increase in depression. Psychological turmoil, initiated by identity threat, may produce emotion regulation deficits that lead to lapses in judgment regarding condom use and then HIV/STI (Weiss, Sullivan, & Stall, 2015). This understanding of the proximal psychological conditions eroding HIV prevention in this population is especially applicable to transwomen involved in the sex trade.

SEX WORK AS AN HIV RISK FACTOR   The predicted effects of sex work on URAI and HIV/STI were found consistently (see Tables 11.1 and 11.5). URAI with a paying partner, while too infrequent to fully analyze, increased in a non-monotonic manner across levels of sex work (7.0%, 23.7%, and 20.8%). Compared to those with no sex work, reports of URAI with committed and casual partners were about two times higher among those with a low level of sex work; this level of risk behavior did not further increase among those with moderate or high levels of sex work. Those with a low level of sex work reported a level of risk behavior that was roughly equivalent to that of those with higher levels of sex work and many more sexual partners.

The predicted effects of sex work on incident HIV/STI were also supported. With potential confounders controlled, the rate of HIV/STI was three times higher among those with a low level of sex work and three to four times higher among those with moderate or high levels of sex work. Mirroring the risk behavior findings, changes in the rates of HIV/STI across levels of sex work do not reflect proportional increases in the number of paying partners. Compared to those with no partners, low-level sex workers were three times more likely to become infected; moderate- and high-level sex workers were three and four times more likely, respectively, to become infected. Those involved in different levels of sex work may be different populations, with different relationships with their paying partners and different work environments.

SEX WORK WITH POTENTIAL MEDIATORS The hypothesized effects of sex work on gender abuse, depressive symptoms, and substance use were also found (see Table 11.2). Levels of sex work were associated with an approximate one-half-point increase on the measure of gender abuse with a range of 0 through 3 (betas from .39 to .54); 11- to 14-point increases in depressive symptoms with a range of 0 through 60 (betas from 10.4 through 14.0); an increased likelihood of using one additional drug (betas from .72 to 1.12); and using drugs one to two more days (betas from .89 to 1.87). On the basis of behavioral sciences norms and substantive effects, these effect sizes may be understood as moderately strong to strong (Valentine & Cooper, 2003).

POTENTIAL MEDIATORS WITH URAI AND HIV/STI The hypothesized effects of gender abuse, depressive symptoms, and substance use (posited mediators) on high-risk sexual behavior and HIV/STI were consistently also found (see Tables 11.3 and 11.6). One-point increments on gender abuse, with a range of 0 through 3, were associated with 60% increases in URAI with all partners. One-point increments on depressive symptoms, with a range of 0 through 60, were associated with 3% increases in URAI. One-point increments in number of days, with a range of 0 through 4, were associated with 51% increases in URAI. One-point increments in drug days, with a range of 0 through 15, were associated with 24% increases in this risk behavior.

Mirroring the risk behavior findings, one-point increments on gender abuse (0–3) were associated with 48% increases in the rate of HIV/STI. One-point increments on depressive symptoms (0–60) were associated with 3% increases in HIV/STI. One-point increments in number of days (0–4) were associated with 19% increases in HIV/STI. One-point increments in drug days (0–15) were associated with 21% increases in infection. Substantively, all of these effects may be characterized as strong in magnitude.

UNDERSTANDING THE EFFECT OF SEX WORK ON HIV The predicted reductions in effects of sex work on URAI and HIV/STI, with controls for hypothesized mediators, were observed as well (see Tables 11.4 and 11.7). Associations of sex work and URAI were almost completely explained by the intervening effects of gender abuse, depressive symptoms, and substance use. Associations of sex work with HIV/STI were significantly, but not completely, explained by these intervening effects. The comparative lack of success in the mediation modeling of HIV/STI may reflect uncontrolled and unmeasured factors associated with becoming infected in the midst of an epidemic. These factors may include variation in infectivity of sexual partners, likelihoods of encountering these individuals as sexual partners, and local differences in the spread of HIV and other STI.

Implications of the Findings

Given the consistently observed and robust associations of sex work with both sexual risk behavior and HIV/STI, there is clearly a critical need for improved HIV prevention among transwomen in the sex trade (Poteat et al., 2015).

HIV prevention initiatives are, of course, needed for transgender women deeply involved in the sex trade, but these initiatives should not exclude recreational sex workers (1 through 4 partners). Low-level sex workers may service a small number of selected clients on a regular basis and perhaps develop a relationship with some degree of intimacy, which has been shown to diminish the motivation for condom use (Jackson et al., 2005). HIV risk associated with such a small clientele approaches the risk associated with moderate and high levels of sex work, and innovative strategies are needed to identify these individuals and motivate them to engage in safe sex.

Failures to use condoms with committed (Operario et al., 2011) and casual sex partners (Reback and Lombardi, 2001) among transwomen have been described, and approaches to HIV prevention (e.g., couples therapy and education) have been proposed. URAI with noncommercial partners, according to this study, is intertwined and increased in conjunction with sex work, and broad-based HIV prevention among transgender women who trade sex should include issues with committed and casual sex partners.

Strengths and Weaknesses of the Study

The findings and conclusions of this study should be understood with an eye toward the study's strengths and weaknesses. Strengths include a prospective research design that incorporated determinations of biologically assessed new cases of HIV/STI and parallel analyses of both high-risk sexual behavior (URAI) and actual HIV/STI. Weaknesses include nonrandom sampling, a failure to include significant numbers of study participants for the full three years of follow-up, and the use of non-HIV sexually transmitted infections as proxies for HIV infection.

NOTE

This research was supported by a grant from the National Institute on Drug Abuse (NIDA) (1 R01 DA018080) (Larry Nuttbrock, principal investigator).

REFERENCES

Baral, S. D., Poteat, T., Strömdahl, S., Wirtz, A. L., Guadamuz, T. E., & Beyer, C. (2013). Worldwide burden of HIV in transgender women: A systematic review and meta-analysis. *Lancet Infectious Diseases, 13,* 216–222.

Baron R. M., & Kenny, D. A. (1986). The moderator-mediator variable distinction in social psychological research: Conceptual, strategic, and statistical considerations. *Journal of Personality and Social Psychology, 51,* 1173–1182.

Clements-Nolle, K., Guzman, R., & Harris, S. G. (2008). Sex trade in a male-to-female population: Psychosocial correlates of inconsistent condom use. *Sexual Health, 5,* 49–54.

Clements-Nolle, K., Marx, R., Guzman, R., & Katz, M. (2001). HIV prevention, risk behaviors, health care use, and mental health status of transgender persons: Implications for public health intervention. *American Journal of Public Health, 91,* 915–921.

Cleves, M. A., Gould, W. W., Gutierrez, R. G., & Marchenko, Y. U. (2008). *An introduction to survival analysis using Stata* (2nd ed.). College Station, TX: Stata Corporation.

Elifson, K. W., Boles, J., Posey, E., Sweat, M., Darrow, W., & Elsea, W. (1993). Male transvestite prostitutes and HIV risk. *American Journal of Public Health, 83,* 260–262.

Hardin, J. R., & Hilbe, J. R. (2012). *Generalized estimating equations* (2nd ed.). New York: CRC Press.

Herbst, J. H., Jacobs, E. D., Finlayson, T. J., McKleroy, V. S., Neumann, M. S., & Crepaz, N., & HIV/AIDS Prevention Research Synthesis Team. (2008). Estimating HIV prevalence and risk behaviors in transgender persons in the United States: A systematic review. *AIDS and Behavior, 12,* 1–17.

Hotton, A. I., Garafalo, R., Kuhns, L. M., & Johnson, A. K. (2013). Substance use as a mediator of the relationship between life stress and sexual risk among transgender women. *AIDS Education & Prevention, 25,* 62–71.

Jackson, L. A., Sowinski, B., Bennett, C. S., & Ryan, D., (2005). Female sex trade workers, condoms, and the public-private divide. In J. T. Parsons (ed.), *Contemporary Research on Sex Work* (pp. 83–106). Binghamton, NY: Haworth Press.

Kellogg, T. A., Clements-Nolle, K., Dilley, J., Katz, M. H., & McFarland, W. (2001). Incidence of human immunodeficiency virus among male-to-female transgendered persons in San Francisco. *Journal of Acquired Immune Deficiency Syndrome, 28,* 380–384.

Laumann, E. O., Gagnon, J. H., Michael, R. T., & Michaels, S. (1994). *The social organization of sexuality: Sexual practices in the United States.* Chicago: University of Chicago Press.

Lazarus, R. S., & Folkman, S. (1984). *Stress, appraisal, and coping.* New York: Springer.

MacKinnon, D. P., Lockwood, C. M., Hoffman J. M., West, S. G., & Sheets, V. (2002). A comparison of methods to test mediation and other intervening variable effects. *Psychological Methods, 7,* 83–104.

Nemoto, T., Luke, D., Mamo, L., Ching, A., & Patria, J. (1999). HIV risk behaviours among male-to-female transgenders in comparison with homosexual or bisexual males and heterosexual females. *AIDS Care, 11,* 297–312.

Nemoto, T., Operario, D., Keatley, J., Han, L., & Soma, T. (2004). HIV risk behaviors among male-to-female transgender persons of color in San Francisco. *American Journal of Public Health, 94,* 1193–1199.

Nemoto, T., Operario, D., Keatley, J., & Villegas, D. (2004). Social context of HIV risk behaviors among male-to-female transgenders of color. *AIDS Care, 16,* 724–735.

Nuttbrock, L., Bockting, W., Rosenblum, A., Hwahng, S., Mason, M., Macri, M., & Becker J. (2014). Gender abuse, depressive symptoms, and substance use among transgender women: A 3-year prospective study. *American Journal of Public Health, 104,* 2199–2206.

———. (2013). Gender abuse, depressive symptoms, and HIV and sexually transmitted infections among male-to-female transgender persons: A 3-year prospective study. *American Journal of Public Health, 103,* 300–307.

Nuttbrock, L., Hwahng, S., Bockting, W., Rosenblum, A., Mason, M., Macri, M., & Becker, J. (2009). Lifetime risk factors for HIV/STI infections among male-to-female transgender persons. *Journal of Acquired Immune Deficiency Syndrome, 52,* 417–421.

Operario, E., Nemoto, T., Iwamoto, M., & Moore, T. (2011). Unprotected sexual behavior and HIV risk in the context of primary partnerships of transgender women. *AIDS and Behavior, 15,* 674–682.

Operario, D., Soma, T., & Underhill K. (2008). Sex work and HIV status among transgender women: Systematic review and meta-analysis. *Journal of Acquired Immune Deficiency Syndrome, 48,* 97–103.

Poteat, T., Wirtz, A. L., Radix, A., Borquez, A., Silva-Santisteban, A., Deatsch, M. B., . . . & Operario, D. (2015). HIV risk and prevention interventions in transgender women sex workers. *Lancet, 385,* 274–286.

Radloff, L. S. (1977). The CES-D scale: A self-report depression scale for research in the general population. *Applied Psychological Measurement, 1*, 385–401.

Reback, C. J., & Lombardi, E. L. (2001). HIV risk behaviors of male-to-female transgenders in a community-based Harm Reduction Program. In W. Bockting and S. Kirk (eds.), *Transgender and HIV: Risks, prevention, and care* (pp. 59–68). Binghamton, NY: Haworth Press.

Reback, C. J., Lombardi, E., Simon, P. A., & Frye, D. M. (2005). HIV seroprevalence and risk behaviors among transgender women who exchange sex in comparison to those who do not. In J. T. Parsons (ed.), *Contemporary Research on Sex Work* (pp. 5–22). Binghamton, NY: Haworth Press.

Robertson, A. M., Syvertsen, J. L., Palinkas, L. A., Vera, A., Rangel, G., Martinez, G., . . . & Strathdee, S. A. (2013). Sex workers' noncommercial male partners who inject drugs report higher-risk sexual risk behaviors. *Sexually Transmitted Diseases, 40*, 801–803.

Sausa, L., Keatley, J., & Operario, D. (2007). Perceived risks and benefits of sex work among transgender women of color in San Francisco. *Archives of Sexual Behavior, 36*, 768–77.

Selvin, S. (2004). *Statistical analysis of epidemiologic data* (3rd ed.). New York: Oxford University Press.

Simon, P. A., Reback, C. J., & Bemis, C. C. (2000). HIV prevalence and incidence among male-to-female transsexuals receiving prevention services in Los Angeles County. *AIDS, 18*, 2953–2955.

Sue, D. W. (2010). *Microaggressions in everyday life: Race, gender, and sexual orientation.* Hoboken, NJ: John Wiley.

Valentine, J. C., & Cooper, H. (2003). *Effect size substantive interpretation guidelines: Issues in the interpretation of effect sizes.* Washington, DC: What Works Clearinghouse.

Weiss, N., Sullivan, T. P., & Stall, M. T. (2015). Explicating the role of emotional dysregulation in risk behavior: A review and synthesis of the literature with direction for future research and clinical practice. *Clinical Opinion in Psychology, 3*, 22–29.

CHAPTER 12

Sex Work and Antiretroviral Therapy among Transwomen of Color Living with HIV in New York City

Larry A. Nuttbrock[1]

1 Previously with the National Development and Research Institutes (NDRI) and currently a private consultant living in New York City.

SUMMARY

Using data from the baseline component of the New York Transgender Project, this chapter presents findings regarding the prevalence and correlates of antiretroviral therapy (ART) among transwomen of color living with HIV in New York City. A significant minority (12.7%) were not receiving ART, and over one-third (37.5%) of those receiving ART self-reported a detectable viral load. Compared to those reporting no sex work, those who were highly involved were 70% less likely to report an undetectable viral load (OR = .30). This likelihood may reflect a lifestyle that is not conducive to adhering to treatment protocols. Better ways of engaging and promoting ART among HIV-positive transgender women highly involved in the sex trade are clearly needed.

KEY TERMS

antiretroviral therapy (ART); sex work; transwomen of color; viral load

The high prevalence of HIV among transwomen in the United States and worldwide, as reviewed in other chapters, means that large numbers of these individuals are living with HIV, and providing them with appropriate medical care, including antiretroviral therapy (ART), is

Nuttbrock, Larry, *Transgender Sex Work and Society*
dx.doi.org/10.17312/harringtonparkpress/2017.11.tsws.012
© 2018 by Harrington Park Press

essential (Gore-Felton et al., 2005). According to current guidelines from the World Health Organization (2015), all newly diagnosed individuals in high-income countries should immediately begin ART with the goal of maintaining an undetectable viral load. Continuous viral load suppression raises the possibility of a life expectancy that is only slightly reduced, combined with a low probability of sexually transmitting the virus to others (World Health Organization, 2015).

The successful application of ART to everyone diagnosed with HIV (including transwomen) is unfortunately limited by the failure of many infected individuals to seek ART and adhere to the often-complex medication regimens (Beer et al., 2012). In some cases, owing to concerns about the development of drug-resistant viral strains associated with inconsistent medication use, some physicians may be reluctant to prescribe this therapy (Beer et al., 2012).

Transwomen living with HIV represent a highly affected population in which the universal and successful application of ART may be especially challenging (Sevelius, Potouhas, et al., 2014). Baseline data from the Healthy Living Project (Gore-Felton et al., 2005), for example, show that HIV-positive transwomen are 23% less likely than their nontransgender counterparts to be receiving ART (Melendez et al., 2005). Follow-up treatment data from the San Francisco Department of Public Health show that the viral loads of transwomen are almost three times higher than those of nontransgender adults (Das et al., 2010). Perhaps most important, data from Das and colleagues' study also showed that HIV-related morbidity and mortality were comparatively higher among transwomen compared to others (San Francisco Department of Public Health, 2008). Later reports by Sevelius and colleagues, mostly based on the Healthy Living Project, have pointed to age, stigma, transphobic experiences, and concerns about including hormone therapy in treatment as correlates of ART adherence and self-reported viral load (Sevelius, Carrico, & Johnson, 2010; Sevelius, Saberi, & Johnson, 2014).

An extensive broader literature now exists on ART in key populations with a high prevalence of HIV (Arnsten et al., 2002). Reviews of this literature have pointed to traumatic events, including abuse (Machtinger et al., 2012) and substance use, especially cocaine (Hinkin et al., 2007; Sharpe et al., 2004), as factors associated with not receiving ART, a failure to adhere to the treatment protocols, and continuing high levels of viral load.

Building on this literature, the current study examined age, nativity, history of abuse, hormone therapy, and cocaine use, in conjunction with sex work, as correlates of health insurance coverage, receipt of ART, knowledge of current viral load, and self-reported viral load among transwomen living with HIV in New York City. Given the low prevalence of HIV among white transwomen in this data set (Nuttbrock et al., 2009), as well as an earlier study of this population in San Francisco (Clements-Nolle et al., 2001), the current analysis was based only on transwomen of color living with HIV.

METHOD

Transgender or gender-variant individuals were actively involved in all aspects and phases of this project, including the design of the instrument, interviewing, data collection, and some of the data analysis. The Institutional Review Board (IRB) of the National Development and Research Institutes (NDRI) approved all the research protocols.

Selection of Study Participants

Transwomen were initially recruited for the baseline component of the New York Transgender Project. The current analysis was based on the subsets of these recruited study participants who were both nonwhite and self-reported as HIV-positive (N = 143). All were medically assigned as male at birth but subsequently did not regard themselves as "completely male" in all situations or roles (reflecting an MTF/transfeminine spectrum). Eligibility criteria also included age of 19 through 59 and absence of psychotic ideation. The study participants were recruited through transgender organizations in the New York metropolitan area, newspaper advertisements, the streets, clubs, referrals of other participants, and paid assistants from transgender communities who worked on a day-to-day basis with the field staff.

Statistical Technique

The data were analyzed with ordinary and multinomial logistic regression as implemented with version 9 of Stata with the effects expressed as odds ratios (OR).

Measurements

Participants completed face-to-face interviews in conjunction with the

Life Review of Transgender Experiences (LRTE). The English version of the LRTE was fully translated to Spanish, and 19% (44/230) were interviewed in Spanish with a fluent interviewer. The study participants were compensated $40 for completing the interview.

AGE was included as a continuous variable from 19 through 59. *Nativity* referred to being born in the United States as compared to those foreign-born. *Ethnicity* was included for descriptive purposes only; the numbers were too low for a full analysis. In this report, with non-Hispanic whites excluded, ethnicity was grouped as Hispanic, non-Hispanic black, and all other categories. *Hormone therapy* was assessed as any lifetime use of hormone supplements or anti-androgen products. *Gender abuse* was defined here as any experience, since the age of ten, of being "physically beaten" as a result of gender identity or presentation. *Cocaine use* was biologically detected in conjunction with an on-site 12-panel T-cup urine analysis (Medimpex United, Inc.) that screens for recent use with a detection window of two through five days.

HEALTH INSURANCE COVERAGE was assessed by the query "Do you currently have any type of private or government-provided health insurance?" *Antiretroviral therapy* reflected a positive response to the query "Are you currently receiving antiviral therapy as a treatment for HIV?" Using five preestablished categories ranging from less than 500 (labeled as "undetectable") to 100,000 or more, study participants were asked to select "your most recent viral load result." Following the reliability study of Kalichman, Rompa, and Cage (2000), self-reported *viral load* was coded as either undetectable (500 or fewer copies/ml of blood) or detectable (more than 500 copies/ml of blood). *Knowledge of viral load* was based on whether respondents indicated knowing their viral load in response to the above query.

Respondents were asked if they had "traded sex for money, drugs, or gifts" during the previous six months; if so, they were asked about the number of different sexual partners. *Sex work* was coded as "none" (no paying partner), "low" (1 through 4 partners), "moderate" (5 through 25 partners), and "high" (26 through 350 partners). Dummy variable coding was used in the analysis; "low," "moderate," and "high" levels of sex work were analyzed with reference to "no" sex work.

RESULTS

Description of the Variables

The participants averaged 35.8 years of age (SD = 8.62). Using census protocols and coding, 60.0% identified as Hispanic; 29.6% were classified as non-Hispanic black; and 10.4% were grouped as some other category. About three-fourths (75.2%) reported being born in the United States. The majority (80.1%) indicated a lifetime use of hormone supplements. Lifetime physical gender abuse, since early adolescence, was 68.0%. Almost half (42.8%) were assayed as recently using cocaine. Most (59.9%) reported no sex work, and 15.8%, 13.8%, and 10.2%, respectively, reported "low," "moderate," and "high" levels of sex work.

As Table 12.1 shows, 94.4% of these HIV-positive transwomen of color reported having some form of health insurance. The vast majority (87.3%) indicated they were receiving ART at that time. Among those receiving ART, 78.0% reported knowing their current viral load. Among those who knew their viral load, 62.5% reported a viral load characterized as undetectable.

TABLE 12.1

Insurance Coverage and Aspects of Successful Antiretroviral Therapy (ART)

	Subsample	Percentage
Health insurance coverage[a]	N = 143	94.4
Currently receiving ART	N = 143	87.3
If currently on ART, viral load known	N = 123	78.0
If viral load known, undetectable viral load[b]	N = 96	62.5

NOTE: Sample of transwomen of color self-reporting a positive HIV status.
[a] Includes any current health insurance coverage, either private or government-subsidized (Medicaid).
[b] Undetectable viral load was determined by self-report and coded as fewer than 500 copies/ml of blood.

As Table 12.2 summarizes, older respondents were more likely to report some type of health insurance (OR = 1.12) and more likely to know their viral load (OR = 1.06). Cocaine users were much less likely to be receiving ART (OR = .26), and if viral load was known, to report an undetectable level (OR = .42). Those classified as engaging in a "high" level of sex work were less likely to have health insurance (OR = .33) and less likely to report an undetectable viral load (OR = .30).

TABLE 12.2

Study Variables with Insurance Coverage and Aspects of Successful Antiretroviral Therapy (ART)

	Health Insurance[a]	Receiving ART [a]	Known Viral Load[b]	Undetectable Viral Load[c]
Age	1.12**	1.05	1.06*	1.03
Nativity	.82	.75	.81	1.03
Lifetime hormone therapy	1.38	.92	.97	.83
Lifetime gender abuse	2.21	.94	.81	1.91
Cocaine use[d]	.23*	.26*	1.52	.42*
Current sex work[e]				
None (reference)	—	—	—	—
Low	1.01	1.90	.77	1.24
Moderate	.50	.83	.42	.46
High	.33*	.89	.77	.30*

NOTE: Odds ratios based on logistic regression.
[a] Sample of 143 transwomen of color self-reporting a positive HIV status.
[b] Subsample of 121 transwomen of color currently receiving ART.
[c] Subsample of 96 transwomen of color with known viral load.
[d] Recent cocaine use as determined by an on-site urine analysis.
[e] Sex work was analyzed with dummy variables for low, moderate, and high sex work compared to no sex work.
*$p < .05$. **$p < .01$.

DISCUSSION

The universal and successful application of ART to transwomen of color living with HIV in New York City, according to these data, is far from achieved. Though almost all these women reported having some type of health insurance, a significant minority (12.7%) were not receiving ART, and over one-third (37.5%) of those receiving ART self-reported a detectable viral load.

Issues with ART were much more problematic in subpopulations of cocaine users and those highly involved in the sex trade. Reflecting earlier studies of broader populations (Hinkin et al., 2007; Sharpe et al., 2004), cocaine users in this sample were 74% less likely to be receiving ART, and if receiving it, 58% less likely to report an undetectable viral load. Recent biologically assayed cocaine use in this population of transwomen living with HIV was surprisingly high (42.8%), and its association with aspects of unsuccessful ART is clearly a public health issue. Better ways of engaging transwomen cocaine users in substance use treatment, and transgender-positive ways of successfully treating them, are critically needed (Nuttbrock, 2012).

Those with a low involvement in the sex trade (recreational sex workers) indicated levels of insurance, ART, and viral load that were roughly the same as the non–sex workers. Lack of associations of levels of sex work with reports of receiving ART, despite a comparative lack of insurance, may reflect the no-cost or Medicaid-pending services and outreach facilities available for persons living with HIV in New York City (Nuttbrock et al., 2003).

Compared to those reporting no sex work, those who were highly involved were 67% (OR = .33) less likely to have any type of health insurance, and if receiving ART, 70% less likely to report an undetectable viral load (OR = .30).[1] This association may reflect a lifestyle that is not conducive to adhering to treatment protocols. Better ways of engaging and promoting ART among HIV-positive transwomen highly involved in the sex trade are clearly needed.

NOTES

This research was supported by a grant from the National Institute on Drug Abuse (NIDA) (1 R01 DA018080) (Larry Nuttbrock, principal investigator).

1. Sevelius, Saberi, & Johnson (2014) found no association between a dichotomous measurement of sex work (no sex work versus any sex work) and viral load. I also observed no associations between dichotomized sex work and the three outcomes in this study.

REFERENCES

Arnsten, J. H., Demas, P. A., Grant, R. W., Gourevitch, M. N., Farzadegan, H., Howard, A. A., & Schoenbaum, E. E. (2002). Impact of active drug use on antiretroviral therapy adherence and viral suppression in HIV-infected drug users. *Journal of General Internal Medicine, 17*, 377–381.

Beer, L., Heffelfinger, J., Frazer, D., Mattson, C., Roter, B., Barash, E., . . . & Valverde, E. (2012). Use of and adherence to antiretroviral therapy in a large U.S. sample of HIV-infected adults in care, 2007–2008. *Open AIDS Journal, 6*, 213–223.

Clements-Nolle, K., Marx, R., Guzman, R., & Katz, M. (2001). HIV prevention, risk behaviors, health care use, and mental health status of transgender persons: Implications for public health intervention. *American Journal of Public Health, 91*, 915–921.

Das, M., Chu, P. L., Santos, G. M., Scheer, S., Vittinghoff, E., McFarland, W., & Colfax, G. N. (2010). Decreases in community viral load are accompanied by reductions in new HIV infections in San Francisco. *PLOS One, 5*, 1068.

Gore-Felton, C., Rotheram-Borus, M. J., Weinhardt, L. S., Kelly, J. A., Lightfoot, M., Kirschenbaum, S. B., . . . & NIMH Health Living Project. (2005). The Healthy Living Project: An individually tailored, multidimensional intervention for HIV-infected persons. *AIDS Education and Prevention, 17*, 21–39.

Hinkin, C. H., Barclay, T. R., Castellon, S. A., Levine, A., Durvasula, R. S., & Marion, S. D. (2007). Drug use and medication adherence among HIV-1 infected individuals. *AIDS and Behavior, 11*, 185–194.

Kalichman, S. C., Rompa, D., & Cage, M. (2000). Reliability and validity of self-reported CD4 lymphocyte count and viral load test results in people living with HIV/AIDS. *International Journal of STD and AIDS, 11*, 579–585.

Machtinger, E., Haberer, J., Wilson T., & Weiss, D. (2012). Recent trauma is associated with antiretroviral failure and HIV transmission risk behavior among HIV-positive women and female-identified transgenders. *AIDS and Behavior, 16*, 2091–2100.

Melendez, R., Exner, T., Ehrhardt, A., Dodge, B., Remien, R., Rotheram-Borus, M., & NIM Healthy Living Project. (2005). Health and health care among male-to-female transgender persons who are HIV-positive. *American Journal of Public Health, 96*, 1034–1037.

Nuttbrock, L. (2012). Culturally competent substance abuse treatment with transgender persons. *Journal of Addictive Diseases, 31,* 236–41.

Nuttbrock, L., Hwahng, S., Bockting, W., Rosenblum, A., Mason, M., Macri, M., & Becker, J. (2009). Lifetime risk factors for HIV/STI infections among male-to-female transgender persons. *Journal of Acquired Immune Deficiency Syndrome, 52,* 417–421.

Nuttbrock, L., McQuistion, H., Rosenblum, A., & Magura, S. (2003). Broadening perspectives on medical outreach to homeless people. *Journal of Health Care for the Poor and Underserved, 14,* 5–16.

Nuttbrock, L., Rosenblum, A., Magura, S., McQuistion, H. L., & Joseph, H. (2000). The association between cocaine use and HIV/STI among soup kitchen attendees in New York City. *Journal of Acquired Immune Deficiency Syndrome, 25,* 86–91.

San Francisco Department of Public Health. (2008). *HIV/AIDS epidemiology annual report.* San Francisco: San Francisco Department of Public Health.

Sevelius, J. M., (2013). Gender affirmation: A framework for conceptualizing risk behavior among transgender women of color. *Sex Roles, 68,* 675–689.

Sevelius, J., Carrico, A., & Johnson, M. (2010). Antiretroviral therapy adherence among transgender women living with HIV. *Journal of the Association of Nurses in AIDS Care, 21,* 256–264.

Sevelius, J., Patouhas, E., Keatley, J., & Johnson, M. (2014). Barriers and facilitators to engagement and retention in care among transgender women living with human immunodeficiency virus. *Annals of Behavioral Medicine, 47,* 5–16.

Sevelius, J. M., Saberi, P., & Johnson, M. O. (2014). Correlates of antiretroviral adherence and antiretroviral load among transgender women living with HIV. *AIDS Care, 26,* 976–982.

Sharpe, T. T., Lee, L. M., Nakashima, A. K., Elam-Evans, L. D., & Fleming, P. L. (2004). Crack cocaine use and adherence to antiretroviral treatment among HIV-infected black women. *Journal of Community Health, 29,* 117.

World Health Organization. (2015). *Guidelines on when to start antiretroviral therapy and on pre-exposure prophylaxis for HIV.* Geneva: World Health Organization.

———. (2013). *Consolidated guidelines on the use of antiretroviral drugs for treating and preventing HIV infection: Recommendations for a public health approach.* Geneva: World Health Organization.

This section examines transgender sex work in different settings around the world with an eye toward the ways the experiences of these individuals are shaped by broader cultural and societal factors. The section begins with a qualitative study of the experiences of transgender women sex workers in Turkey. This is followed by a current review of sex work among *hijras*/transgender women in India. Next is an examination of transgender sex work in Brazil with a reprint of Kulick's classic study of transgendered prostitutes in that country. This chapter is followed by a current and broad-based discussion of transgender sex work in Brazil written by an international lawyer with deep knowledge of this population. This is followed by discussions and empirical studies of transgender sex work in Malaysia, Thailand, the Andean region of South America, and China.

CHAPTER 13

Sex Work in Turkey

Experiences of Transwomen

Ceylan Engin[1]

1 Doctoral candidate in the Department of Sociology at Texas A&M University.

SUMMARY

Most research that is available on transgender sex workers focuses on Western nations, and research on the status of transgender sex workers in non-Western societies remains limited. This chapter focuses on transwomen who participate in sex work in Turkish society. Turkey presents a unique example as a predominantly Muslim society where prostitution is legal in the form of state-run brothels, also known as *genelevler*. I posit that the current *genelev* system marginalizes transgender sex workers by allowing only biological women to work as registered sex workers. I then perform a content analysis of the experiences of transwomen, drawing from 53 previously collected interviews and testimonials. I argue that indoor prostitution in the form of *genelevler* would provide a superior working environment for transgender sex workers and could alleviate some of the hazards associated with street prostitution.

KEY TERMS

genelevler; registered sex workers; sex workers; transgender; Turkey

Until the late nineteenth century, it was illegal for Muslim women to participate in prostitution, and only non-Muslim minorities were formally allowed to work in the profession. Nevertheless, illegal prostitution was present during that period in some Muslim areas of Istanbul,

Nuttbrock, Larry, *Transgender Sex Work and Society*
dx.doi.org/10.17312/harringtonparkpress/2017.11.tsws.013
© 2018 by Harrington Park Press

including Aksaray, Kadıköy, and Üsküdar (Sevengil, 1927). Prostitution became more commonplace and visible in Istanbul after World War I (Rasım, 2005). During this time, the spread of syphilis and other STDs became a major problem and led to the establishment of the first state-regulated brothels (Temel, 2002).

Turkey remains one of the few democratic and predominantly Muslim countries to allow state-regulated prostitution, along with Kazakhstan and Bangladesh (2007 Country Reports, 2008). Turkey currently has around 3,000 licensed sex workers operating within its borders, all of whom work in 56 state-run brothels, also known as genelevler ("Seks işçileri ve Yasalar," 2011). A genelev is an indoor prostitution area where only registered unmarried women over the age of eighteen are allowed to work. Once women are registered as sex workers, they are not allowed to seek employment outside the sex industry without first notifying the police. The government requires registered sex workers to undergo regular health examinations. This state-regulated system recognizes this work as a legitimate form of employment and provides the workers with state pensions for healthcare and social security (Zengin, 2011). Despite the existence of legal brothels, most sex workers in Turkey operate outside the genelev system and number around 100,000 ("Seks işçileri ve Yasalar," 2011). These individuals work in private escort agencies and illegal brothels, as streetwalkers, and as individuals who sell sexual services from their homes. Sex workers who operate outside the legal brothel sector are subject to criminal charges.

A growing body of research recognizes the varied ways in which sex work is arranged, regulated, and experienced by workers, clients, and other third-party members across time, space, and sector (Weitzer, 2012). Despite this broadening outlook, the literature on sex work lacks sufficient data on the ways in which the commercial sex trade functions in Turkey. Turkish scholars who have attempted to collect data on the culture of prostitution often express their frustration with the silence surrounding sexual discourse and the difficulty of speaking to research participants. For instance, in her book, İktidarın Mahremiyeti: İstanbul'da Hayat Kadınları, Seks İşçiliği ve Şiddet (Istanbul's Prostitutes, Sex Work, and Violence), Zengin (2011) discusses how challenging it was to reach women who engaged in prostitution in Istanbul, a difficulty that resulted in her securing only five interviewees (two former brothel workers and three street workers). Zengin focuses on the relationship between the state and sex workers, arguing that legal prostitution in Turkey is related to the control of sex workers' bodies. Drawing from her interviews, she argues that state policies to regulate prostitution exert tremendous control over women's bodies, influencing the experiences and working conditions of sex workers by way of the legalized brothel system.

Both empowering and oppressive conditions can be present in sex work, but these situations fluctuate and differ with selected types of prostitution and control mechanisms that are put in place to regulate the sex industry. A prominent sex work scholar, Ronald Weitzer (2012), describes this phenomenon as the *polymorphous paradigm*. The two most commonly held perspectives that describe the nature of sex work are the empowerment and oppression paradigms. Those who embrace the oppression paradigm hold the viewpoint that sex work is a product of patriarchal gender relations that result in the subjugation and exploitation of women. This perspective denies human agency in sex work and assumes that female sex workers are always victims of violence (Weitzer, 2012).

In contrast, the empowerment paradigm considers sex work to be a legitimate line of work that involves human agency. This viewpoint posits that sex work can be empowering for workers and provide better socioeconomic opportunities than many other jobs. Both empowering and oppressive situations can take place in the sex industry. One-dimensional and monolithic paradigms, such as the oppression and empowerment paradigms, lack the complexity to fully explain the intricacies of how the sex industry functions, particularly in Turkish society. Weitzer (2012) points out that "victimization, exploitation, agency, job satisfaction, self-esteem, and other dimensions should be treated as variables (not constants) that differ between types of sex work, geographical locations, and other structural conditions" (p. 18).

The ways in which indoor and street prostitution differ have been examined by other researchers in the developed world. Recent research suggests that indoor prostitution has potential advantages over street prostitution (Church, Henderson, & Barnard, 2001; Lowman & Fraser, 1995; Plumridge & Abel, 2001; Weitzer, 2012). Previously collected research on how victimization rates differ among indoor and street prostitutes shows that street workers are more likely to experience being robbed, assaulted, and raped. In their work, Porter and Bonilla (2010) illustrate that street prostitution differs from indoor prostitution to various degrees, depending on race, drug use, and location within the United States.

Porter and Bonilla (2010) conclude in their study that one-third of those who participate in street prostitution used drugs. Most of these street workers were drug users before they started working in the sex industry. In addition, street workers tend to stay in the industry in order to support their drug habits, and they participate in survival sex such as sex in exchange for drugs, food, or other goods. Because they use drugs and engage in sexual activities in precarious environments more often than indoor sex workers, they are more prone to suffer from STDs. Exploitation by third-party managers can be present in both indoor and street prostitution; however, those who work in indoor environments are less likely to have experienced exploitation by their clients.

Even though Porter and Bonilla (and other researchers) focus on Western systems of indoor and street prostitution, the characteristics of street prostitution in the developed world can be applied to the characteristics of prostitution in Turkey. Though indoor prostitution in Turkey exists under harsher conditions than in other developing countries, the *genelev* system still provides a safer and superior work environment than street prostitution. *Genelev* workers are less vulnerable to being assaulted, robbed, or killed compared to street workers. In a *genelev* setting if a client becomes abusive, other workers or managers are able to intervene. Because *genelevler* are less visible to the community, they also draw less attention and complaints from nearby residents. Those who work in a *genelev* are also less likely to suffer from sexually transmitted diseases. Clients of both brothel and street prostitutes pressure workers to engage in unprotected sex. However, *genelev* workers have more agency to decline clients who seek unprotected sex. In addition, because they are required to attend state-provided mandatory health screenings, they are also more likely to get treatment and STD protection than street workers (Ördek, 2014b).

TRANSGENDER SEX WORK IN TURKEY

Street workers in Turkey tend to conduct their sexual encounters in more dangerous and precarious environments than indoor workers, much like street workers elsewhere in the developed world. As a result, street workers are more likely to be subjected to violence and abuse from clients and are prone to arbitrary arrests (Ördek, 2014b). While the *genelev* system has advantages over street prostitution, legalized prostitution in Turkey directly disadvantages transwomen because the current brothel system allows only biological women to register as sex workers. Accordingly, Turkish transgender sex workers are discriminated against because of their gender identity and are forced to work on the street. According to the Human Resource Development Foundation's (IKGV) 2011 report, around 4,000 transgender sex workers work in Istanbul, constituting 15% of the total number of sex workers. Overall, a total of 8,000 to 10,000 transwomen work as sex workers in major cities of Turkey (Ördek, 2014b).

Transgender sex workers offer sexual services in riskier settings and are unable to benefit from government assistance and healthcare. They are left with few avenues other than to participate in illegal sex work outside the *genelev* system so that they can simultaneously earn enough money to support themselves and express their gender identity. Because Turkish transgender sex workers have to work outside the legal *genelev* system, they also become subject to criminalization. Government policies that criminalize street work lead to more economic and social deprivation of transgender women.

Transgender individuals are often ostracized by their family members and friends once they reveal their nonconforming gender identity. A lack of employment opportunities combined with the absence of family support leads most transwomen to participate in sex work (Lambda Istanbul, 2012; Kulick, 1998; Sausa, Keatley, & Operario, 2007). However, transwomen do not participate in prostitution solely because of a lack of economic opportunities. Recent research on the sex industry (Abbott, 2010; Hausbeck & Brents, 2010; Kulick, 1998) shows that sex workers can feel high self-esteem and empowerment while participating in various types of sex work. For instance, Kulick (1998) finds that receiving compliments and validation by men can be gratifying for most Brazilian *travestis* who participated in sex work. His respondents also reported that prostitution provided them with a high level of personal self-worth, self-confidence, and self-esteem. A study conducted by Hausbeck and Brents (2010) of Nevada's legal brothels also demonstrates that it was the women's choice to enter sex work because it provided them with better socioeconomic opportunities than other service industry jobs.

In Turkish society, where masculinity and heteronormativity are glorified, transwomen lose power and status after their transition from male to female, and they consequently become subject to more unequal treatment and discrimination. As a result of both their gender identity and their sex worker status, transwomen are often subjected to discrimination and extreme forms of physical, sexual, and verbal violence from clients and the police. Between 2008 and 2015, 37 transgender homicides were committed in Turkey, the highest of any European country. These homicides included shootings, stabbings, strangling, and battery ("Alarming Figures," 2015). Seventeen transwomen were murdered in Turkey from 2011 to 2015, all of whom were identified as sex workers ("17 Trans Women Killed," 2015).

A study of 116 transgender women conducted by Lambda (Lambda Istanbul, 2012), an LGBT rights organization, found that 82.8% of the respondents were either currently working as sex workers or had participated in sex work in the past. The same study showed that 79.3% of transwomen reported experiencing physical violence from people they did not know, and 89.7% experienced verbal and sexual assault. Violence from police officials is also commonly experienced by transwomen. Of the respondents, 90.5% reported experiencing physical violence, and 92.2% had experienced verbal assault from the police (Lambda Istanbul, 2012). The Turkish government fails to protect the rights of transgender individuals. Although having a transgender status is not banned by law in Turkish society, there are no antidiscrimination laws that prohibit discrimination on the basis of gender identity and sexual orientation. Moreover, perpetrators of discrimination and hate crimes against transgender women are seldom investigated. In cases in which offenders are caught, they often receive reduced sentences by the Turkish legal system, receiving small fines or minor jail time (Karakaş, 2014; Söyle, 2011).

BACKLASH IN ATTITUDES TOWARD PROSTITUTION

Over the last decade, Turkey has experienced a resurgence of traditionalism in regard to sexual mores, creating a moral conflict on issues related to sex work. Since the election of the conservative and right-wing Justice and Development Party (JDP) in 2001, there has been a shift in the attitude of policy makers and government officials toward the regulation of prostitution and brothels. As a result, state control over prostitution has become much stricter. The current legislators consider prostitution immoral and sinful behavior because, according to Islamic religion, sex outside marriage is forbidden. As a result, policy makers often portray those who participate in sex work as individuals who denigrate societal and traditional family values. When the mayor of Ankara was elected, he stated: "I will cancel their licenses and take the *genelevler* out of the city" (Susmann, 2012). By 2008 the mayor had managed to close down half of the city's brothels, forcing 330 women onto the streets. One reason for the many unregistered sex workers in Turkey is that the government stopped issuing new permits to sex workers and brothel owners in 2001, rendering most of the sex industry illegal and dangerously unregulated (Ördek, 2014b; Susmann, 2012).

The police routinely perform raids on brothels in an attempt to eliminate prostitution altogether. Recently, numerous closures of legal brothels in the red-light districts of Turkey have occurred without legal justification. By eliminating safe spaces for sex workers without providing any long-term solutions to help them obtain other forms of employment, government policies further add to their stigmatization and marginalization. Stricter prostitution legislation and criminalization also negatively influence transgender sex workers. By not legalizing sex work regardless of gender identity, the government forces transgender sex workers to labor in dangerous, unhealthy environments, where they become vulnerable to robbery, assault, rape, and violence (Ördek, 2014b).

METHODS

In this study I perform a content analysis of previously collected interviews and testimonials of 53 transgender women in Turkey. Among these, the majority revealed that they either were currently participating or had participated in sex work in the past. The data are derived from three different secondary sources. Translations of most testimonials were available; however, I translated them as a native Turkish speaker if they were not accessible. Forty-seven of the testimonials were published in LGBTI News Turkey, a volunteer-run organization that provides English translations on issues related to LGBTI individuals. While most of these testimonials include transwomen's first names, some of them include only their initials. These testimonials focus particularly on the physical violence transgender sex workers experience from clients and the police in addition to Turkish governments' discriminatory practices against them. Interviews with three of the transwomen—Mehtap, Gülay, and Şevval—were conducted by the journalist and columnist Ayse Arman. Her interviews illustrate these women's perspectives on transitioning and sex work. Finally, three of the interviews were compiled by Kemal Ördek and the Red Umbrella Sexual Health and Human Rights Association. This set of interviews focuses on transgender sex workers' intimate life stories. More specifically, it includes their relationships with their families and their entry into sex work in addition to their experiences with discrimination and violence. The names of the subjects were kept anonymous in this set of interviews. Instead, they were given pseudonyms that represent their life story as a whole.

FINDINGS

Entry into Sex Work

A majority of transwomen are ostracized by their family members and friends from an early age once they reveal their nonconforming gender identities. Transwomen often express "feeling like a girl stuck in a boy's body," which makes them unhappy with the bodies they have. Instead of finding support from their primary social networks, they face threats and violence if they exhibit "feminine" behavior (Ördek, 2014a). "Rebellion" explains the violence one transwoman has experienced from her family: "They used to resort to violence so many times. They imprisoned me at home. They chained me to a chair and all that stuff. . . . I fainted and I was in a coma with blood all over me, but they wouldn't even let me go to a hospital" (Ördek, 2014a, p. 56). Similarly, Sinem noted: "Once your trans identity comes out, you draw all bad reactions upon yourself. It was the same with me as well. My family gave a verdict of death on me and were discussing where to bury me. So I was kidnapped by someone from my family who understood me. I had already been subjected to violence; I was covered in bruises all over. I had to abandon my home in the last grade of high school in that state. After that, I did not see my family for years" (Eroğlu, 2012b, para. 12).

Though not every Turkish transwoman's family resorts to violence, very seldom do they support their children's transitioning process. This lack of support leads transwomen to leave their hometowns for bigger cities with the hopes of finding greater acceptance and opportunities. Instead, however, they often experience economic deprivation combined with lack of family support. This in turn frequently leads transwomen to participate in sex work. Demet, a transgender sex worker, describes her experience:

> I thought that someone like me could work in the tourism industry, that I wouldn't encounter people judging me. I graduated and soon found out that this would not be the case. Not a single hotel would hire me as an intern. I couldn't find an internship. Then, a close friend of mine arranged for me to start interning at a five-star hotel. During my internship, both the hotel clients and the staff harassed me incessantly. People kept offering sexual relations in a way that could be considered harassment. That's when I understood that if you are a trans individual, you have to be a sex worker. If you are employed in other lines of work, you will be harassed much more so than biological females. People see you as a potential sex doll. When men get boners, they see you like sex dolls they could use to satisfy themselves. (Tar, 2014, para. 6)

Another transgender sex worker, Sinem, also stresses the difficulty of continuing her education after undergoing endless harassment and violence from her peers: "When I realized that my identity was obvious even when I tried to hide it, I decided to dress the way I wanted to. I was walking around with my ripped pants and wearing earrings in a place like Erzincan [a town in eastern Turkey]. They were fed up with me and would say, 'We are sick of beating you but you are not sick of getting beaten up'" (Eroğlu, 2012b, para. 20).

Shortly after becoming a teacher, Sinem also experienced endless pressures from multiple schools. She returned to sex work after struggling to remain a teacher for four years. She said: "I struggled so much until 1998 but I resigned in 1999. Because I knew I would have to go back to sex work, I tried to endure but it turned into torture. I resigned in tears; I loved my job and my place of appointment" (Eroğlu, 2012b, para. 29). Though a majority of transwomen feel they are forced to participate in street prostitution because of economic pressures, a few of them asserted that they chose to work in the sex industry. For instance, accordingly to "Solidarity," sex work provided better economic outcomes than other types of work: "Obviously, I cannot earn to the extent that I earn in sex work. My hair extensions, hormone treatment, house rent, and other needs cost much more as compared to normal people's. . . . Therefore, our life is more difficult as compared to normal people's. I would have concerns about how to make both ends meet if I worked in a normal job" (Ördek, 2014a, p. 491).

Some women also expressed having thought that sex work would be a viable choice when they first started, without being aware of the dangers associated with it. For instance, Sevval said: "When my trans friend said, 'You can stay with me but being a woman comes with a price. We are all doing sex work; you need to be prepared to be able to deal with that,' I was twenty years old. I told myself, 'So many handsome men, plus I get to get paid.' I was very young and stupid. For me, sex work meant flirting with pretty men. I had a life like this for a year and a half. . . . I realized how difficult and calamitous it can be much later" (Arman, 2011, para. 104).

"Compassion" spoke of having a similar experience: "I was a student and had no money. I was living with the money my parents gave me. It was tempting to both sleep with someone and get paid for that in that time. That was the starting point, and then with the stipulation of my friends, I found myself in an environment full of sex workers and I started doing it as well. . . . I was 18 when I first started. Back then, it was all like a game to me. I wasn't aware of the seriousness of the situation and what I actually was doing" (Ördek, 2014a, p. 417).

Experiences with Clients

As I previously mentioned, the current *genelev* system allows only biological women to work legally as sex workers. As a result, most transgender women cannot participate in the legalized *genelevler* in Turkey. This leads transgender sex workers to be more vulnerable to violent attacks by their clients because they participate in street prostitution. In the past year, there have been 125 violent attacks against transwomen in Turkey. Of these women, 95% were also sex workers, and their attackers presented themselves as clients ("Son Bir Yılda," 2016). In May 2015 a transgender sex worker, Migel, was brutally injured by a client. She was beaten and had deep knife wounds all over her body. The same night another transgender sex worker, Işil, was assaulted by a group of men. The attackers broke her jaw ("Two Transphobic

Attacks," 2015). In August 2015 Ada Su, also a transgender sex worker, was robbed and stabbed three times by two men after she declined to provide sexual services ("Knife Attack," 2015). In November 2015 a client strangled a 33-year-old transgender sex worker, Nilay, with a bathrobe after stabbing her multiple times ("Trans Woman Stabbed," 2015).

Transwomen in Turkey experience severe forms of violence as a result of both their gender identity and their sex worker status. By conducting sex work in dangerous environments, they become even more vulnerable to physical, emotional, and verbal violence. For instance, two clients of one transgender sex worker, Eylül, attempted to rob her. One man stabbed her three times when she resisted, causing her large intestine to be ruptured ("Transphobic Violence," 2015). Görkem, a transwoman, had a similar experience:

> I am a sex worker because I have to work. I work especially on side streets. I do not really think I am worth this little, but I have to do it. I am subjected to violence when I am working as a sex worker. This past July, I got into a car and made a deal. We went to his place. He did not pay the price I wanted; we argued. I slammed the door and got out. Because my outfit was revealing, two drunk people who were passing by said, "Come, stay with us." I sensed they were going to do something nasty. Whether I stayed or not, something bad was going to happen to me. So I sprayed their eyes and got into a cab immediately. I had also been drinking during that time. Somehow the cab turned round and round and took me back to the people I was running away from. . . . The only thing that I can remember is the people I had argued with taking me out of the car. They attacked me immediately. They wounded me on the face, arm and leg with a knife. (Eroğlu, 2012a, para. 4)

Legal Injustice

On numerous occasions, transwomen talked about experiencing unjust treatment and discrimination from the police, legal administrators, and healthcare officials. For instance, Görkem asserted in regard to filing a complaint after experiencing a violent attack: "If you are a trans individual, I learned that it is useless for you to complain. . . . The police threatened me and said, 'Withdraw your complaint, this business will take a long time, you will be the one who is sorry'" (Eroğlu, 2012a, para. 2–24). Serap, another transgender sex worker, recalled not being assigned a lawyer from the Bar Association in the courthouse for her complaint after being subjected to armed assault by a client. The clerks at the courthouse told her, "We do not assign lawyers to transvestites" ("Bar Association," 2014, para. 3).

Moreover, other transwomen criticized the hypocrisy of the lack of prosecution and punishment of crimes that are committed against transgender sex workers. There are frequent instances in which attacks against transgender women result in reduced sentences for the perpetrators. Most of the time, the cases are closed without even being investigated. Regarding sentence reductions, the lawyer Fırat Söyle, who was representing Seda, a transwoman who was beaten to death, said: "This is a verdict far from justice. The felon's statement is not an unheard-of defense. Courts find such statements as 'they propositioned,' or 'they propositioned for anal sex,' or 'I thought they were a woman' all as entirely reasonable defenses that warrant reduced sentences. If the murderers do not confess to their crimes, it is even possible that they may still be acquitted" (Karakaş, 2014, para. 7).

The current sex work legislation also disadvantages transgender sex workers, especially after the implementation of the Misdemeanor Law No. 5326, in 2005, along with a bonus system introduced by the Istanbul chief of police as a means to "combat" prostitution. The bonus system assigns points to police officers for the number of arrests and fines they issue to lawbreakers (Ördek, 2014b; "Turkey: Change Law of Misdemeanors," 2009). Because street prostitution is illegal, transgender sex workers are frequently arrested by the police under the broad sweep of this law. As a result, transgender sex workers regularly report receiving fines (ranging from 50 to 140 liras [$20 to $50]), detention, extortion, and brutality from the police ("Turkey: Change Law of Misdemeanors," 2009). The present system, which criminalizes sex workers, involves specific attempts to discourage and eliminate prostitution. A current sex worker and activist, Sinem, protests against the government's criminalization policies, arguing that criminalization through fines and arrests leads only to more economic and social deprivation of transwomen (Eroğlu, 2012b). Demet also explains how difficult it is to survive as a sex worker in Turkey: "It turns out that to be a prostitute in this country, I had to pay money to the state within the framework of the Law of

Misdemeanors. To find clients on the street, I had to pay off the mafia [pimps]. Moreover, I had to sleep with the mafia for free from time to time. And the police too. . . . Some policemen would just flip their dicks out, telling me 'come on suck it.' It is not so easy being a prostitute. Actually, it's harder than some 'honorable professions'" (Tar, 2014, para. 9).

Transwomen also experience discrimination in health services and often do not have the economic means to afford medical care. Turkey lacks medical staff and physicians trained in the needs of transgender individuals. As a result, transgender individuals lack information about the potential risks and benefits associated with gender-reassignment surgeries, hormone therapies, and other treatment. Transgender individuals often report experiencing gender bias from health providers (doctors, nurses, and paramedics) who refuse to treat them, make fun of them, or pay little attention to their immediate needs. For instance, in December 2015 a doctor refused to examine a transwoman, H.C., stating, "It is not my specialty; I will not do the examination. You are a man, I do not condone your situation" ("Court Sentences," 2015, para. 7). Görkem also discussed her experience in hospitals:

> Most of the doctors treat you differently from the normal patients. Some of them do not see it as a problem, but some of them do not even want to touch you. Because I earn money as a sex worker, I have to accept certain things that happen to me. I go there because of the violence I experience on the streets, on top of it I get discriminated against by health workers. Doctors should begin their careers by knowing that they have to serve the entire community; if they are going to be discriminative, they should not be doctors in the first place. (Eroğlu, 2012a, para. 16)

The current state legislation also leaves those who participate in street prostitution unprotected against sexually transmitted diseases. The government lacks inexpensive and accessible services for transgender sex workers that focus on protection, prevention, diagnosis, and treatment. Unlike those who work in the *genelev* system, street prostitutes are unable to benefit from public healthcare and have less agency to negotiate condom use with their clients. In regard to this issue, Red Umbrella Sexual Health and Human Rights Association made the following statement:

Sex workers working on the streets do not have the chance to negotiate on the use of condoms with their clients because of the fear of police raids. Sex workers who have to work on the streets and elsewhere since the closure of brothels do not have access to protection means. Sex workers who grapple with poverty and who are constantly imposed punitive fines based on the Law of Misdemeanors cannot resist their clients' demands for not using condoms because of the fact that they need to earn money. The regulations leave sex workers unprotected against HIV and other sexually transmitted diseases. ("Regulations Leave Sex Workers Unprotected against HIV," 2013, para. 7)

Overall, this study describes the common experiences of Turkish transgender individuals who participate in street prostitution. The findings demonstrate that an overwhelming majority of transgender women in Turkey participate in sex work as a result of lack of employment opportunities they experience after being ostracized by their family members. Moreover, the current legalized *genelev* system marginalizes transgender women by allowing only biological women to work as registered sex workers. The legal system thus leads transgender women to labor in precarious environments that make them vulnerable to robbery, rape, and violent assaults. Because transgender sex workers cannot benefit from government healthcare that imposes mandatory health checkups and treatment, they also become more vulnerable to STDs and often do not have resources to afford treatment. The Turkish government's criminalization policies, combined with a lack of civil rights, perpetuates economic deprivation, social marginalization, and violence against transgender sex workers.

CONCLUSION

Transgender sex workers in non-Western societies remain an understudied phenomenon. In this chapter, I examine the current sex work policy in Turkey, a predominantly Muslim society where prostitution is legal in the form of state-run brothels, or *genelevler*. I specifically analyze the status of transgender sex workers and how it is influenced by the current *genelev* system. This study consists of a content analysis of previously collected interviews and testimonials of 53 transgender women. More specifically, it examines these women's entry into sex work and their experiences with clients, the police, healthcare, and the legal system.

Though Turkey is often considered an example of a modern democracy compared to other Middle Eastern societies that are run by dictatorships, traditional Islamic values continue to be a prominent aspect of Turkish life. Even though having a deviant gender identity is not banned by law in Turkey, there are also no antidiscrimination laws that prohibit discrimination on the basis of gender identity or sexual orientation. Moreover, individuals who do not conform to socially accepted gender norms experience stigmatization, discrimination, and violence. The findings of this study demonstrate that the majority of transwomen in Turkey participate in the sex industry because of a lack of employment opportunities available to them. The current *genelev* system, in allowing only biological women to participate, also pushes transgender sex workers to engage in street prostitution, where violence is commonplace. As a result of laboring in dangerous environments, transwomen regularly suffer from discrimination and violence from clients, the police, and the state.

The discrimination and violence that transgender sex workers experience are not unique to Turkey. The findings of this study correlate with previously collected research on transgender sex workers in other countries (Grant et al., 2011; Kulick, 1998; Sausa, Keatley, & Operario, 2007). Recent studies also reveal that many transwomen participate in the sex industry because of employment discrimination they experience, whereas others report choosing to participate in sex work because they find it empowering. Accordingly, sex work scholars often promote decriminalization of sex work and argue that criminalization places sex workers at a greater risk for violence, poor sexual health, and incarceration (Harcourt, Egger, & Donovan, 2005; Weitzer, 2012).

Various policy changes need to be adopted by the Turkish constitution to reduce discrimination and violence experienced by transgender sex workers. The numerous instances of hate crimes against transwomen show the failure of the Turkish justice system. The adoption of an equality law that prevents discrimination on the basis of sexual orientation, gender identity, and gender expression is essential to alleviate the inequalities that transgender individuals experience economically, legally, and socially. It is also vital to revise the current sex work policy and regulations in Turkey. Although sex work is regulated in the form of *genelevler*, the majority of sex workers labor outside the system.

Because the majority of sex work policy makers consider sex work immoral behavior, their attitudes toward sex work have also been strict in their push to eliminate prostitution. The current system marginalizes and criminalizes those who participate in street prostitution instead of protecting them.

The criminalization policies of the government are not an effective way of curbing prostitution; rather, they further marginalize transgender sex workers and force them to operate in more dangerous environments. Because *genelevler* provide a safer working environment for sex workers than street prostitution, legalizing indoor prostitution regardless of sexual orientation and gender identity can ameliorate some of the problems of transgender sex workers by allowing them to benefit from government healthcare and social security. Health professionals who can effectively address the needs of transgender individuals without gender bias are also crucial for securing transwomen's well-being. Implementing programs that provide legal and social support is a fundamental requirement for improving the working and living conditions of transgender sex workers in the long term.

REFERENCES

Abbott, S. (2010). Motivations for pursuing a career in pornography. *In* R. Weitzer (ed.), *Sex for sale: Prostitution, pornography, and the sex industry* (pp. 47–66). New York: Routledge.

Alarming figures: Over 1,700 trans people killed in the last 7 years. (2015, May 8). *Transgender Europe*. Retrieved from http://transrespect.org/en/transgender-europe-idahot-tmm-2015/.

Arman, A. (2011, May 1). "Trans"larla 3 gün. *Gecce*. Retrieved from https://gecce.com/haber-ayse-arman-translarla-3-gun-gecirdi.

The Bar Association: "We do not assign lawyers to transvestites." (2014, October 9). *LGBTI News Turkey*. Retrieved from http://lgbtinewsturkey.com/2014/10/10/bar-association-discrimination/.

Church, S., Henderson, M., & Barnard, M. (2001). Violence by clients towards female prostitutes in different work settings. *British Medical Journal, 32*, 524–526.

Court sentences trans woman who was denied access to health care. (2015, December 8). *LGBTI News Turkey*. Retrieved from http://lgbtinewsturkey.com/2015/12/09/court-sentences-trans-woman-who-was-denied-access-to-health-care/.

Eroğlu, D. (2012a, December 12). If you are a trans individual, I learned that it is useless for you to complain. *LGBTI News Turkey*. Retrieved from https://lgbtinewsturkey.com/2013/08/23/if-you-are-a-trans-individual-i-learned-that-it-is-useless-for-you-to-complain.

———. (2012b, December 22). I was forced to resign from teaching because of my gender identity. *LGBTI News Turkey*. Retrieved from http://lgbtinewsturkey.com/2013/09/06/forced-to-resign-for-gender-identity/.

Grant, M. J., Mottet, A. L., Tanis, J., Harrison, J., Herman, L. J., & Keisling, M. (2011). *Injustice at every turn: A report of the national transgender discrimination survey.* Washington, DC: National Center for Transgender Equality and National Gay and Lesbian Task Force. Retrieved from www.thetaskforce.org/downloads/reports/reports/ntds_full.pdf.

Harcourt, C., Egger, S., & Donovan, B. (2005). Sex work and the law. *Sex Health, 2* (3), 121–128.

Hausbeck, K., & Brents, B. G. (2010). Nevada's legal brothels. In R. Weitzer (ed.), *Sex for sale: Prostitution, pornography, and the sex industry* (pp. 255–284). New York: Routledge.

Karakaş, B. (2014, June 3). Killing a trans is reason for reduced sentences. *LGBTI News Turkey*. Retrieved from http://lgbtinewsturkey.com/2014/06/05/killing-a-trans-is-reason-for-reduced-sentences/.

Knife attack on young trans woman in Istanbul's Şişli district. (2015, August 10). *LGBTI News Turkey*. Retrieved from http://lgbtinewsturkey.com/2015/08/16/knife-attack-on-young-trans-woman-in-istanbuls-sisli-district/.

Kulick, D. (1998). *Travesti: Sex, gender, and culture among Brazillian transgendered prostitutes.* Chicago: University of Chicago Press.

Lambda Istanbul. (2012). *"İt iti ısırmaz!" Bir alan araştırması: İstanbul'da yaşayan trans kadınların sorunları.* Lambdaistanbul LGBTT Dayanışma Derneği. Retrieved from www.spod.org.tr/turkce/eskisite/wp-content/uploads/2012/12/Trans_Anket_Kitab%C4%B1_Grafikli.pdf.

Lowman, J., & Fraser., L. (1995). *Violence against persons who prostitute: The experience in British Columbia.* Ottawa, Canada: Department of Justice.

Ördek, K. (2014a). *"Those women": Violence stories from sex workers trans women.* Istanbul: Ayrinti Publishing House. Retrieved from www.kirmizisemsiye.org/Dosyalar/THOSE WOMEN_BASKI.pdf.

———. (2014b). *Violence directed towards sex worker trans women in Turkey: A struggle for existence caught between crossfire of invisibility and impunity.* Ankara: Red Umbrella Sexual Health and Human Rights Association.

Plumridge, E. W., & Abel, G. (2001). A "segmented" sex industry in New Zealand: Sexual and personal safety of female sex workers. *Australian and New Zealand Journal of Public Health, 25* (1), 78–83.

Porter, J., & Bonilla, L. (2010). The ecology of street prostitution. In R. Weitzer (ed.), *Sex for sale: Prostitution, pornography, and the sex industry* (pp. 163–186). New York: Routledge.

Rasım, A. (2005). *Fuhs-i atik.* Istanbul: Üc Harf.

Regulations leave sex workers unprotected against HIV. (2013, December 2). *LGBTI News Turkey*. Retrieved from http://lgbtinewsturkey.com/2013/12/04/turkeys-regulations-leave-sex-workers-unprotected-against-hiv/.

Sausa, L. A., Keatley, J., & Operario, D. (2007). Perceived risks and benefits of sex work among transgender women of color in San Francisco. *Archives of Sexual Behavior, 3* (6), 768–777. http://doi.org/10.1007/s10508-007-9210-3.

Seks işçileri ve yasalar: Türkiye'de yasaların seks işçilerine etkileri ve öneriler. (2011). Retrieved from www.kadinkapisi.org/kaynak/Seks Iscileri ve Yasalar.pdf.

Sevengil, R. A. (1927). *İstanbul nasl eğleniyordu?* Istanbul: İletişim Yayınları.

17 trans women killed in Turkey in last 4.5 Years. (2015, November 20). Bianet. Istanbul. Retrieved from http://bianet.org/english/lgbti/169421-17-trans-women-killed-in-turkey-in-last-4-5-years.

Son bir yılda trans kadınlara yönelik 125 saldırı gerçekleşti! (2016, January 3). *T24.* Retrieved from http://t24.com.tr/haber/son-bir-yilda-trans-kadinlara-yonelik-125-saldiri-gerceklesti,322745.

Söyle, F. (2011, October 12). Yargı homofobik mi? *BIA Haber Merkezi.* Istanbul. Retrieved from http://www.bianet.org/biamag/diger/133985-yargi-homofobik-mi.

Susmann, A. L. (2012, May 14). The brothel next door: Turkey is cracking down on the sex trade. What's next? *Foreign Policy.* Retrieved from http://foreignpolicy.com/2012/05/14/the-brothel-next-door/.

Tar, Y. (2014, September 16). Demet Yanardağ: "Turns out I had to pay off the state to be a prostitute." *LGBTI News Turkey.* Retrieved from http://lgbtinewsturkey.com /2014/09/17/demet-yanardag-turns-out-i-had-to-pay-off-the-state-to-be-a-prostitute/.

Temel, M. (2002). Osmanlı Devleti'nin son döneminde fuhuş ve frengi ile mücadele. *Türkler Yeni Türkiye Yay, 14,* 169–172.

Transphobic violence in Istanbul on 23 May. (2015, May 24). *LGBTI News Turkey.* Retrieved from http://lgbtinewsturkey.com/2015/06/04/transphobic-violence-in-istanbul-on-23-may/.

Trans woman stabbed and strangled to death. (2015, November 24). *LGBTI News Turkey.* Retrieved from http://lgbtinewsturkey.com/2015/11/24/trans-woman-stabbed-and-strangled-to-death/.

Turkey: Change Law of Misdemeanors to end abuse of trans people. (2009). *LGBTNews Turkey.* Retrieved from http://iglhrc.org/content/turkey-change-law-misdemeanors-end-abuse-trans-people.

Two transphobic attacks in Istanbul on 12 May. (2015, May 13). *LGBTI News Turkey.* Retrieved from http://lgbtinewsturkey.com/2015/05/14/two-transphobic-attacks-in-istanbul-on-12-may/.

US Department of State. (2008). *2007 country reports on human rights practices.* Retrieved from http://www.state.gov/j/drl/rls/hrrpt/2007/index.htm.

Weitzer, R. (2012). *Legalizing prostitution: From illicit vice to lawful business.* New York: New York University Press.

Zengin, A. (2011). *İktidarın mahremiyeti: İstanbulda hayat kadınları, seks işçiliği ve şiddet.* Istanbul: Metis Yayinlari.

CHAPTER 14

Hijras/Transwomen and Sex Work in India

From Marginalization to Social Protection

Venkatesan Chakrapani[1]
Peter A. Newman[2]
Ernest Noronha[3]

1 Founder and chairperson of the Centre for Sexuality and Health Research and Policy in Chennai, India.
2 Professor, University of Toronto, Factor-Inwentash Faculty of Social Work, and Canada Research Chair in Health and Social Justice.
3 Policy analyst for human rights at the UNDP Bangkok Regional Hub.

SUMMARY

Transgender people have been evident in India for centuries, a fact reflected in descriptions in the *Kama Sutra,* an ancient Sanskrit text more than 1,500 years year old. Descriptions of transgender men and women are also found in major Sanskrit epics of India (Pattanaik, 2014), among the oldest surviving epic poems on earth, and images of transgender people are depicted in many ancient Indian temple carvings. In the sixteenth and seventeenth centuries, when the Mughal Empire controlled most of the Indian subcontinent, trans people attained special status in the king's court as political advisers, administrators, and generals; they also served as guardians of women in harems (Reddy, 2005). Thus, the concepts of a third gender, that some male-born and female-born individuals desire to identify with a gender different from that assigned at birth, and that trans-women may engage in sex work, have been relatively well known in India for centuries. From this perspective, transgender people in India have a longer documented history than they do in most other nations on earth.

KEY TERMS

hijras; HIV; sex work; third gender; transwomen

Nuttbrock, Larry, *Transgender Sex Work and Society*
dx.doi.org/10.17312/harringtonparkpress/2017.11.tsws.014
© 2018 by Harrington Park Press

Traditionally, *hijras* have been described as male-born individuals who are "neither man nor woman" (Herdt, 1991). However, *hijras* belong to a complex and heterogeneous group that includes male-to-female trans persons who may want to live sometimes or all of the time as women, and both those who desire a sex change operation (or at least removal of male genitalia) and those who don't want such an operation (Chakrapani, 2015). Some hijra-identified people want to undergo modern sex-reassignment surgery, including the construction of a vagina (Chakrapani, 2015; Singh et al., 2014).

Recently, the term *third gender* has been used in the mainstream media to denote transgender people—although some transgender activists in India oppose this term for a variety of reasons. First, not all trans people wish to be recognized as "third gender," as some may aspire to be recognized as men or women. Second, some gender-queer-identified people feel that this term merely reinforces mutually exclusive categories of gender, moving from a gender binary to three genders. Third, the term may presuppose that both transmen and transwomen wish to be combined under the single category "third gender." Fourth, and relatedly, "third gender" is equated with visible transwomen/hijras, further marginalizing transmen. Finally, there is a hierarchy and devaluation implicit in the term *third gender:* first gender being man, second being woman/ biological female, and the last, "third gender."

Although the term *hijras* is known to most trans people throughout India, there are several other indigenous terms by which trans people, especially transwomen, self-identify. These terms vary by regions in India: *kinnars, thirunangai* (or *aravanis*) in Tamil Nadu, *mangalmuki* in Karnataka, *shivshakti* in Andhra Pradesh, and *jogappa* or *jogta* in parts of Karnataka and Maharashtra (Chakrapani et al., 2007).

A significant commonality across most of these indigenous trans communities in India is the presence of a hierarchical social structure. Among hijra communities, under a *guru* (master) there are several *chelas* (disciples), and they belong to a *gharana* (clan) that is headed by a *nayak* (supreme leader). Hijras usually belong to one of seven gharanas headed by seven nayaks. In some states of India, there may be fewer or different gharanas (e.g., in Hyderabad, there are only two gharanas, Bade Haveli and Chotte Haveli). In general, the gharanas are divided according to the nature of the work done by their members. Accordingly, sex work is engaged in mainly by members of a particular gharana (Chakrapani et al., 2007). A recent study conducted in 17 states of India estimated about 62,000 transgender women and that about 62% of them engage in occasional or full-time sex work (Subramanian et al., 2015).

Among these 17 states, the five states reporting the highest proportions of transwomen involved in sex work were Uttar Pradesh (84%), Rajasthan (73%), Karnataka (72%), Jharkhand (66%), and Chhattisgarh (66%). Overall, 72% of all gharana-based hijras/transwomen were reported to be involved in sex work (National Institute of Epidemiology [NIE], 2014). The government of India's 2011 census reports that there were 480,000 persons who identified not as "male" or "female," but as "other" (Government of India, 2011); however, information on their self-identifications and how many engage in sex work is not available. Nevertheless, extrapolating from the 17-state data reported and the proportion engaged in sex work to the Indian census data, the numbers suggest roughly 300,000 trans people in sex work. As is the case with any marginalized and stigmatized population, in which some individuals are unlikely to represent themselves openly to government authorities or researchers, these reports probably represent the lower bound of trans people, and transwomen in sex work, in India.

This chapter reviews and summarizes the multiple sources of vulnerability among transwomen in sex work, including the contexts and pathways of entry into sex work, and introduces a transformative social protection framework. For this chapter, quantitative and qualitative data based on academic and gray literature were synthesized. Academic literature was systematically searched in three databases (PubMed, PsycINFO, and Web of Science) using key words such as *hijras, transgender, India, sex work, prostitution, social protection, HIV,* and *risk.* Relevant gray literature, including government reports, was included. Data from quantitative, qualitative, and mixed-methods studies were synthesized in an integrative manner (Gough, Oliver, & Thomas, 2012).

LEGAL AND POLICY CONTEXTS

A variety of national and state laws and policies exert a profound influence on the lives of trans people in India, and important changes have to be considered. The Immoral Traffic (Prevention) Act (ITPA) of 1956 in India has been unilaterally applied to female, male, and transgender sex workers—even if they report having voluntarily entered into sex work (Gupta, 2005). ITPA was enacted after India ratified the United

Nations Convention for the Suppression of the Traffic in Persons and of the Exploitation of the Prostitution of Others in 1949. Under this act, sex workers are prevented from supporting their families or anyone else. Hijra gurus who support hijra chelas who engage in sex work are also at risk of being arrested for living on income generated by sex work. Several human rights reports in India indicate that trans people in sex work are frequently charged and arrested not under ITPA or Section 377 (criminal law against consensual nonvaginal sex), but under other laws related to public indecency or nuisance, petty theft, and various state-level acts against begging in public (Gupta, 2005; People's Union for Civil Liberties, Karnataka [PUCL-K], 2003).

The presence of these laws and acts contributes to documented human rights violations against hijra sex workers from police themselves, including physical and sexual abuse, wrongful confinement, and extortion of money (PUCL-K, 2003; Shaw et al., 2012). The lack of specific antidiscrimination laws for violations against trans people remains a significant gap in legal protections. Recently the Transgender Persons (Protection of Rights) Bill, 2016 has been approved by the Indian cabinet (Express News Service, 2016) and is currently before the lower house of the Indian Parliament (Lok Sabha) for consideration. This bill includes clauses that focus on protection of trans people against discrimination and violence, although many trans community members find this bill to be inadequate or feel it has many flaws (Trivedi, 2016).

The recent Supreme Court judgment in *National Legal Services Authority v. Union of India* (Supreme Court of India, 2014) supported the rights of trans people in general. The judgment also explicitly mentioned "sex work," although it did not include specific recommendations for trans people in sex work. Somewhat ironically, that judgment emerged shortly after Section 377, which criminalizes any consensual sexual act between same-sex adults, was reinstated in December 2013 by the Supreme Court (Sarin, 2014). The 2014 judgment recommended establishing an allocation of a certain number (not yet determined) of jobs reserved for transgender people (Supreme Court of India, 2014), a measure to remedy pervasive employment discrimination.

The Ministry of Social Justice and Empowerment (MSJE) is considering measures to prevent people, including trans people, from begging on the streets, and it is also planning to introduce livelihood and income-generation opportunities for trans people (Srivastava et al., 2014). Reactions to "anti-beggary" measures are mixed, however; in addition to concerns about their constitutionality in general (Goel, 2010), trans activists are worried about their causing harm in criminalizing the livelihood of some transwomen who rely on begging, leaving only the option of sex work. The Tamil Nadu transgender welfare board has been a pioneer in relation to supporting livelihood opportunities for transwomen by providing seed money for small businesses to self-help groups of trans people and to individuals, and by providing educational loans to expand employment opportunities (Chakrapani, 2012) — adopting a rehabilitative rather than a punitive (i.e., "anti-beggary") approach, as professed by the MSJE. Other state governments — such as Maharashtra (Menon, 2014), Andhra Pradesh (Varma, 2014), Kerala (Mandhani, 2015) — are establishing transgender welfare boards along similar lines to expand business and employment opportunities for transwomen.

SEX WORK AMONG HIJRAS AND OTHER TRANSWOMEN

Traditionally, hijras earned their livelihood by blessing newborn babies and newlywed couples (*Badhai*), and by dancing in festivals and marriage ceremonies (Chakrapani et al., 2007). Gradually, a decline in the number of people who support hijras in these ways has led many hijras to engage in occasional or full-time sex work — which hijras refer to as *dhanda*, literally, "work" — and to collect money from shops (*mangti*) according to the areas allocated to different gharanas, and even to beg at traffic signals and from the general public (Chakrapani et al., 2007; Kalra, 2012). Salman Rushdie (2008) quotes John Irving (1994), who has written, "In Bombay, fewer and fewer hijras were able to support themselves by conferring blessings or by begging; more and more of them were becoming prostitutes." Rushdie writes: "Fourteen years later, these words are still accurate. And consequently the world of the hijras, already beset by the larger world's distrust, dislike, and distaste, is now also threatened by the increasing danger of HIV infection, and so of AIDS." It is important to understand sex work among hijras in these evolving legal, policy, and social contexts.

Sex Work Settings, Clients, and Other Sexual Partners

Clients of hijras/transwomen in sex work are almost exclusively men, who represent the breadth of the socioeconomic spectrum. Qualitative studies have described a range of male clients of transgender sex workers, including truck drivers, rickshaw pullers, *coolies* (daily wage laborers), and professionals, as any "masculine" male is seen as a potential sexual partner (called *panthi* or *giriya*) (Chakrapani et al., 2007; Chakrapani et al., 2008). Both public spaces within urban areas (e.g., beaches, parks) and outside urban areas (e.g., highways, bushes) are frequented by street-based transwomen in sex work to meet potential male paying partners. Sex may take place in these same sites or at hotels, lodges, or private rooms. In Bangalore, bathing places called *hammams* are frequented by hijras to meet potential male paying partners (Phillips et al., 2010). In Kolkata and Mumbai, a proportion of transgender sex workers, like female sex workers, are brothel-based, in addition to those engaging in street-based sex work. Hijras in brothels as well as street-based trans sex workers usually are required, following tradition, to give a significant part of their earnings to their gurus, and gurus usually take care of the needs of their chelas (these needs include accommodation, food, and security). Seasonal sex work by hijras (and *kothi*-identified men who have sex with men) has been reported in northern India, when they move from one state to another (Bihar and Uttar Pradesh) to perform *"launda* dance" in marriage ceremonies (Lahiri & Kar, 2007).

In addition to male paying partners, hijras in sex work are reported to have regular male partners (who may be lovers or husbands), casual male partners, and male partners whom they pay (National AIDS Control Organisation [NACO], 2015b). Sometimes if a male partner is considered good-looking and is chosen by a hijra in sex work, payment for services is waived. Finally, although having female partners is seen as taboo, some hijras or transwomen may have been married before they formally joined the hijra community, often owing to family pressure — as family members may see heterosexual marriage as a potential "cure" for transgenderism or what they construe as homosexuality (Chakrapani et al., 2007; Chakrapani et al., 2008).

Sexual Practices and Safer Sex Barriers

Hijras in sex work have been reported to engage primarily in receptive anal sex or receptive oral sex, depending on their gender role expectations. As a risk-reduction strategy, some hijras allow their clients to have only "thigh sex" (Chakrapani et al., 2007; Chakrapani et al., 2008) or trick them into engaging in thigh sex while the clients may believe that they are engaging in anal sex. Hijras in sex work appear to understand the high risk of HIV acquisition from unprotected anal sex and the importance of using condoms. However, as in other populations, several challenges have been reported to consistent use of condoms (Chakrapani et al., 2007; Chakrapani, Shunmugam, et al., 2015): not wanting to lose clients and income (if clients do not want to use condoms); being under the influence of alcohol (self or client or both); if the partner is good-looking; and situations of forced sex (by "thugs" and police).

Among HIV-positive hijras in sex work, fear of discrimination and violence, and loss of livelihood, may prevent them from revealing their HIV status, which sometimes results in unprotected sex. Fear of discrimination from other hijras is another factor influencing HIV-positive hijras not to disclose their HIV status, because hijra community members are the main source of psychological and emotional support, given the general absence of support from their family members (Chakrapani, Shunmugam, et al., 2015).

HIV EPIDEMIC AND HIJRAS/TRANSWOMEN IN SEX WORK

Hijras and other transwomen populations are disproportionately affected by the HIV epidemic in India. The national average HIV prevalence among transwomen is 7.5% (95% CI = 6.2%–9.0%) (NACO, 2015b). This is nearly two times higher than that among men who have sex with men (4.3%). Several studies of HIV risk among transwomen included a high proportion of those in sex work (55%–62%) (Brahmam et al., 2008; Chakrapani, Newman, et al., 2015; Shaikh et al., 2016), and it is likely that hijras/transwomen in sex work have higher HIV prevalence compared with those who do not engage in sex work. This increased risk of HIV acquisition among transwomen in general, and transwomen in sex work in particular, is a result of factors on multiple levels (Chakrapani et al., 2007; Chakrapani et al., 2008; Chakrapani, Newman, et al., 2015): inconsistent condom use owing to a variety of contextual barriers, survival sex, lack of supportive legal and social environments, rampant stigma and discrimination toward transgender people and sex workers, and forced sex by thugs and police (PUCL-K, 2003; Shaw et al., 2012).

In general, HIV preventive interventions for hijras/transwomen (including those in sex work), including condom distribution, are conducted through peer outreach. Current HIV prevention projects supported by the Indian National AIDS Control Organisation (NACO), however, have achieved coverage of only 34% (as of September 2015) among transwomen, as compared to the 77% coverage achieved among female sex workers (NACO, 2016). A specific HIV prevention focus on hijras/transwomen was initiated only at the beginning of the fourth phase of the National AIDS Control Programme, in 2012.

Until then, hijras/transwomen were combined with men who have sex with men as one target population (NACO, 2007) and reached through "core-composite" interventions—not an ideal strategy to address the population-specific risks and needs of transwomen. The low coverage of hijras/transwomen through these combined HIV prevention programs led to a NACO mandate to rapidly scale up tailored HIV preventive interventions. A recent mapping and size estimation study of transwomen recommended that the priority for HIV prevention should be to cover at least all hijras/transwomen in sex work (NIE, 2014; Subramanian et al., 2015).

While recent NACO (2015a) operational guidelines on implementing HIV prevention programs for hijras/transwomen describe different models of intervention—hotspot-based (i.e., areas to meet sex partners), festival-based, and gharana-based—hotspot-based intervention through physical outreach is the predominant model. Increasing evidence indicates that some hijras/transwomen also seek out and identify potential sexual partners using cell phones and the Internet (dating websites), but current HIV interventions largely do not use these technologies to reach hijras in sex work with prevention messages or for HIV prevention outreach.

CONTEXTS AND PATHWAYS OF ENTRY INTO SEX WORK

A social exclusion framework has been used to explain why and how hijras and transwomen in India are marginalized and barred from social and cultural participation (e.g., from family and education), economic participation (e.g., from the workforce), and political participation (e.g., restricted rights as citizens) (Chakrapani, 2010). This large-scale exclusion from economic participation in both formal and informal employment sectors explains why many hijras/transwomen enter into sex work.

Though poverty is an important impetus for sex work, several inter-connected pathways and contexts facilitate transwomen's entry into and remaining in sex work (see Figure 14.1): lack of family support secondary to society's negative attitudes toward trans people; joining a hijra com-munity because of lack of family support and lack of education; need for money for gender transition–related expenses; connection between sex work and gender affirmation; and lack of economic opportunities in informal and formal work sectors.

Lack of Family Support

Many trans people realize at a very early age that their physical sex is incongruent with their psychological gender. When they express gender-variant behaviors or mannerisms, these are often noticed by parents and siblings. Trans people have reported stigma and even violence from their family members—especially fathers and elder male siblings—in their efforts to coerce trans persons to conform to expected gender norms (Chakrapani & Dhall, 2011). Consequently, many gender-variant children and youths are forced to leave their parental home to avoid embarrassment to their family members or to avoid violence, or they are evicted from their parents' home. According to one hijra-identified person: "I was caught red-handed when I was standing with [other hijras] in a cinema theatre queue. My brother saw me and he created a lot of prob-lems. He wounded my hand and scolded me a lot" (Chakrapani & Dhall, 2011, p. 17).

Gender-nonconforming males are easily noticed by teachers and other students in schools, which often leads to bullying by other stu-dents and long-term microaggressions such as name-calling. These recurring incidents ultimately lead many gender-variant children and youths to lose interest in their studies, and they are forced to drop out of school (C-SHaRP & TAI-VHS, 2014). A nonsupportive environment at school as well as at home leads many trans youths ultimately to decide to leave home and go some place where they are accepted—often in the homes of other trans people. Joining a hijra community becomes a primary option.[1] Some trans youths may come out as trans persons when they are studying in college; the consequences may range from loss of support from friends and families to eviction from home. As a result, many do not finish college, which further limits employment opportunities in the formal work sector.

FIGURE 14.1

Hijras/transwomen in sex work: contexts and pathways of entry into sex work.

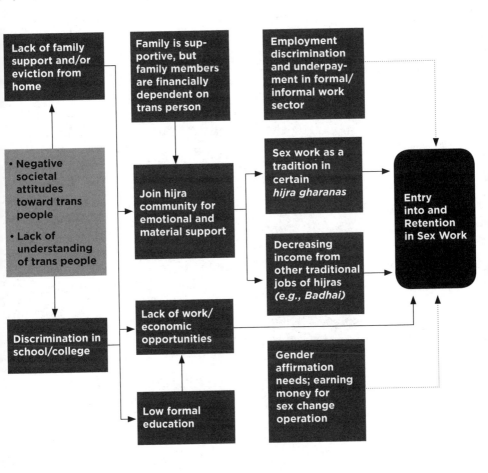

Notes. Badhai: blessing newborn babies and newlywed couples. Gharana: clan headed by a nayak (supreme leader) under which gurus (masters) and chelas (disciples) are organized.

Joining a Hijra Community

Lack of family support and lack of education often lead transwomen to engage in sex work—either working alone on the streets or joining a hijra community. Even though in hijra communities only certain gharanas are supposed to engage in sex work, individuals in other gharanas also may become involved in sex work without the knowledge of their hijra gurus or with their passive acceptance, given income-generating capacity (Chakrapani et al., 2007).

In gharanas where sex work is allowed, hijras may either engage in sex work on the streets or work in brothels (as in some parts of Kolkata and Mumbai)—although both kinds of trans sex workers face risks of violence and extortion by thugs and police as a result of the criminalization of this work. Because hijras who opt not to engage in sex work can move to other gharanas, although they have to pay a fine or "compensation" to their current hijra guru for doing so, theoretically there seems to be no particular peer pressure or coercion to remain in sex work (Kalra, 2012; Reddy, 2005), although, again, lack of education and other opportunities to earn their livelihood pose substantial constraints.

Gender Transition and Sex Work

One of the reasons reported by hijras for engaging in sex work is to save money to undergo proper sex-reassignment surgery (also referred to by activists as "gender-affirmative surgery") or at least to remove their male sexual organs, that is, "to become a *nirvan*" (Chakrapani, 2015; Singh et al., 2014). The cost for sexual organ removal by unqualified medical practitioners (quacks) is often at least INR 10,000 (about US $150, or several months' income, presuming that one has steady employment), and that for proper sex-reassignment surgery in a private hospital may range from INR 40,000 to 100,000, depending on the nature of the operation (Singh et al., 2014)—roughly equivalent to a full year's per capita income in India. Those hijras who cannot afford sex-reassignment surgery by a qualified surgeon go to either a quack or a senior hijra (called *dai amma* or *daima*), who removes male external genitalia in a ritual ceremony (Chakrapani, 2015; Rushdie, 2008; Singh et al., 2014).

Some hijras may prefer *dai amma*, believing that the traditional way of removing male genitalia is better than that conducted by a quack or even a qualified surgeon (Singh et al., 2014). Postoperative complications (urethral obstruction, multiple openings or fistulas) have been documented after some of these crude operations (Chakrapani, 2015). Sometimes the cost for the crude *nirvan* operation by quacks is paid by the hijra guru, and the hijra who underwent the operation later repays the debt by engaging in sex work. It is also reported that after the operation—whether crude or proper surgery—trans sex workers can earn more, though this is reported as an added benefit rather than a primary reason for undergoing sex-reassignment surgery (C-SHaRP & TAI-VHS, 2014).

Some transwomen who have completed high school or college and who have undergone sex-reassignment surgery or who live as a woman face difficulties in finding suitable employment. This is often due to either a mismatch in the name or gender on their educational certificate and current identity documents or a lack of understanding or apathy among employers in government and private institutions (C-SHaRP & TAI-VHS, 2014; Chakrapani & Narrain, 2012). This means that even among trans people who have completed formal schooling or college, some are forced to take up sex work for survival.

Gender Affirmation and Sex Work

Another dimension of the impetus for some transwomen to engage in sex work, as reported in studies from India (Chakrapani et al., 2007; Chakrapani et al., 2008) and other countries (Reisner et al., 2015), is that having multiple male partners and engaging in sex work affirms their gender identity as women. Despite the risks of sex work, if many men are willing to have sex with them, that fact indicates that men appreciate them as women. This illustrates interconnections between transwomen's gender identity, need for gender affirmation, sexual-reassignment surgery, and engagement in sex work.

Lack of Economic Opportunities and Underpayment in Regular Jobs

Lack of education as well as gender minority status mean most transwomen have trouble getting any kind of employment, even in the informal work sector. If they do find employment, should they find a supportive employer, for example, transwomen have been reported to leave those jobs because of ongoing lack of support and stigma from their coworkers. One study reported lack of formal mechanisms for redress, perceptions of being underemployed and underpaid, and psychological stress and negative life attitude as factors that affected transwomen's inability to sustain employment (C-SHaRP & TAI-VHS, 2014). During periods in which they lack a regular job, hijras/transwomen may be driven back to occasional or full-time sex work. According to one hijra: "When a hijra is in male attire, they can at least get some job, but when a male [here refers to hijra] is in female attire, nobody would be willing to give even a housemaid job. No options are opened to her [other than going to sex work]" (Chakrapani et al., 2008, p. 26).

In addition, restrictions that are based on dress codes and lower wages when compared to other staff (men and women) lead many transwomen eventually to leave their employment in the informal or formal work sector. This is especially true for those transwomen who had earned an adequate income through sex work, but for whom the income from a regular job is insufficient to cover their living expenses. According to a thirunangai: "They did that [low payment] in both the companies. When I asked about it, they said no one will offer you a job; we are offering you. So just take what we pay you" (C-SHaRP & TAI-VHS, 2014). Interventions that support or provide alternative employment opportunities or encourage trans people to complete their formal education need to take these contexts and factors into account in order to support their effectiveness.

SOCIAL PROTECTION AND TRANSWOMEN IN SEX WORK: A LIFE-STAGE APPROACH

In light of the many contexts of stigma and marginalization faced by transwomen across multiple sectors and the risks of engaging in sex work—particularly as a sole option for earning one's livelihood, undertaken in a discriminatory social climate—we describe a social protection approach for transwomen in sex work in India. Social protection aims to ensure a life of dignity for everyone, including trans people in sex work, and affirms the need for the state to allocate and distribute resources to those who are most in need, in addition to protection of their human rights (Waring et al., 2013).

On the basis of the "Operational Social Protection" definition used by Devereux and Sabates-Wheeler (2004), social protection for trans people (including those in sex work) needs to cover all formal and informal initiatives that provide:

Social assistance (e.g., old-age pension)

Social services (e.g., assistance in getting entitlements)

Social insurance to protect people against the risks and consequences of livelihood shocks (e.g., self-help groups)

Social equity to protect people against social risks such as discrimination and abuse (e.g., formal mechanisms for redress, antidiscrimination laws)

Social protection for transgender sex workers needs to be rights-based, gender sensitive, transformative (i.e., addressing discrimination and inequities), and anticipatory (e.g., anticipating economic vulnerabilities and risks at particular stages in life). Accordingly, a transformative and anticipatory framework for social protection for trans people (including those in sex work), based on a life stage approach, is presented in Figure 14.2. This figure and the approach detailed below are not meant to be comprehensive or exhaustive, but to indicate possible strategies and activities that can be implemented. A transformative framework, which emphasizes reduction of stigma, discrimination, and violence against hijras/transwomen in sex work, is appropriate given evidence that social exclusion and discrimination against sexual and gender minorities, including trans people, negatively affect economic development in India (Badgett, 2014), and evidence for the connection between gender minority status and poverty (Dhall & Boyce, 2015).

Life Stage Approach

CHILDHOOD As the family's lack of acceptance of their transgender child or sibling often leads trans people to leave their family of origin and abandon their education, educational and counseling interventions to promote acceptance of gender-variant children and youths by family members are needed. Programs to promote understanding of trans people among school and college authorities and students also may support acceptance of trans people, thus removing a barrier to completion of education. Ideally, nondiscrimination policies on gender-variant children and youths should be enacted to strengthen these sensitization and educational initiatives.

YOUTH AND WORKING AGE While the fundamental human rights of those transwomen who voluntarily enter into sex work should be pro-

FIGURE 14.2

Social protection framework using a life-stage approach.

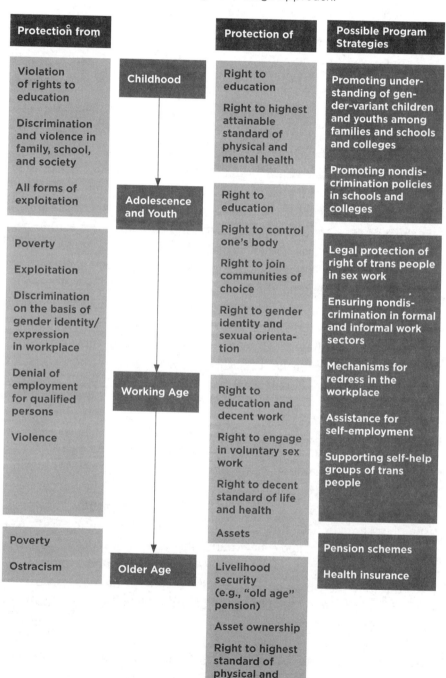

tected, transwomen who would like to take up other work should be provided adequate opportunities that are in line with their qualifications and abilities. Additionally, transwomen should be supported in building their capacities and skills to meet the requirements of their desired employment. Unemployment benefits (a stipend for the unemployed—both able-bodied and differently abled persons) should also be considered in line with this broader emerging trend in some states (e.g., Tamil Nadu [*The Hindu*, 2008]) in India.

Like some of the initiatives of the Tamil Nadu Transgender Welfare Board (Chakrapani, 2012), assistance to individual trans people and to self-help groups of transwomen for starting and running small-scale business enterprises may provide important support to those seeking self-employment or group employment. Furthermore, development of official mechanisms for redress and measures to ensure accountability for workplace issues in at least the formal work sector may be integral to preventing workplace discrimination and thereby to promoting sustained employment of transwomen.

OLDER AGE Once hijras in sex work become older, they are less likely to be able to sustain their income through an adequate number of clients. They are more likely to become gurus, depending on their chelas (disciples) who engage in sex work to support them. There is a need to support older hijras, including those who are current or former sex workers. Providing an old-age pension is one possibility.[2] Increasingly state governments have started providing old-age pensions for hijras/transwomen (e.g., Delhi, Tamil Nadu, Kerala, Odisha), although the amount of financial support is seen as inadequate by trans communities.

CONCLUSION

Transwomen in sex work are highly vulnerable to HIV infection, harassment, and violence, and they face pervasive stigma and discrimination across multiple life domains and life stages. It is important that programs aiming to improve their health and well-being take into account long-standing sociocultural and historical contexts of transwomen/hijras in India to ensure that their rights are protected, and opportunities in education and employment are expanded, without coercing them to engage in jobs other than sex work.

At present, many community-based organizations of hijras and other transwomen in India are supported by the government only for HIV prevention work. However, a few initiatives have begun to explicitly improve social protection of transwomen on a pilot basis—either as stand-alone projects or as part of larger projects (e.g., Svavritti [SAATHII, 2016], Utkarsh [Swasti, 2013], Pehchan [Shaikh et al., 2016]). The lessons from these initiatives will be useful in further refining and scaling up social protection programs for transwomen, including those in sex work. Although building on the work of HIV program infrastructures in community-based organizations offers one viable pathway for rapid scale-up of social protection for trans people in need, it is important that other means of reaching trans people—for example, by supporting and strengthening trans community organizations that are not currently implementing HIV prevention projects—are also considered and integrated to achieve more comprehensive programming.

Emerging strategies and initiatives for the provision of social protection to transwomen in India, while a positive development, seem to exist only under the Ministry of Social Justice and Empowerment. Other government ministries, such as the Ministry of Women and Children, Law Ministry, and Ministry of Education and Human Resource Development, should also be involved in bringing the breadth of their expertise and experience to support comprehensive social protection programs for transwomen in sex work. This broader approach may also serve to reduce the marginalization that is characteristic of the experience of many transwomen in sex work.

Importantly, many transwomen in sex work do not explicitly assume or articulate identification as sex workers, and as a result their unique needs may not be addressed. In some regions and cities such as Kolkata and Mumbai, a sex worker identity may be equally present among transwomen in sex work and other women in sex work, which may help transwomen in working together with women in sex work to realize and protect their collective rights. Elsewhere in India, consciousness-raising in relation to sex work among trans people may offer one pathway to better address the unmet social protection needs of transwomen in sex work.

Finally, engagement and ongoing involvement of trans communities in India in initiatives designed to support their health and well-being are critical from multiple perspectives. For one, such engagement is an important mechanism for reducing pervasive stigma and discrimination faced by transwomen from the broader society. Second, engagement of the trans community, including sex workers, serves to actively support empowerment of transwomen in sex work, a key component of reducing vulnerability. Third, measures for greater social inclusion, with expanded opportunities in education and employment, help render sex work a choice rather than a pathway imposed because of a lack of other choices to earn a livelihood. And fourth, the design, development, evaluation, and monitoring of programs designed to support trans communities have a greater likelihood of being acceptable and effective if they address the expressed needs of the population.

Although trans people, and transwomen in sex work in particular, are marginalized populations—across family, work, social, legal, health, and community domains—the thousands of years of culture and history of trans people in India suggest enduring strengths and mechanisms for community survival that should be integrated in effective social protection programs and government responses in the future.

ACKNOWLEDGMENTS

Dr. Chakrapani's contribution was supported in part by UNDP India. Dr. Newman was supported in part by the Canada Research Chairs Program.

NOTES

1. In community consultations, trans activists who are living with their parents claimed that because of their supportive parents they did not join a hijra community, although they do have close ties with hijra activists.
2. The Lawyers Collective notes that the Pension Parishad, a national movement to mandate a universal old-age pension, has demanded relaxation of the eligibility age to 45 years for highly vulnerable groups, including transwomen in sex work.

REFERENCES

Badgett, M. V. L. (2014, October 3). *The economic cost of stigma and the exclusion of LGBT people: A case study of India*. World Bank. Retrieved from http://documents .worldbank.org/curated/en/527261468035379692/The-economic-cost-of-stigma-and-the-exclusion-of-LGBT-people-a-case-study-of-India.

Brahmam, G. N., Kodavalla, V., Rajkumar, H., Rachakulla, H. K., Kallam, S., Myakala, S. P., . . . & IBBA Study Team. (2008). Sexual practices, HIV, and sexually transmitted infections among self-identified men who have sex with men in four high HIV prevalence states of India. *AIDS, 22* (Suppl. 5), S45–S57.

Butler, J. (1990). *Gender trouble: Feminism and the subversion of identity.* New York: Routledge.

Chakrapani, V. (2015). Sex change operation and feminizing procedures for transgender women in India: Current scenario and way forward. In A. Narrain & V. Chandran (eds.), *Nothing to fix: Medicalisation of sexual orientation and gender identity: A human rights resource book.* New Delhi, India: SAGE Yoda Press.

———. (2012). *The case of Tamil Nadu Transgender Welfare Board: Insights for developing practical models of social protection programmes for transgender people in India.* New Delhi, India: United Nations Development Programme.

———. (2010). *Hijras/transgender women in India: HIV, human rights, and social exclusion.* New Delhi, India: United Nations Development Programme.

Chakrapani, V., & Dhall, P. (2011). *Family acceptance among self-identified men who have sex with men (MSM) and transgender people in India.* Mumbai, India: Family Planning Association of India.

Chakrapani, V., Mehta, S., Buggineni, P., & Barr, F. (2008). *Sexual and reproductive health of males-at-risk in India: Service needs, gaps, and barriers.* New Delhi, India: India HIV/AIDS Alliance.

Chakrapani, V., & Narrain, A. (2012). *Legal recognition of gender identity of transgender people in India: Current situation and potential options.* United Nations Development Programme, 2012. Retrieved from www.undp.org/content/dam/india/docs/HIV_and_development/legal-recognition-of-gender-identity-of-transgender-people-in-in.pdf.

Chakrapani, V., Newman, P. A., Mhaprolkar, H., & Kavi, A. R. (2007). *Sexual and social networks of MSM and hijras in India: A qualitative study.* Mumbai, India: The Humsafar Trust.

Chakrapani, V., Newman, P. A., Shunmugam, M., Logie, C. H., & Samuel, M. (2015). Syndemics of depression, alcohol use, and victimisation, and their association with HIV-related sexual risk among men who have sex with men and transgender women in India. *Global Public Health.* Advance online publication. doi:10.1080/17441692.2015.1091024.

Chakrapani, V., Shunmugam, M., Newman, P. A., Kershaw, T., & Dubrow, R. (2015). HIV status disclosure and condom use among HIV-positive men who have sex with men and hijras (male-to-female transgender people) in India: Implications for prevention. *Journal of HIV/AIDS & Social Services, 14* (1), 26–44.

C-SHaRP & TAI-VHS. (2014). *Getting a job and keeping it: Issues faced by thirunangai (transgender people) and kothis in Tamil Nadu in getting and retaining employment.* Chennai, India: Tamil Nadu AIDS Initiative—Voluntary Health Services (TAI-VHS).

Daniélou, A., trans. (1993). *The complete Kama Sutra: The first unabridged modern translation of the classic Indian text.* Rochester, VT: Inner Traditions.

Devereux, S., & Sabates-Wheeler, R. (2004). *Transformative social protection.* IDS Working Paper 232. Brighton, UK: Institute of Development Studies.

Dhall, P., & Boyce, P. (2015). *Livelihood, exclusion and opportunity: Socioeconomic welfare among gender and sexuality non-normative people in India*. Evidence Report Number 106: Sexuality, poverty and law. Brighton, UK: Institute of Development Studies.

Express News Service. (2016, July 22). Cabinet approves bill to empower transgenders: Harassment will entail punishment, proposes draft law. *Indian Express*. Retrieved from http://indianexpress.com/article/india/india-news-india/transgender-persons-bill-passed-approve-empowerment-2926551/.

Goel, A. (2010). Indian anti-beggary laws and their constitutionality through the prism of fundamental rights, with special reference to Ram Lakham v. State. *Asian Pacific Journal of Human Rights and the Law, 11* (1), 23–38.

Gough, D., Oliver, S., & Thomas, J. (2012). *An introduction to systematic reviews*. London: Sage.

Government of India. (2011). *Transgender in India*. Census 2011. Retrieved from www.census2011.co.in/transgender.php.

Gupta, I. S. (2005). *Human rights of minority and women's: Transgender human rights*. New Dehli, India: Gyan.

Herdt, G. (1991). Review of Neither man nor woman: The hijras of India, by Serena Nanda. *American Anthropologist, 93* (1), 199–200.

The Hindu. (2008, November 9). Government stipend for unemployed youth. Retrieved from www.thehindu.com/todays-paper/tp-national/tp-tamilnadu/government-stipend-for-unemployed-youth/article1372248.ece.

Irving, J. (1994). *A son of the circus*. New York: Random House.

Kalra, G. (2012). Hijras: The unique transgender culture of India. *International Journal of Culture and Mental Health, 5* (2), 121–126.

Lahiri, A., & Kar, S. (2007). *Dancing boys: Traditional prostitution of young males in India*. New Delhi, India: United Nations Develoment Programme.

Mandhani, A. (2015, November 14). Transgender welfare boards, 24 × 7 helpline, monthly pension, self employment grants: Kerala Govt. releases historic transgender policy. *Live Law*. Retrieved from www.livelaw.in/transgender-welfare-boards-24×7-helpline-monthly-pension-self-employment-grants-kerala-govt-releases-historic-transgender-policy/.

Menon, M. (2014, August 28). Maharashtra forms board for transgender welfare. *The Hindu*. Retrieved from www.thehindu.com/news/national/national-policy-on-transgenders-still-awaited/article6360734.ece.

National AIDS Control Organisation (NACO). (2016). *National AIDS Control Organisation — Annual report 2015–16*. New Delhi, India: National AIDS Control Organisation.

———. (2015a). *Operational guidelines for implementing HIV targeted interventions among hijras/transgender people in India*. New Delhi, India: National AIDS Control Organisation.

———. (2015b). *National Integrated Biological and Behavioural Surveillance (IBBS), India 2014–15: High risk groups*. New Delhi, India: National AIDS Control Organisation.

———. (2007). *Targeted interventions under NACP III: Operational guidelines, vol. 1, Core high risk groups.* New Delhi, India: National AIDS Control Organisation.

National Institute of Epidemiology (NIE). (2014). *Technical report: Mapping and size estimation of hijras and other transgender populations in 17 states of India.* Chennai, India: National Institute of Epidemiology.

Pattanaik, D. (2014). *Shikhandi and other tales they don't tell you.* New Delhi, India: Zubaan and Penguin Books.

People's Union for Civil Liberties, Karnataka (PUCL=K). (2003). *Human rights violations against the transgender community: A study of kothi and hijra sex workers in Bangalore, India.* Bangalore, India: People's Union for Civil Liberties, Karnataka.

Phillips, A. E., Lowndes, C. M., Boily, M. C., Garnett, G. P., Gurav, K., Ramesh, B. M., . . . & Alary, M. (2010). Men who have sex with men and women in Bangalore, South India, and potential impact on the HIV epidemic. *Sexually Transmitted Infections, 86* (3), 187–192.

Reddy, G. (2005). *With respect to sex: Negotiating hijra identity in South India.* Chicago: University of Chicago Press.

Reisner, S. L., White Hughto, J. M., Pardee, D., & Sevelius, J. (2015). Syndemics and gender affirmation: HIV sexual risk in female-to-male trans masculine adults reporting sexual contact with cisgender males. *International Journal of STDs and AIDS, 27* (11), 955–966.

Rushdie, S. (2008). The half-woman god. *In* N. Akhavi (ed.), *AIDS Sutra: Untold stories from India.* New York: Anchor Books.

Sarin, A. (2014). On criminalisation and pathology: A commentary on the Supreme Court judgment on Section 377. *Indian Journal of Medical Ethics, 11* (1), 5–7.

Shaikh, S., Mburu, G., Arumugam, V., Mattipalli, N., Aher, A., Mehta, S., & Robertson, J. (2016). Empowering communities and strengthening systems to improve transgender health: Outcomes from the Pehchan programme in India. *Journal of the International AIDS Society, 19* (3 Suppl. 2), 208–209.

Shaw, S. Y., Lorway, R. R., Deering, K. N., Avery, L., Mohan, H. L., Bhattacharjee, P., . . . & Blanchard, J. F. (2012). Factors associated with sexual violence against men who have sex with men and transgendered individuals in Karnataka, India. *PLoS One, 7* (3), e31705.

Singh, Y., Aher, A., Shaikh, S., Mehta, S., Robertson, J., & Chakrapani, V. (2014). Gender transition services for hijras and other male-to-female transgender people in India: Availability and barriers to access and use. *International Journal of Transgenderism, 15* (1), 1–15.

Solidarity and Action against the HIV Infection in India (SAATHII). (2016, May 9). Community literacy: Schemes and legal services. Retrieved from www.saathii.org/node/199.

Srivastava, A. K., & Expert Committee of Ministry of Social Justice & Empowerment. (2014). *Report of the Expert Committee on the issues relating to transgender persons.* New Delhi: Ministry of Social Justice and Empowerment, Government of India. Retrieved from socialjustice.nic.in/writereaddata/UploadFile/Binder2.pdf.

Subramanian, T., Chakrapani, V., Selvaraj, V., Noronha, E., Narang, A., & Mehendale, S. (2015). Mapping and size estimation of hijras and other trans-women in 17 states of India: First level findings. *International Journal of Health Sciences and Research, 5* (10), 1–10.

Supreme Court of India. (2014, April 15). National Legal Services Authority v. Union of India and others (Writ Petition no. 400 of 2012 with Writ Petition no. 604 of 2013). Judgment. Retrieved from http://supremecourtofindia.nic.in/outto day/wc40012.pdf.

Swasti-Health Resource Centre. (2013). *Utkarsh.* Swasti, 2013. Retrieved from www .swasti.org/utkarsh.

Tiwari, E. (2014). Distortion of "tritya prakriti" (third nature) by colonial ideology in India. International Journal of Literature and Art, 2, 19–24.

Trivedi, D. (2016, November 11). A flawed bill. *Frontline* (India). Retrieved from www .frontline.in/social-issues/a-flawed-bill/article9266479.ece.

Varma, P. S. (2014, December 18). Welfare board to protect transgender rights planned. *The Hindu.* Retrieved from www.thehindu.com/todays-paper/tp-national/tp -andhrapradesh/welfare-board-to-protect-transgender-rights-planned/article 6703220.ece.

Waring, M., Mukherjee, A. N., Reid, E., & Shivdas, M. (2013). *Anticipatory social protection: Claiming dignity and rights.* London: Commonwealth Secretariat.

CHAPTER 15

Transgender Sex Work in Brazil

Historico-Cultural Perspectives

Don Kulick[1]

1 Distinguished University Professor of Anthropology at Uppsala University in Sweden.

SUMMARY

This is a new introduction to Harrington Park Press's reprint of "The Gender of Brazilian Transgendered Prostitutes" (article originally published in *American Anthropologist* 99 (3), 574–585, September 1997).

KEY TERMS

Brazil; sex work; transgender; transgender prostitutes; travestis

The following article was originally published twenty years ago. It is a summary of the main argument I make in my book *Travesti: Sex, Gender, and Culture among Brazilian Transgendered Prostitutes*, which was published a year after the article (Kulick, 1998). The article and the book appeared during what we might call the second wave of social science research on trans people. Some excellent and enduring research had been done earlier: classics such as the sociologist Harold Garfinkel's meditations on Agnes, a young man who managed to obtain sex-reassignment surgery in the 1950s by convincing an entire UCLA medical team that he had been born with an intersexed body (Garfinkel, 1967); the anthropologist Esther Newton's astonishingly *avant la lettre* ethnography of drag queens in Chicago (*Mother Camp*, 1972); and some of the anthropological work on Native American berdaches, or Two-Spirit people (Whitehead, 1981, is an example). But the theoretical tsunami that set off the 1990s wave was the

Nuttbrock, Larry, *Transgender Sex Work and Society*
dx.doi.org/10.17312/harringtonparkpress/2017.11.tsws.015
© 2018 by Harrington Park Press

advent of queer theory. Two books especially—the literature scholar Eve Kosofsky Sedgwick's 1990 *Epistemology of the Closet*, and the philosopher Judith Butler's *Gender Trouble*, published that same year—authorized and legitimized nonclinical academic research into trans people's lives in a way that had not happened before.

My own research among travestis in Salvador, Brazil, in the mid-1990s wasn't inspired by queer theory; it was inspired by a chance encounter. In *Travesti* I describe how I came upon travestis during a brief holiday visit to Brazil. I first saw travestis one night when a city bus I was on stopped in a traffic jam in front of one of the corners where travestis liked to stand and work. At the time, I spoke no Portuguese, I knew next to nothing about Brazil, and I had no idea at all who the raucous, scantly clad, irresistibly defiant individuals I saw from the bus might be. But they hooked me. I remember feeling a warm flush of awe that they were flaunting themselves so shamelessly, and I liked their throaty laughter.

The research I ended up doing with travestis revolved around two seemingly simple questions: Who in the world are these people, and why do they do what they do? The answers to those questions were not obvious. Most Brazilians who had written about travestis seemed to believe that travestis wanted to be women, and that travestis were condemned to a marginalized existence and participation in sex work and petty crime.

It took me almost no time at all to figure out that travestis did not want to be women. They had no desire to undergo surgery to remove their penises. On the contrary—every travesti I came to know loved her penis and delighted in the pleasure that copious quantities of sex afforded her. Travestis didn't want to be women; what they wanted, they readily told me and anyone else who might have taken a moment to listen, was to become beautiful gays. The reason travestis modify their comportment and their bodies with high heels, miniskirts, braids, hormones, pluckings, cosmetics, and industrial silicone is that they want to be attractive to the men they are attracted to: specifically, masculine, heterosexual macho men who desire women, but who might be persuaded to go for a feminine gay person if she is beautiful and sexy, and if she has enough money to support her man so that he might live a life of utter indolence.

My description of travesti subjectivity appeared at a time when relatively little had been written about trans people outside Western Europe or North America; certainly there were almost no ethnographies that detailed the lives of non-Western trans people. The intimacy with which I came to know travestis' lives allowed me to both exemplify queer theories about the relationship between gender and sexuality, and extend those theories to suggest that ruminations about third genders in fact protect and reinforce gender binaries, instead of questioning or complicating them.

After this article and *Travesti* were published, I had intended to continue doing ethnographic fieldwork among travestis. I made grand plans for what I announced to my friends would be a "Travesti Trilogy." I was going to go to Italy, to live there with Brazilian travestis who had smuggled themselves into the country. That would be volume 2. Then I planned to return to Brazil and write a third book about what happened to those travestis who were deported from Europe, or who returned to Brazil voluntarily, and how the travesti traffic between Brazil and Europe had affected the culture, ambitions, working practices, and lives of travestis who never left Brazil in the first place.

I did go to Milan in the early 2000s, and I lived among Brazilian travestis there for four months. But I ended up abandoning my travesti trilogy. Despite the success of the book, I was never able to secure research funding for my transnational research project. More consequential, though, was the fact that my fieldwork in Milan changed my relationship with travestis. Working conditions for travestis in Italy were much harsher than they were in Salvador. Travestis were in Italy illegally. (As Brazilian citizens, they needed visas, which they didn't have; all had crossed the border clandestinely from Austria or Switzerland.)

No travesti was ever "trafficked" to Italy against her will; on the contrary, every travesti in Italy had worked hard to get there. But most travestis arrived in Italy already in substantial debt to the travesti brokers who had financed their trip across the Atlantic. They were kept in debt by having to pay those other, already established travestis exorbitant prices for a room to stay in (or, more usually, a bed to sleep on, in a room shared by other travestis); the right to sell sex on a particular stretch of sidewalk or motorway; transportation to and from work; food; and appropriately sexy clothing. In short, they were made to pay a lot of money for everything. They worked long hours and seemed much more stressed and unhappy than I had known them to be in Brazil.

The anxiety that many travestis found themselves experiencing in Italy resulted in the worst aspects of their culture flaring up and taking over their lives. In *Travesti* I document how the travestis I knew, who could be helpful and sympathetic to one another, more usually undermined, bad-mouthed, and deceived one another. I interpreted that destructive sociality as an expression of the fact that the most valued assets among travestis are not friendliness, solidarity, and kindness. What counts most for travestis is youth, beauty, and money. Furthermore, for various reasons (most of which have to do with boyfriends and clients), all those things are regarded as limited goods that travestis imagine themselves to be forever competing for with one another.

Whatever social buffers are in place in Brazil to help ensure that travestis, despite all the competition, can still form relatively coherent and even supportive communities—none of that existed in Italy. I was horrified to see how badly travestis treated one another, and how cutthroat their lives seemed to become, as soon as they arrived in Milan.

The relative brutality of travestis' treatment of one another in Milan made it difficult for me to write about them. My four months in Milan left me not liking travestis very much. This is a debilitating problem for an anthropologist, because anthropologists for the most part write only about people we like. I know, for example, that one of the reasons my work on Brazil is still read is that I seem to have managed to convey my vast respect for, and delight in, travestis.

In Italy, though, I was flummoxed by how rude, disrespectful, mean, deceitful, and hurtful Brazilian travestis were *to one another*. I am a seasoned and jaded fieldworker, so it isn't as if I didn't understand that the ultimate source of the cruelty was the exploitative situation in which travestis found themselves (within the larger context of stigma and marginalization, but also in a situation perpetuated and controlled by other, more well-established travestis). But I was not imaginative enough at the time to figure out how I might write empathetically and compellingly about people I had come to frankly dislike.

Perhaps some day I will pick up the pieces of my research on travestis and try again to write my travesti trilogy, or at least some fragment of it. Certainly when I reread this article for this collection, I experienced a sharp pang of longing for travesti company and travesti laughter. One thing I find myself wanting to know more about is the situation of old travestis—the few who remain alive from when I was in Salvador, for example. What has happened to them? Nobody seems to care much about old travestis—not other travestis, who care only about youth, and, as far as I know, not other social scientists, who also tend to be dazzled (as I was) by travesti self-fashioning in the blossom of youth. But old travestis exist today in greater numbers than ever before, thanks to better and more accessible healthcare in Brazil, a markedly more humanitarian (although, as I write this, alas rapidly deteriorating) political situation, and a stronger and more vocal trans-activism in Brazil that has succeeded in achieving recognition and progress that was unimagined during the time of my fieldwork in Salvador twenty years ago.

To the extent that this article still has any value, in my view, it is to remind readers of this book that there are people in the world who have radically different understandings of gender and sexuality from what they probably are used to or expect. Those understandings of gender and sexuality are not primitive, deficient, confused, or defective. They are — on the contrary — complex, trellised, and lovely.

And the people who hold them are savvy, thoughtful, funny, and beautiful.

REFERENCES

Butler, J. (1990). *Gender trouble: Feminism and the subversion of identity*. New York: Routledge.

Garfinkel, H. (1967). *Studies in ethnomethodology*. Englewood Cliffs, NJ: Prentice-Hall.

Kulick, D. (1998). *Travesti: Sex, gender, and culture among Brazilian transgendered prostitutes*. Chicago: University of Chicago Press.

Newton, E. (1972). *Mother camp: Female impersonators in America*. Chicago: University of Chicago Press.

Sedgwick, E. K. (1990). *Epistemology of the closet*. Berkeley: University of California Press.

Whitehead, H. (1981). The bow and the burden strap: A new look at institutionalized homosexuality in Native North America. *In* S. Ortner and H. Whitehead (eds.), *Sexual meanings: The cultural construction of gender and sexuality* (pp. 80–115). Cambridge: Cambridge University Press.

THE GENDER OF BRAZILIAN
TRANSGENDERED PROSTITUTES

This historic document is reprinted from *American Anthropologist*, n.s., *99* (3) (1997): 574–585, under the title "The Gender of Brazilian Transgendered Prostitutes." Originally published by Wiley on behalf of the American Anthropological Association. It is presented here as it was originally published.

Males who enjoy being anally penetrated by other males are, in many places in the world, an object of special cultural elaboration. Anywhere they occur as a culturally recognized type, it is usually they who are classified and named, not the males who penetrate them (who are often simply called "men"). Furthermore, to the extent that male same-sex sexual relations are stigmatized, the object of social vituperation is, again, usually those males who allow themselves to be penetrated, not the males who penetrate them. Anywhere they constitute a salient cultural category, men who enjoy being penetrated are believed to think, talk, and act in particular, identifiable, and often cross-gendered manners. What is more, a large number of such men do in fact behave in these culturally intelligible ways. So whether they are the *mahus, hijras, kathoeys, xaniths,* or *berdaches* of non-Western societies, or the mollies and fairies of our own history, links between habitual receptivity in anal sex and particular effeminate behavioral patterns structure the ways in which males who are regularly anally penetrated are perceived, and they structure the ways in which many of those males think about and live their lives.[1]

One area of the world in which males who enjoy being anally penetrated receive a very high degree of cultural attention is Latin America. Any student of Latin America will be familiar with the effervescent figure of the effeminate male homosexual. Called *maricón, cochón, joto, marica, pajara, loca, frango, bicha,* or any number of other names depending on where one finds him (see Murray and Dynes 1987 and Dynes 1987 for a sampling), these males all appear to share certain behavioral characteristics and seem to be thought of, throughout Latin America, in quite similar ways.[2]

One of the basic things one quickly learns from any analysis of Latin American sexual categories is that sex between males in this part of the world does not necessarily result in both partners being perceived as homosexual. The crucial determinant of a homosexual classification is not so much the fact of sex as it is the role performed during the sexual act. A male who anally penetrates another male is generally not considered to be homosexual. He is considered, in all the various local idioms, to be a "man"; indeed, in some communities, penetrating another male and then bragging about it is one way in which men demonstrate their masculinity to others (Lancaster 1992:241; cf. Brandes 1981:234). Quite different associations attach themselves to a male who allows himself to be penetrated. That male has placed himself in what is understood to be an unmasculine, passive position. By doing so, he has forfeited manhood and becomes seen as something other than a man. This cultural classification as feminine is often reflected in the general comportment, speech practices, and dress patterns of such males, all of which tend to be recognizable to others as effeminate.

A conceptual system in which only males who are penetrated are homosexual is clearly very different from the modern heterosexual-homosexual dichotomy currently in place in countries such as the United States, where popular understanding generally maintains that a male who has sex with another male is gay, no matter how carefully he may restrict his behavior to the role of penetrator.[3] This difference between Latin American and northern Euro-American understandings of sexuality is analyzed with great insight in the literature on male same-sex relations in Latin America, and one of the chief merits of that literature is its sensitive documentation of the ways in which erotic practices and sexual identities are culturally organized.

Somewhat surprisingly, the same sensitivity that informs the literature when it comes to sexuality does not extend to the realm of gender. A question not broached in this literature is whether the fundamental differences that exist between northern Euro-American and Latin American regimes of sexuality might also result in, or be reflective of, different regimes of gender. This oversight is odd in light of the obvious and important links between sexuality and gender in a system where a simple act of penetration has the power to profoundly alter a male's cultural definition and social status. Instead of exploring what the differences in the construction of sexuality might mean for differences in the construction of gender, however, analysis in this literature falls back on familiar concepts. So just as gender in northern Europe and North America consists of men and women, so does it consist of men and women in Latin America, we are told. The characteristics ascribed to and the behavior expected of those two different types of people are not exactly the same in these two different parts of the world, to be sure, but the basic gender categories are the same.

This article contests that view. I will argue that the *sexual division* that researchers have noted between those who penetrate and those who are penetrated extends far beyond sexual interactions between males to constitute the basis of the *gender division* in Latin America. Gender, in this particular elaboration, is grounded not so much in sex (like it is, for example, in modern northern European and North American cultures) as it is grounded in sexuality. This difference in grounding generates a gender configuration different from the one that researchers working in Latin America have postulated, and it allows and even encourages the elaboration of cultural spaces such as those inhabited by effeminate male homosexuals. Gender in Latin America should be seen not as consisting of men and women, but rather of men and not-men, the latter being a category into which both biological females and males who enjoy anal penetration are culturally situated. This specific situatedness provides individuals—not just men who enjoy anal penetration, but everyone—with a conceptual framework that they can draw on in order to understand and organize their own and others' desires, bodies, affective and physical relations, and social roles.

THE BODY IN QUESTION

The evidence for the arguments developed here will be drawn from my fieldwork in the Brazilian city of Salvador, among a group of males who enjoy anal penetration. These males are effeminized prostitutes known throughout Brazil as *travestis* (a word derived from *transvestir*, to cross-dress).[4]

Travestis occupy a strikingly visible place in both Brazilian social space and in the Brazilian cultural imaginary.[5] All Brazilian cities of any size contain travestis, and in the large cities of Rio de Janeiro and São Paulo, travestis number in the thousands. (In Salvador, travestis numbered between about 80 and 250, depending on the time of year.)[6] Travestis are most exuberantly visible during Brazil's famous annual Carnival, and any depiction or analysis of the festival will inevitably include at least a passing reference to them, because their gender inversions are often invoked as embodiments of the Carnival spirit. But even in more mundane contexts and discourses, travestis figure prominently. A popular Saturday afternoon television show, for example, includes a spot in which female impersonators, some of whom are clearly travestis, get judged on how beautiful they are and on how well they mime the lyrics to songs sung by female vocalists. Another weekly television show regularly features Valéria, a well-known travesti. *Tieta*, one of the most popular television *novelas* in recent years, featured a special guest appearance by Rogéria, another famous travesti. And most telling of the special place reserved for travestis in the Brazilian popular imagination is the fact that the individual widely acclaimed to be the most beautiful woman in Brazil in the mid-1980s was . . . a travesti. That travesti, Roberta Close, became a household name throughout the country. She regularly appeared on national television, starred in a play in Rio, posed nude (with demurely crossed legs) in *Playboy* magazine, was continually interviewed and portrayed in virtually every magazine in the country, and had at least three songs written about her by well-known composers. Although her popularity declined when, at the end of the 1980s, she left Brazil to have a sex-change operation and live in Europe, Roberta Close remains extremely well-known. As recently as 1995, she appeared in a nationwide advertisement for Duloren lingerie, in which a photograph of her passport, bearing her male name, was transposed with a photograph of her looking sexy and chic in a black lace undergarment. The caption read, "Você não imagina do que uma Duloren é capaz" (You can't imagine what a Duloren can do).

Regrettably, the fact that a handful of travestis manage to achieve wealth, admiration, and, in the case of Roberta Close, an almost iconic cultural status says very little about the lives of the vast majority of travestis. Those travestis, the ones that most Brazilians only glimpse occasionally standing along highways or on dimly lit street corners at night or read about in the crime pages of their local newspapers, comprise one of the most marginalized, feared, and despised groups in Brazilian society. In most Brazilian cities, travestis are so discriminated against that many of them avoid venturing out onto the street during the day. They are regularly the victims of violent police brutality and murder.[7] The vast majority of them come from very poor backgrounds and remain poor throughout their lives, living a hand-to-mouth existence and dying before the age of 50 from violence, drug abuse, health problems caused or exacerbated by the silicone they inject into their bodies, or, increasingly, AIDS.

The single most characteristic thing about travestis is their bodies. Unlike the drag performers examined by Esther Newton (1972) and recently elevated to the status of theoretical paragons in the work of postmodernist queer scholars such as Judith Butler (1990), travestis do not merely don female attributes. They incorporate them. Sometimes starting at ages as young as 10 or 12, boys who self-identify as travestis begin ingesting or injecting themselves with massive doses of female hormones in order to give their bodies rounded features, broad hips, prominent buttocks, and breasts. The hormones these boys take either are medications designed to combat estrogen deficiency or are contraceptive preparations designed, like "the pill," to prevent pregnancy. In Brazil such hormones are cheap (a month's supply, which would be consumed by a travesti in a week or less, costs the equivalent of only a few dollars) and are sold over the counter in any pharmacy.

Boys discover hormones from a variety of sources. Most of my travesti friends told me that they learned about hormones by approaching adult travestis and asking them how they had achieved the bodies they had. Others were advised by admirers, boyfriends, or clients, who told them that they would look more attractive and make more money if they looked more like girls.

Hormones are valued by travestis because they are inexpensive, easy to obtain, and fast working. Most hormones produce visible results after only about two months of daily ingestion. A problem with them, however, is that they can, especially after prolonged consumption, result in chronic nausea, headaches, heart palpitations, burning sensations in the legs and chest, extreme weight gain, and allergic reactions. In addition, the doses of female hormones required to produce breasts and wide hips make it difficult for travestis to achieve erections. This can be quite a serious problem, since a great percentage of travestis' clients want to be penetrated by the travesti (a point to which I shall return below). What usually happens after several years of taking hormones is that most individuals stop, at least for a while, and begin injecting silicone into their bodies.

Just as hormones are procured by the individual travestis themselves, without any medical intervention or interference, so is silicone purchased from and administered by acquaintances or friends. The silicone available to the travestis in Salvador is industrial silicone, which is a kind of plastic normally used to manufacture automobile parts such as dashboards. Although it is widely thought to be illegal for industrial outlets to sell this silicone to private individuals, at least one or two travestis in any city containing a silicone manufacturing plant will be well connected enough to be able to buy it. Whenever they sense a demand, these travestis contact their supplier at the plant and travel there in great secrecy to buy several liters. They then resell this silicone (at a hefty profit) to other travestis, who in turn pay travestis who work as *bombadeiras* (pumpers) to inject it directly into their bodies.

Most travestis in Salvador over the age of 17 have some silicone in their bodies. The amount of silicone that individual travestis choose to inject ranges from a few glasses to up to 18 liters. (Travestis measure silicone in liters and water glasses *(copos)*, six of which make up a liter.) Most have between two and five liters. The majority have it in their buttocks, hips, knees, and inner thighs. This strategic placement of silicone is in direct deference to Brazilian aesthetic ideals that consider fleshy thighs, expansive hips, and a prominent, teardrop-shaped *bunda* (buttocks) to be the hallmark of feminine beauty. The majority of travestis do *not* have silicone in their breasts, because they believe that silicone in breasts (but not elsewhere in the body) causes cancer, because they are satisfied with the size of the breasts they have achieved through hormone consumption, because they are convinced that silicone injections into the chest are risky and extremely painful, or because they are waiting for the day when they will have enough money to pay for silicone implants *(prótese)* surgically inserted by doctors. A final reason for a general disinclination to inject silicone into one's breasts is that everyone knows that this silicone shifts its position very easily. Every travesti is acquainted with several unfortunate others whose breasts have either merged in the middle, creating a pronounced undifferentiated swelling known as a "pigeon breast" *(peito de pomba)*, or whose silicone has descended into lumpy protrusions just above the stomach.

THE BODY IN PROCESS

Why do they do it? One of the reasons habitually cited by travestis seems self-evident. Elizabeth, a 29-year-old travesti with 1½ liters of silicone in her hips and one waterglass of silicone in each breast, explained it to me this way: "To mold my body, you know, be more feminine, with the body of a woman." But why do travestis want the body of a woman?

When I first began asking travestis that question, I expected them to tell me that they wanted the body of a woman because they felt themselves to be women. That was not the answer I received. No one ever offered the explanation that they might be women trapped in male bodies, even when I suggested it. In fact, there is a strong consensus among travestis in Salvador that any travesti who claims to be a woman is mentally disturbed. A travesti is not a woman and can never be a woman, they tell one another, because God created them male. As individuals, they are free to embellish and augment what God has given them, but their sex cannot be changed. Any attempt to do so would be disastrous. Not only do sex-change operations not produce women (they produce, travestis say, only *bichas castradas*, castrated homosexuals), they also inevitably result in madness. I was told on numerous occasions that, without a penis, semen cannot leave the body. When trapped, it travels to the brain, where it collects and forms a "stone" that will continue to increase in size until it eventually causes insanity.

So Roberta Close notwithstanding, travestis modify their bodies not because they feel themselves to be women but because they feel themselves to be "feminine" (*feminino*) or "like a woman" (*se sentir mulher*), qualities most often talked about not in terms of inherent predispositions or essences but rather in terms of behaviors, appearances, and relationships to men.[8] When I asked Elizabeth what it meant when she told me she felt feminine, for example, she answered, "I like to dress like a woman. I like when someone—when men—admire me, you know? . . . I like to be admired, when I go with a man who, like, says: 'Sheez, you're really pretty, you're really feminine.' That . . . makes me want to be more feminine and more beautiful every day, you see?" Similar themes emerged when travestis talked about when they first began to understand that they were travestis. A common response I received from many different people when I asked that question was that they made this discovery in connection with attraction and sexuality. Eighteen-year-old Cintia told me that she understood she was a travesti from the age of seven:

> I already liked girls' things, I played with dolls, played with . . . girls' things; I only played with girls. I didn't play with boys. I just played with these two boys; during the afternoon I always played with them . . . well, you know, rubbing penises together, rubbing them, kissing on the mouth. [*Laughs.*]

Forty-one-year-old Gabriela says that she knew that she was a travesti early on largely because "since childhood I always liked men, hairy legs, things like that, you know?" Banana, a 34-year-old travesti, told me "the [understanding that I was a] travesti came after, you know, I, um, eight, nine years, ten years old, I felt attracted, really attracted to men."

The attraction that these individuals felt for males is thus perceived by them to be a major motivating force behind their self-production as travestis, both privately and professionally. Travestis are quick to point out that, in addition to making them feel more feminine, female forms also help them earn more money as prostitutes. At night when they work on the street, those travestis who have acquired pronounced feminine features use them to attract the attention of passing motorists, and they dress (or rather, undress) to display those features prominently.

But if the goal of a travesti's bodily modifications is to feel feminine and be attractive to men, what does she think about her male genitals?

The most important point to be clear about is that virtually every travesti values her penis: "There's not a better thing in the whole world," 19-year-old Adriana once told me with a big smile. Any thought of having it amputated repels them. "Deus é mais" (God forbid), many of them interject whenever talk of sex-change operations arises. "What, and never cum (i.e., ejaculate, *gozar*) again?!" they gasp, horrified.

Despite the positive feelings that they express about their genitals, however, a travesti keeps her penis, for the most part, hidden, "imprisoned" (*presa*) between her legs. That is, travestis habitually pull their penises down between their legs and press them against their perineums with their underpanties. This is known as "making a cunt" (*fazer uma buceta*). This cunt is an important bodily practice in a travesti's day-to-day public appearance. It is also crucial in another extremely important context of a travesti's life, namely in her relationship to her *marido* (live-in boyfriend). The maridos of travestis are typically attractive, muscular, tattooed young men with little or no education and no jobs. Although they are not pimps (travestis move them into their rooms because they are impassioned [*apaixonada*] with them, and they eject them when the passion wears thin), maridos are supported economically by their travesti girlfriends. All these boyfriends regard themselves, and are regarded by their travesti girlfriends, as *homens* (men) and, therefore, as nonhomosexual.

One of the defining attributes of being a *homem* (man) in the gender system that the travestis draw on and invoke is that a man will not be interested in another male's penis. A man, in this interpretative framework, will happily penetrate another male's anus. But he will not touch or express any desire for another male's penis. For him to do so would be tantamount to relinquishing his status as a man. He would stop being a man and be reclassified as a *viado* (homosexual, faggot), which is how the travestis are classified by others and how they see themselves.

Travestis want their boyfriends to be men, not viados. They require, in other words, their boyfriends to be symbolically and socially different from, not similar to, themselves. Therefore, a travesti does not want her boyfriend to notice, comment on, or in any way concern himself with her penis, even during sex. Sex with a boyfriend consists, for the most part, of the travesti sucking the boyfriend's penis and of her boyfriend penetrating her, most often from behind, with the travesti on all fours or lying on her stomach on the bed. If the boyfriend touches the travesti at all, he will caress her breasts and perhaps kiss her. But no contact with the travesti's penis will occur, which means, according to most travestis I have spoken to, that travestis do not usually have orgasms during sex with their boyfriends.

What surprised me most about this arrangement was that the ones who are the most adamant that it be maintained are the travestis themselves. They respect their boyfriends and maintain their relationships with them only as long as the boyfriends remain "men." If a boyfriend expresses interest in a travesti's penis, becomes concerned that the travesti ejaculate during sex, or worst of all, if the boyfriend expresses a desire to be anally penetrated by the travesti, the relationship, all travestis told me firmly, would be over. They would comply with the boyfriend's request, they all told me, "because if someone offers me their ass, you think I'm not gonna take it?" Afterward, however, they were agreed, they would lose respect for the boyfriend. "You'll feel disgust (*nojo*) toward him," one travesti put it pithily. The boyfriend would no longer be a man in their eyes. He would, instead, be reduced to a viado. And as such, he could no longer be a boyfriend. Travestis unfailingly terminate relationships with any boyfriend who deviates from what they consider to be proper manly sexuality.

This absolute unwillingness to engage their own penises in sexual activity with their boyfriends stands in stark contrast to what travestis do with their penises when they are with their clients. On the street, travestis know they are valued for their possession of a penis. Clients will often request to see or feel a travesti's penis before agreeing to pay for sex with her, and travestis are agreed that those travestis who have large penises are more sought after than those with small ones. Similarly, several travestis told me that one of the reasons they stopped taking hormones was because they were losing clients. They realized that clients had begun avoiding them because they knew that the travesti could not achieve an erection. Travestis maintain that one of the most common sexual services they are paid to perform is to anally penetrate their clients.

Most travestis enjoy this. In fact, one of the more surprising findings of my study is that travestis, in significant and highly marked contrast to what is generally reported for other prostitutes, enjoy sex with clients.[9] That is not to say they enjoy sex every time or with every client. But whenever they talk about thrilling, fulfilling, or incredibly fun sex, their partner is always either a client or what they call a *vício*, a word that literally means "vice" or "addiction" and that refers to a male, often encountered on the street while they are working, with whom they have sex for free. Sometimes, if the vício is especially attractive, is known to have an especially large penis, or is known to be especially versatile in bed, the travesti will even pay *him*.

THE BODY IN CONTEXT

At this point, having illustrated the way in which the body of a travesti is constructed, thought about, and used in a variety of contexts, I am ready to address the question of cultural intelligibility and personal desirability. Why do travestis want the kind of body they create for themselves? What is it about Brazilian culture that incites and sustains desire for a male body made feminine through hormones and silicone?

By phrasing that question primarily in terms of culture, I do not mean to deny that there are also social and economic considerations behind the production of travesti bodies and subjectivities. As I noted above, a body full of silicone translates into cash in the Brazilian sexual marketplace. It is important to understand, however—particularly because popular and academic discourses about prostitution tend to frame it so narrowly in terms of victimization, poverty, and exploitation—that males do not become travestis because they were sexually abused as children or just for economic gain. Only one of the approximately 40 travestis in my close circle of acquaintances was clearly the victim of childhood sexual abuse. And while the vast majority of travestis (like, one must realize, the vast majority of people in Brazil) come from working-class or poor backgrounds, it is far from impossible for poor, openly effeminate homosexual males to find employment, especially in the professions of hairdressers, cooks, and housecleaners, where they are quite heavily represented.

Another factor that makes it problematic to view travestis primarily in social or economic terms is the fact that the sexual marketplace does not require males who prostitute themselves to be travestis. Male prostitution (where the prostitutes, who are called *michês*, look and act like men) is widespread in Brazil and has been the topic of one published ethnographic study (Perlongher 1987). Also, even transgendered prostitution does not require the radical body modifications that travestis undertake. Before hormones and silicone became widely available (in the mid-1970s and mid-1980s, respectively) males dressed up as females, using wigs and foam-rubber padding *(pirelli)*, and worked successfully as prostitutes. Some males still do this today.

Finally, it should be appreciated that travestis do not need to actually have sex with their clients to earn money as prostitutes. A large percentage (in some cases, the bulk) of a travesti's income from clients is derived from robbing them. In order to rob a client, all that is required is that a travesti come into close physical proximity with him. Once a travesti is in a client's car or once she has begun caressing a passerby's penis, asking him seductively if he *"quer gozar"* (wants to cum), the rest, for most travestis, is easy. Either by pickpocketing the client, assaulting him, or if she does have sex with him, by threatening afterward to create a public scandal, the travesti will often walk away with all the client's money (Kulick 1996a). Thus it is entirely possible to derive a respectable income from prostitution and still not consume hormones and inject silicone into one's body.

In addition to all those considerations, I also phrase the question of travestis in terms of culture because, even if it were possible to claim that males who become travestis do so because of poverty, early sexual exploitation, or some enigmatic inner psychic orientation, the mystery of travestis as a sociocultural phenomenon would remain unsolved. What is it about the understandings, representations, and definitions of sexuality, gender, and sex in Brazilian society that makes travesti subjectivity imaginable and intelligible?

Let me begin answering that question by noting an aspect of travesti language that initially puzzled me. In their talk to one another, travestis frequently refer to biological males by using feminine pronouns and feminine adjectival endings. Thus the common utterance *"ela ficou doida"* (she was furious) can refer to a travesti, a woman, a gay male, or a heterosexual male who has allowed himself to be penetrated by another male. All of these different people are classified by travestis in the same manner. This classificatory system is quite subtle, complex, and context sensitive; travestis narrating their life stories frequently use masculine pronouns and adjectival endings when talking about themselves as children but switch to feminine forms when discussing their present-day lives. In a similar way, clients are often referred to as "she," but the same client will be referred to with different gendered pronouns depending on the actions he performs. When a travesti recounts that she struggled with a client over money or when she describes him paying, for example, his gender will often change from feminine to masculine. The important point here is that the gender of males is subject to fluctuation and change in travesti talk. Males are sometimes referred to as "she" and sometimes as "he." Males, in other words, can shift gender depending on the context and the actions they perform. The same is not true for females. Females, even the several extremely brawny and conspicuously unfeminine lesbians who associate with the travestis I know, are never referred to as "he" (Kulick 1996b). So whereas the gender of females remains fixed, the gender of males fluctuates and shifts continually.

Why can males be either male or female, but females can only be female? The answer, I believe, lies in the way that the gender system that the travestis draw on is constituted. Debates about transgendered individuals such as 18th-century mollies, Byzantine eunuchs, Indian hijras, Native American berdaches, U.S. transsexuals, and others often suggest that those individuals constitute a third, or intermediate, gender, one that is neither male nor female or one that combines both male and female.[10] Journalists and social commentators in Brazil sometimes take a similar line when they write about travestis, arguing that travestis transcend maleness and femaleness and constitute a kind of postmodern androgyny.

My contention is the opposite. Despite outward physical appearances and despite local claims to the contrary, there is no third or intermediate sex here; travestis only arise and are only culturally intelligible within a gender system based on a strict dichotomy. That gender system, however, is structured according to a dichotomy different from the one with which many of us are familiar, anchored in and arising from principles different from those that structure and give meaning to gender in northern Europe and North America.

The fundamental difference is that, whereas the northern Euro-American gender system is based on sex, the gender system that structures travestis' perceptions and actions is based on sexuality. The dominant idea in northern Euro-American societies is that one is a man or a woman because of the genitals one possesses. That biological difference is understood to accrete differences in behavior, language, sexuality, perception, emotion, and so on. As scholars such as Harold Garfinkel (1967), Suzanne Kessler and Wendy McKenna (1985 [1978]), and Janice Raymond (1979) have pointed out, it is within such a cultural system that a transsexual body can arise, because here biological males, for example, who do not feel or behave as men should, can make sense of that difference by reference to their genitals. They are not men; therefore they must be women, and to be a woman means to have the genitals of a female.

While the biological differences between men and women are certainly not ignored in Brazil, the possession of genitals is fundamentally conflated with what they can be used for, and in the particular configuration of sexuality, gender, and sex that has developed there, the determinative criterion in the identification of males and females is not so much the genitals as it is the role those genitals perform in sexual encounters. Here the locus of gender difference is the act of penetration. If one *only* penetrates, one is a man, but if one gets penetrated, one is not a man, which, in this case, means that one is either a viado (a faggot) or a mulher (a woman). Tina, a 27-year-old travesti, makes the parallels clear in a story about why she eventually left one of her ex-boyfriends:

1. *Tina*: For three years [my marido] was a man for me. A total man (*foi homíssimo*). Then I was the man, and he was the faggot (viado).

2. *Don:* What?

3. *Tina:* Do you see?

4. *Don:* Yes. . . . But no, how?

5. *Tina:* For three years he was a man for me, and after those three years he became a woman (*ele foi mulher*). I was the man, and he was the woman. The first three years I was together with him, do you see, he penetrated me (*ele me comia*) and I sucked [his penis]. I was his woman.

6. *Don:* Yeah . . .

7. *Tina:* And after those three years, I was his man. Do you understand now? Now you get it.

8. *Don:* But what happened? What, what made him . . .

9. *Tina:* Change?

10. *Don:* Change, yeah.

11. *Tina:* It changed with him touching my penis. . . . He began doing other kinds of sex things. "You don't have to cum [i.e., have orgasms] on the street [with clients]" [he told me], "I can jerk you off (*eu bato uma punhetinha pra você*). And later on we can do other new things." He gives me his ass, he gave me his ass, started to suck [my penis], and well, there you are.

Note how Tina explains that she was her boyfriend's woman, in that "he penetrated me and I sucked [his penis]" (line 5). Note also how Tina uses the words *viado* (faggot) and *mulher* (woman) interchangeably (lines 1 and 5) to express what her boyfriend became after he started expressing an interest in her penis and after he started "giving his ass" to her. This discursive conflation is similar to that used when travestis talk about their clients, the vast majority of whom are believed by travestis to desire to be anally penetrated by the travesti—a desire that, as I just explained, disqualifies them from being men and makes them into viados, like the travestis themselves. Hence they are commonly referred to in travestis' talk by the feminine pronoun *ela* (she).

Anal penetration figures prominently as an engendering device in another important dimension of travestis' lives, namely, their self-discovery as travestis. When I asked travestis to tell me when they first began to understand that they were travestis, the most common response, as I noted earlier, was that they discovered this in connection with attraction to males. Sooner or later, this attraction always led to sexuality, which in practice means that the travesti began allowing herself to be penetrated anally. This act is always cited by travestis as crucial in their self-understanding as travestis.

A final example of the role that anal penetration plays as a determining factor in gender assignment is the particular way in which travestis talk about gay men. Travestis frequently dismiss and disparage gay men for "pretending to be men" (*[andar/passar] como se fosse homem),* a phrase that initially confounded me, especially when it was used by travestis in reference to me. One Sunday afternoon, for example, I was standing with two travesti friends eating candy in one of Salvador's main plazas. As two policemen walked by, one travesti began to giggle. "They see you standing here with us," she said to me, "and they probably think you're a man." Both travestis then collapsed in laughter at the sheer outrageousness of such a profound misunderstanding. It took me, however, a long time to figure out what was so funny.

I finally came to realize that as a gay man, a viado, I am assumed by travestis to *dar* (be penetrated by men). I am, therefore, the same as them. But I and all other gay men who do not dress as women and modify their bodies to be more feminine disguise this sameness. We hide, we deceive, we pretend to be men, when we really are not men at all. It is in this sense that travestis can perceive themselves to be more honest, and much more radical, than "butch" *(machuda)* homosexuals like myself. It is also in this sense that travestis simply do not understand the discrimination that they face throughout Brazil at the hands of gay men, many of whom feel that travestis compromise the public image of homosexuals and give gay men a bad name.

What all these examples point to is that for travestis, as reflected in their actions and in all their talk about themselves, clients, boyfriends, vícios, gay men, women, and sexuality, there are two genders; there is a binary system of opposites very firmly in place and in operation. But the salient difference in this system is not between men and women. It is, instead, between those who penetrate *(comer,* literally "to eat" in Brazilian Portuguese) and those who get penetrated *(dar,* literally "to give"), *in a system where the act of being penetrated has transformative force.* Thus those who *only* "eat" (and *never* "give") in this system are culturally designated as "men"; those who give (even if they *also* eat) are classified as being something else, a something that I will call, partly for want of a culturally elaborated label and partly to foreground my conviction that the gender system that makes it possible for travestis to emerge and make sense is one massively oriented towards, if not determined by, male subjectivity, male desire, and male pleasure, as those are culturally elaborated in Brazil: "not men." What this particular binarity implies is that females and males who enjoy being penetrated belong to the same classificatory category, they are on the same side of the gendered binary. They share, in other words, a gender.

This sharing is the reason why the overwhelming majority of travestis do not self-identify as women and have no desire to have an operation to become a woman even though they spend their lives dramatically modifying their bodies to make them look more feminine. Culturally speaking, travestis, because they enjoy being penetrated, are structurally equivalent to, even if they are not biologically identical to, women. Because they already share a gender with women, a sex-change operation would (again, culturally speaking) give a travesti nothing that she does not already have. All a sex-change operation would do is rob her of a significant source of pleasure and income.

It is important to stress that the claim I am making here is that travestis share a gender with women, not that they *are* women (or that women are travestis). Individual travestis will not always or necessarily share individual women's roles, goals, or social status. Just as the worldviews, self-images, social statuses, and possibilities of, say, a poor black mother, a single mulatto prostitute, and a rich white businesswoman in Brazil differ dramatically, even though all those individuals share a gender, so will the goals, perspectives, and possibilities of individual travestis differ from those of individual women, even though all those individuals share a gender. But inasmuch as travestis share the same gender as women, they are understood to share (and feel themselves to share) a whole spectrum of tastes, perceptions, behaviors, styles, feelings, and desires. And one of the most important of those desires is understood and felt to be the desire to attract and be attractive for persons of the opposite gender.[11] The desire to be attractive for persons of the opposite gender puts pressure on individuals to attempt to approximate cultural ideals of beauty, thereby drawing them into patriarchal and heterosexual imperatives that guide aesthetic values and that frame the direction and the content of the erotic gaze.[12] And although attractive male bodies get quite a lot of attention and exposure in Brazil, the pressure to conform to cultural ideals of beauty, in Brazil as in northern Euro-American societies, is much stronger on females than on males. In all these societies, the ones who are culturally incited to look (with all the subtexts of power and control that that action can imply) are males, and the ones who are exhorted to desire to be looked *at* are females.

In Brazil, the paragon of beauty, the body that is held forth, disseminated, and extolled as desirable—in the media, on television, in popular music, during Carnival, and in the day-to-day public practices of both individual men and women (comments and catcalls from groups of males at women passing by, microscopic string bikinis, known throughout the country as *fio dental* [dental floss], worn by women at the beach)—is a feminine body with smallish breasts, ample buttocks, and high, wide hips. Anyone wishing to be considered desirable to a man should do what she can to approximate that ideal. And this, of course, is precisely what travestis do. They appropriate and incorporate the ideals of beauty that their culture offers them in order to be attractive to men: both real men (i.e., boyfriends, some clients, and vícios), and males who publicly "pretend to be men" (clients and vícios who enjoy being penetrated).

CONCLUSION: PENETRATING GENDER

What exactly is gender and what is the relationship between sex and gender? Despite several decades of research, discussion, and intense debate, there is still no agreed-upon, widely accepted answer to those basic questions. Researchers who discuss gender tend to either not define it or, if they do define it, do so by placing it in a seemingly necessary relationship to sex. But one of the main reasons for the great success of Judith Butler's *Gender Trouble* (and in anthropology, Marilyn Strathern's *The Gender of the Gift*) is surely because those books called sharp critical attention to understandings of gender that see it as the cultural reading of a precultural, or prediscursive, sex. "And what is 'sex' anyway?" asks Butler in a key passage:

> Is it natural, anatomical, chromosomal, or hormonal, and how is a feminist critic to assess the scientific discourses which purport to establish such "facts" for us? Does sex have a history? Does each sex have a different history, or histories? Is there a history of how the duality of sex was established, a genealogy that might expose the binary options as variable construction? Are the ostensibly natural facts of sex discursively produced by various scientific discourses in the service of other political and social interests? If the immutable character of sex is contested, perhaps this construct called "sex" is as culturally constructed as gender; indeed, perhaps it was always already gender, with the consequence that the distinction between sex and gender turns out to be no distinction at all. [1990:6–7]

It is only when one fully appreciates Butler's point and realizes that sex stands in no particularly privileged, or even necessary, relation to gender that one can begin to understand the various ways in which social groups can organize gender in different ways. My work among travestis has led me to define gender, more or less following Eve Sedgwick (1990:27–28), as a social and symbolic arena of ongoing contestation over specific identities, behaviors, rights, obligations, and sexualities. These identities and so forth are bound up with and productive of male and female persons, in a hier-archically ordered cultural system in which the male/female dichotomy functions as a primary and perhaps a model binarism for a wide range of values, processes, rela-tionships, and behaviors. Gender, in this rendering, does not have to be about "men" and "women." It can just as probably be about "men" and "not-men," a slight but extremely significant difference in social classification that opens up different social configurations and facilitates the production of different identities, understandings, relationships, and imaginings.

One of the main puzzles I have found myself having to solve about Brazilian travestis is why they exist at all. Turning to the rich and growing literature on homo-sexuality in Latin America was less helpful than I had hoped, because the arguments developed there cannot account for (1) the cultural forces at work that make it seem logical and reasonable for some males to permanently alter their bodies to make them look more like women, even though they do not consider themselves to be women and (2) the fact that travestis regularly (not to say daily) perform both the role of pen-etrator and penetrated in their various sexual interactions with clients, vícios, and boyfriends. In the first case the literature on homosexuality in Latin America indicates that it should not be necessary to go to the extremes that Brazilian travestis go to (they could simply live as effeminate, yet still clearly male, homosexuals), and in the second case, the literature leads one to expect that travestis would restrict their sexual roles, by and large, to that of being penetrated.[13] Wrong on both counts.

What is lacking in this literature, and what I hope this essay will help to provide, is a sharper understanding of the ways in which sexuality and gender configure with one another throughout Latin America. My main point is that for the travestis with whom I work in Salvador, gender identity is thought to be determined by one's sexual behavior.[14] My contention is that travestis did not just pull this understanding out of thin air; on the contrary, I believe that they have distilled and clarified a relationship between sexuality and gender that seems to be widespread throughout Latin America. Past research on homosexual roles in Latin America (and by extension, since that literature builds on it, past research on male and female roles in Latin America) has perceived the links to sexuality and gender to which I have drawn attention (see, for example, Parker 1986:157; 1991:43–53, 167), but it has been prevented from theorizing those links in the way I have done in this article because it has conflated sex and gender. Researchers have assumed that gender is a cultural reading of biological males and females and that there are, therefore, two genders: man and woman. Effeminate male homosexuals do not fit into this particular binary; they are clearly not women, but culturally speaking they are not men either. So what are they? Calling them "not quite men, not quite women," as Roger Lancaster (1992:274) does in his analysis of Nicaraguan cochones, is hedging: a slippage into "third gender" language to describe a society in which gender, as Lancaster so carefully documents, is structured according to a powerful and coercive binary. It is also not hearing what cochones, travestis, and other effeminate Latin American homosexuals are saying. When travestis, maricas, or cochones call each other "she" or when they call men who have been anally penetrated "she," they are not just being campy and subcultural, as analyses of the language of homosexual males usually conclude; I suggest that they are perceptively and incisively reading off and enunciating core messages generated by their cultures' arrangements of sexuality, gender, and sex.

I realize that this interpretation of travestis and other effeminate male homosexuals as belonging to the same gender as women will seem counterintuitive for many Latin Americans and students of Latin America. Certainly in Brazil, people generally do not refer to travestis as "she," and many people, travestis will be the first to tell you, seem to enjoy going out of their way to offend travestis by addressing them loudly and mockingly as "o senhor" (sir or mister).[15] The very word *travesti* is grammatically masculine in Brazilian Portuguese (*o travesti*), which makes it not only easy but logical to address the word's referent using masculine forms.[16]

There are certainly many reasons why Brazilians generally contest and mock individual travestis' claims to femininity, not least among them being travestis' strong associations with homosexuality, prostitution, and AIDS—all highly stigmatized issues that tend to elicit harsh condemnation and censure from many people. Refusal to acknowledge travestis' gender is one readily available way of refusing to acknowledge travestis' right to exist at all. It is a way of putting travestis back in their (decently gendered) place, a way of denying and defending against the possibilities that exist within the gender system itself for males to shift from one category to the other.[17]

During the time I have spent in Brazil, I have also noted that the harshest scorn is reserved for unattractive travestis. Travestis such as Roberta Close and some of my own acquaintances in Salvador who closely approximate cultural ideals of feminine beauty are generally not publicly insulted and mocked and addressed as men. On the contrary, such travestis are often admired and regarded with a kind of awe. One conclusion I draw from this is that the commonplace denial of travestis' gender as not-men may not be so much a reaction against them as gender crossers as it is a reaction against unattractiveness in people (women and other not-men), whose job it is to make themselves attractive for men. Seen in this light, some of the hostility against (unattractive) travestis becomes intelligible as a reaction against them as failed women, not failed men, as more orthodox interpretations have usually argued.

Whether or not I am correct in claiming that the patterns I have discussed here have a more widespread existence throughout Latin America remains to be seen. Some of what I argue here may be specific to Brazil, and some of it will inevitably be class specific. In a large, extraordinarily divided, and complex area like Latin America, many different and competing discourses and understandings about sexuality and gender will be available in different ways to different individuals. Those differences need to be investigated and documented in detail. My purpose here is not to suggest a monolithic and immutable model of gender and sexuality for everyone in Latin America. I readily admit to having close firsthand understanding only of the travestis with whom I worked in Salvador, and the arguments presented in this essay have been developed in an ongoing attempt to make sense of their words, choices, actions, and relationships.

At the same time, though, I am struck by the close similarities in gender and sexual roles that I read in other anthropologists' reports about homosexuality and male-female relations in countries and places far away from Salvador, and I think that the points discussed here can be helpful in understanding a number of issues not explicitly analyzed, such as why males throughout Latin America so violently fear being anally penetrated, why men who have sex with or even live with effeminate homosexuals often consider themselves to be heterosexual, why societies like Brazil can grant star status to particularly fetching travestis (they are just like women in that they are not-men, and sometimes they are more beautiful than women), why women in a place like Brazil are generally not offended or outraged by the prominence in the popular imagination of travestis like Roberta Close (like women, travestis like Close are also not-men, and hence they share women's tastes, perceptions, feelings, and desires), why many males in Latin American countries appear to be able to relatively unproblematically enjoy sexual encounters with effeminate homosexuals and travestis (they are definitionally not-men, and hence sexual relations with them do not readily call into question one's self-identity as a man), and why such men even pay to be penetrated by these not-men (for some men being penetrated by a not-man is perhaps not as status- and identity-threatening as being penetrated by a man; for other men it is perhaps more threatening, and maybe, therefore, more exciting). If this essay makes any contribution to our understanding of gender and sexuality in Latin America, it will be in revitalizing exploration of the relationship between sexuality and gender and in providing a clearer framework within which we might be able to see connections that have not been visible before.

NOTES

Acknowledgments. Research support for fieldwork in Brazil was generously provided by the Swedish Council for Research in the Humanities and Social Sciences (HSFR) and the Wenner-Gren Foundation for Anthropological Research. The essay has benefited immensely from the critical comments of Inês Alfano, Lars Fant, Mark Graham, Barbara Hobson, Kenneth Hyltenstam, Heather Levi, Jerry Lombardi, Thaïs Machado-Borges, Cecilia McCallum, Stephen Murray, Bambi Schieffelin, Michael Silverstein, Britt-Marie Thurén, David Valentine, Unni Wikan, and Margaret Willson. My biggest debt is to the travestis in Salvador with whom I work and, especially, to my teacher and coworker, Keila Simpsom, to whom I owe everything.

1. Chauncey 1994; Crisp 1968; Jackson 1989; Nanda 1990; Trumbach 1989; Whitehead 1981; Wikan 1977.
2. See, for example, Almaguer 1991, Carrier 1995, Fry 1986, Guttman 1996, Lancaster 1992, Leiner 1994, Murray 1987, 1995, Parker 1991, Prieur 1994, and Trevisan 1986.
3. One of the few contexts in which ideas similar to Latin American ones are preserved in North American and northern European understandings of male sexuality is prisons. See, for example, Wooden and Parker 1982.
4. This article is based on 11 months of anthropological fieldwork and archival research and more than 50 hours of recorded speech and interviews with travestis between the ages of 11 and 60 in Salvador, Brazil's third-largest city, with a population of over 2 million people. Details about the fieldwork and the transcriptions are in Kulick n.d.
5. Travestis are also the subject of two short anthropological monographs in Portuguese: de Oliveira 1994 and Silva 1993. There is also an article in English on travestis in Salvador: Cornwall 1994. As far as I can see, however, all the ethnographic data on travestis in that article are drawn from de Oliveira's unpublished master's thesis, which later became her monograph, and from other published sources. Some of the

information in the article, such as the author's claim that 90 percent of the travestis in Salvador are devotees of the Afro-Brazilian religion Candomblé, is also hugely inaccurate.

6. In the summer months leading up to Carnival, travestis from other Brazilian cities flock to Salvador to cash in on the fact that the many popular festivals preceding Carnival put men in festive moods and predispose them to spend their money on prostitutes.

7. de Oliveira 1994; Kulick 1996a; Mott and Assunção 1987; Silva 1993.

8. The literal translation of *se sentir mulher* is "to feel woman," and taken out of context, it could be read as meaning that travestis feel themselves to be women. In all instances in which it is used by travestis, however, the phrase means "to feel like a woman," "to feel as if one were a woman (even though one is not)." Its contrastive opposite is *ser mulher* (to be woman).

9. In her study of female prostitutes in London, for example, Day explains that "a prostitute creates distinctions with her body so that work involves very little physical contact in contrast to private sexual contacts. Thus . . . at work . . . only certain types of sex are acceptable while sex outside work involves neither physical barriers nor forbidden zones" (1990:98). The distinctions to which Day refers here are inverted in travesti sexual relationships.

10. Bornstein 1994; Elkins and King 1996; Herdt 1994.

11. One gendered, absolutely central, and culturally incited desire that is almost entirely absent from this picture is the desire for motherhood. Although some readers of this article have suggested to me that the absence of maternal desires negates my thesis that travestis share a gender with women, I am more inclined to see the absence of such desire as yet another reflex of the famous Madonna-Whore complex: travestis align themselves, exuberantly and literally, with the Whore avatar of Latin womanhood, not the Mother incarnation. Also, note again that my claim here is not that travestis *are* women. The claim is that the particular configurations of sex, gender, and sexuality in Brazil and other Latin American societies differ from the dominant configurations in northern Europe and North America, and generate different arrangements of gender, those that I am calling men and not-men. Motherhood is indisputably a crucial component of female roles and desires, in that a female may not be considered to have achieved full womanhood without it (and in this sense, travestis [like female prostitutes?] can only ever remain incomplete, or failed, women). I contend, however, that motherhood is not *determinative* of gender in the way that I am claiming sexuality is.

12. I use the word *heterosexuality* purposely because travesti-boyfriend relationships are generally considered, by travestis and their boyfriends, to be *hetero*sexual. I once asked Edilson, a 35-year-old marido who has had two long-term relationships in his life, both of them with travestis, whether he considered himself to be hetero-

sexual, bisexual, or homosexual. "I'm heterosexual; I'm a man," was his immediate reply. "I won't feel love for another heterosexual," he continued, significantly, demonstrating how very lightly the northern Euro-American classificatory system has been grafted onto more meaningful Brazilian ways of organizing erotic relationships: "[For two males to be able to feel love], one of the two has to be gay."

13. One important exception to this is the Norwegian sociologist Annick Prieur's (1994) sensitive work on Mexican *jotas*.

14. Note that this relationship between sexuality and gender is the *opposite* of what George Chauncey reports for early-20th-century New York. Whereas Chauncey argues that sexuality and gender in that place and time were organized so that "one's sexual behavior was necessarily thought to be determined by one's gender identity" (1994:48), my argument is that for travestis in Salvador, and possibly for many people throughout Latin America, one's gender identity is necessarily thought to be determined by one's sexual behavior.

   One more point here. I wish to note that Unni Wikan, upon reading this paper as a reviewer for the *American Anthropologist*, pointed out that she made a similar claim to the one I argue for here in her 1977 article on the Omani xanith. Rereading that article, I discovered this to be true (see Wikan 1977:309), and I acknowledge that here. A major difference between Wikan's argument and my own, however, is that it is never entirely clear whether Omanis (or Wikan) conceptualize(s) xaniths as men, women, or as a third gender. (For a summary of the xanith debate, see Murray 1997.)

15. The exceptions to this are boyfriends, who often—but, interestingly, not always—use feminine grammatical forms when speaking to and about their travesti girlfriends, and clients, who invariably use feminine forms when negotiating sex with travestis.

16. In their day-to-day language practices, travestis subvert these grammatical strictures by most often using the grammatically feminine words *mona* and *bicha* instead of *travesti*.

17. The possibility for males to shift gender—at least temporarily, in (hopefully) hidden, private encounters—seems to be one of the major attractions that travestis have for clients. From what many different travestis told me, it seems clear that the erotic pleasure that clients derive from being anally penetrated is frequently expressed in very specific, heavily gender-saturated, ways. I heard numerous stories of clients who not only wanted to be penetrated but also, as they were being penetrated, wanted the travesti to call them *gostosa* (delicious/sexy, using the feminine grammatical ending) and address them by female names. Stories of this kind are so common that I find it hard to escape the conclusion that a significant measure of the erotic delight that many clients derive from anal penetration is traceable to the fact that the sexual act is an engendering act that shifts their gender and transforms them from men into not-men.

REFERENCES CITED

Almaguer, Tomás

1991 Chicano Men: A Cartography of Homosexual Identity and Behavior. Differences 3:75–100.

Bornstein, Kate

1994 Gender Outlaw: On Men, Women and the Rest of Us. London: Routledge.

Brandes, Stanley

1981 Like Wounded Stags: Male Sexual Ideology in an Andalusian Town. In Sexual Meanings: The Cultural Construction of Gender and Sexuality. S. B. Ortner and H. Whitehead, eds. Pp. 216–239. Cambridge: Cambridge University Press.

Butler, Judith

1990 Gender Trouble: Feminism and the Subversion of Identity. London: Routledge.

Carrier, Joseph

1995 De los Otros: Intimacy and Homosexuality among Mexican Men. New York: Columbia University Press.

Chauncey, George

1994 Gay New York: Gender, Urban Culture and the Making of the Gay Male World, 1890–1940. New York: Basic Books.

Cornwall, Andrea

1994 Gendered Identities and Gender Ambiguity among Travestis in Salvador, Brazil. In Dislocating Masculinity: Comparative Ethnographies. A. Cornwall and N. Lindisfarne, eds. Pp. 111–132. London: Routledge.

Crisp, Quentin

1968 The Naked Civil Servant. New York: New American Library.

Day, Sophie

1990 Prostitute Women and the Ideology of Work in London. In Culture and AIDS. D. A. Feldman, ed. Pp. 93–109. New York: Praeger.

de Oliveira, Neuza Maria

1994 Damas de paus: O jogo aberto dos travestis no espelho da mulher. Salvador, Brazil: Centro Editorial e Didático da UFBA.

Dynes, Wayne

1987 Portugayese. In Male Homosexuality in Central and South America. S. O. Murray, ed. Pp. 183–191. San Francisco: Instituto Obregón.

Elkins, Richard, and Dave King

1996 Blending Genders: Social Aspects of Cross-dressing and Sex-changing. London: Routledge.

Fry, Peter

1986 Male Homosexuality and Spirit Possession in Brazil. In The Many Faces of Homosexuality: Anthropological Approaches to Homosexual Behavior. E. Blackwood, ed. Pp. 137–153. New York: Harrington Park Press.

Garfinkel, Harold

1967 Studies in Ethnomethodology. Englewood Cliffs, NJ: Prentice-Hall.

Guttman, Matthew C.

1996 The Meanings of Macho: Being a Man in Mexico City. Berkeley: University of California Press.

Herdt, Gilbert, ed.

1994 Third Sex, Third Gender: Beyond Sexual Dimorphism in Culture and History. New York: Zone Books.

Jackson, Peter A.

1989 Male Homosexuality in Thailand: An Interpretation of Contemporary Thai Sources. New York: Global Academic Publishers.

Kessler, Suzanne J., and Wendy McKenna

1985 [1978] Gender: An Ethnomethodological Approach. Chicago: University of Chicago Press.

Kulick, Don

1996a Causing a Commotion: Public Scandals as Resistance among Brazilian Transgendered Prostitutes. Anthropology Today 12 (6):3–7.

1996b Fe/male Trouble: The Unsettling Place of Lesbians in the Self-images of Male Transgendered Prostitutes in Salvador, Brazil. Paper presented at 95th annual meeting of the American Anthropological Association, San Francisco.

n.d. Practically Woman: The Lives, Loves and Work of Brazilian Travesti Prostitutes. Manuscript under review.

Lancaster, Roger N.

1992 Life Is Hard: Machismo, Danger, and the Intimacy of Power in Nicaragua. Berkeley: University of California Press.

Leiner, Marvin

1994 Sexual Politics in Cuba: Machismo, Homosexuality and AIDS. Boulder, CO: Westview Press.

Mott, Luis, and Aroldo Assunção

1987 Gilete na carne: Etnografia das automutilações dos travestis da Bahia. Revista do Instituto de Medicina Social de São Paulo 4 (1):41–56.

Murray, Stephen O.

1997 The Sohari Khanith. In Islamic Homosexualities: Culture, History, and Literature. S. O. Murray and W. Roscoe. Pp. 244–255. New York: New York University Press.

Murray, Stephen O., ed.

1995 Latin American Male Homosexualities. Albuquerque: University of New Mexico Press.

1987 Male Homosexuality in Central and South America. San Francisco: Instituto Obregón.

Murray, Stephen O., and Wayne Dynes

1987 Hispanic Homosexuals: Spanish Lexicon. In Male Homosexuality in Central and South America. S. O. Murray, ed. Pp. 170–182. San Francisco: Instituto Obregón.

Nanda, Serena

1990 Neither Man nor Woman: The Hijras of India. Belmont, CA: Wadsworth Publishing.

Newton, Esther

1972 Mother Camp: Female Impersonators in America. Englewood Cliffs, NJ: Prentice-Hall.

Parker, Richard G.

1986 Masculinity, Femininity, and Homosexuality: On the Anthropological Interpretation of Sexual Meanings in Brazil. In The Many Faces of Homosexuality: Anthropological Approaches to Homosexual Behavior. E. Blackwood, ed. Pp. 155–163. New York: Harrington Park Press.

1991 Bodies, Pleasures and Passions: Sexual Culture in Contemporary Brazil. Boston: Beacon Press.

Perlongher, Nestor

1987 O negócio do michê: Prostituição viril em São Paulo. São Paulo: Editora Brasiliense.

Prieur, Annick

1994 Iscensettelser av kjønn: Tranvestitter og machomenn i Mexico by. Oslo: Pax Forlag.

Raymond, Janice

1979 The Transsexual Empire. London: Women's Press.

Sedgwick, Eve Kosofsky

1990 Epistemology of the Closet. Berkeley: University of California Press.

Silva, Hélio R. S.

1993 Travesti: A invenção do feminino. Rio de Janeiro: Relume-Dumará.

Strathern, Marilyn

1988 The Gender of the Gift: Problems with Women and Problems with Society in Melanesia. Berkeley: University of California Press.

Trevisan, João Silvério

1986 Perverts in Paradise. London: Gay Men's Press.

Trumbach, Randolph

1989 The Birth of the Queen: Sodomy and the Emergence of Gender Equality in Modem Culture, 1660–1750. In Hidden from History: Reclaiming the Gay and Lesbian Past. M. B. Duberman, M. Vicinus, and G. Chauncey Jr., eds. Pp. 129–140. New York: New American Library.

Whitehead, Harriet

1981 The Bow and the Burden Strap: A New Look at Institutionalized Homosexuality in Native North America. In Sexual Meanings: The Cultural Construction of Gender and Sexuality. S. B. Ortner and H. Whitehead, eds. Pp. 80–115. Cambridge: Cambridge University Press.

Wikan, Unni

1977 Man Becomes Woman: Transsexualism in Oman as a Key to Gender Roles. Man, n.s., 12:304–319.

Wooden, Wayne S., and Jay Parker
1982 Men behind Bars: Sexual Exploitation in Prison. New York: Da Capo Press.

CHAPTER 16

The Changing Landscape of Transgender Sex Work, Pimping, and Trafficking in Brazil

Barry M. Wolfe[1]

1 International lawyer, criminologist, and human rights activist.

SUMMARY

This chapter presents an international legal framework for transgender trafficking and sexual exploitation. Particular aspects of the social and cultural environment typically associated with transgender sex work in Brazil will be depicted; transgender pimping structures and processes will be mapped; factors that lead transgender sex workers to accept exploitation will be explored; human trafficking structures and processes will be described; and conclusions about the limits of law enforcement will be presented. The chapter is based on more than ten years of experience interacting and working with Brazilian transgender sex workers. I also founded SOS Dignity, a nongovernmental project that is part of an established AIDS NGO. This organization has defended numerous transgender sex workers in civil and criminal cases ranging from improper arrests to charges of homicide. My conclusions are based on academic qualifications in the fields of international law and criminology; ten years of experience as a specialist in international immigration law; assistance with cases involving human trafficking; and personal involvement.

KEY TERMS

Brazil; human trafficking; immigration law; sexual exploitation; transgender people

Nuttbrock, Larry, *Transgender Sex Work and Society*
dx.doi.org/10.17312/harringtonparkpress/2017.11.tsws.016
© 2018 by Harrington Park Press

The Brazilian transgender scene would appear to be changing in fundamental ways. Until about 2010, the vast majority of these individuals were apparently involved in the sex trade; many of them were exploited by pimps; and many were victims of human trafficking. Those who work closely with these individuals nonetheless perceive a change. There would appear to be a gradual but perceptible trend away from sex work. Among those who take up sex work, there would appear to be a growing tendency to be independent and not to accept being exploited by pimps.

The key to understanding issues associated with Brazilian transgender sex work is *consent:* the willingness to undertake sex work and to submit to exploitation and trafficking, and consequently, a disinclination to see one's self as a "victim." When Brazilian transgender sex workers are trafficked within Brazil or abroad for sexual exploitation, they are aware that they will be engaged in sex work and that those who finance their voyage will take advantage of them in certain ways. Not only do they consent to being trafficked, but they often actively seek out the traffickers, believing that they offer the opportunity of a lifetime. This applies both to adults and to children.

Herein lies the difference between trafficking of women—and men—for sexual exploitation and transgender trafficking. In the case of trafficking of girls and boys for sexual exploitation, the victims are in general duped into believing that, depending on the proposed destination, they will work as domestic servants, dancers, models, or actresses. However, upon their arrival, their passports are confiscated and they discover that they are held prisoners and forced to work in nightclubs and brothels. They are kept in debt bondage indefinitely, cut off from their families. They may be threatened that their families will suffer if they attempt to escape. Not so with transgender trafficking. The same factors that lead transwomen to sex work also make them vulnerable to exploitation by pimps and to becoming a trafficking victim.

PRELIMINARY COMMENTS ON THE CHARACTERIZATION OF HUMAN TRAFFICKING

International Legal Definition

The international legal definition of human trafficking is contained in the Protocols of the 2000 United Nations Convention against Transnational Organized Crime (UNTOC). Article 3 of the Protocol to Prevent, Suppress, and Punish Trafficking in Persons defines trafficking in persons as follows:

> (a) "Trafficking in persons" shall mean the recruitment, transportation, transfer, harboring or receipt of persons, by means of the twhreat or use of force or other forms of coercion, of abduction, of fraud, of deception, of the abuse of power or of a position of vulnerability or of the giving or receiving of payments or benefits to achieve the consent of a person having control over another person, for the purpose of exploitation. Exploitation shall include, at a minimum, the exploitation of the prostitution of others or other forms of sexual exploitation, forced labor or services, slavery or practices similar to slavery, servitude or the removal of organs;

> (b) The consent of a victim of trafficking of persons to the intended exploitation set forth in subparagraph (a) of this article shall be irrelevant where any of the means set forth in subparagraph (a) have been used;

> (c) The recruitment, transportation, transfer, harboring or receipt of a child for the purposes of exploitation shall be considered "trafficking in persons" even if this does not involve any of the means set forth in subparagraph (a) of this article;

> (d) "Child" shall mean any person under eighteen years of age.

Human Trafficking in Practice

In practical terms, trafficking in adults involves three basic elements:

ACTION	recruitment, transportation, transfer, harboring or receipt which is achieved by a
MEANS TO CONTROL	threat or use of force, coercion, abduction, fraud, deception, abuse of power or vulnerability for the purpose of

EXPLOITATION	sexual exploitation, forced labor or domestic servitude, slavery, financial exploitation, illegal adoption, removal of organs

In the case of child trafficking, control is not required. There are two basic components: action and exploitation.

ACTION	recruitment, transportation, transfer, harboring, or receipt
EXPLOITATION	sexual exploitation, forced labor or domestic servitude, slavery, financial exploitation, illegal adoption, removal of organs

Specific Aspects Relating to Transgender Trafficking

Human trafficking normally involves an element of movement, whether national or cross-border. However, characterization as trafficking does not necessarily require the victim to be physically transported from one place to another. Harboring and receiving are sufficient, provided the other elements of control and exploitation are present for adults, and exploitation is present for children. According to the US Department of State: "Human trafficking can include but does not require movement. People may be considered trafficking victims regardless of whether they were born into a state of servitude, were transported to the exploitative situation, previously consented to work for a trafficker, or participated in a crime as a direct result of being trafficked. At the heart of this phenomenon is the traffickers' goal of exploiting and enslaving their victims and the myriad coercive and deceptive practices they use to do so" (US Department of State, 2015, p. 6). For adults, consent is irrelevant if there exists control and exploitation. For children, consent is irrelevant if there is exploitation. Arranging for or facilitating the movement of a person from one country to another, where there is neither control nor exploitation, is human smuggling and not human trafficking.

GENERAL COMMENTS ON THE SITUATION OF TRANSGENDER PEOPLE IN BRAZIL

Brazilian Transgender Terminology

The term *transgender* encompasses all gender-variant individuals, including female-to-male transsexuals, drag queens and kings, and intersex individuals. Notwithstanding the discussion of nonbinary gender identity that increasingly dominates Brazilian academic and transgender discourse, the vast majority of Brazilian transgender sex workers perceive themselves as belonging to one of two general categories: *transvestites* and *transsexuals*, although for many the two terms may be interchangeable. The study by Kulick (reprinted in Chapter 15) suggests that *travestis* are a distinct category in Brazil and certain other parts of South America (also see Chapter 3). These are biological males who present themselves as females in the context of sex work. They want to be seen as attractive women, but, unlike transsexuals, they do not want to become women. They may use hormones and silicone implants to look like women, but they do not seek genital-reassignment surgery (GRS) to alter their genitalia because they wish to remain functional as males. Because they do not seek GRS, it is my experience that these individuals typically describe themselves as transvestites, and I will describe them as such here. In practice, many transvestites and almost all transsexual women make commitments to living and dressing exclusively as women, and they are accordingly distinguished from *transformistas* or "drags" (i.e., classic transvestites) in two respects. First, drags dress and appear as men in normal life and only "mount" themselves as women in specific situations. Second, transvestites and transsexuals generally make significant changes to their bodies, often through massive hormone intake, silicone enhancement, plastic surgery, and, sometimes, sex-reassignment surgery, whereas "drags" do not.

Marginalization, Discrimination, and Sex Work
Transwomen in Brazil may face discrimination and humiliation, which may begin in early childhood. Many have low levels of education and are from poorer neighborhoods and regions in Brazil. Homophobic crimes are notorious in Brazil, and transgender people are frequently the targets.

Dreams, Narratives, and Transforming the Body
Traditionally, many young transgender people have grown up with a limited vision of the future. Many dream of traveling to the big city to earn money that will enable them to transform their bodies. This, in turn, will enable them to become candidates to travel to or be sent to Europe, which opens the possibility of earning money to buy a car or a house. This situation is slowly changing. Transwomen are aware that their

beauty will not last long. They may live for the present and discount risks associated with criminal behavior, drugs, and sexually transmitted diseases, including HIV.

To achieve their dreams, transgender people may transform their bodies in three ways:

(a) Hormone treatment

(b) Breast implants and facial surgery

(c) Silicone pumping, by which buttocks, legs, and sometimes breasts and faces are transformed, is a staple of many transvestites' lives, especially those who engage in sex work. Some transvestites become specialists, known as *bombardeiras* (pumpers), in pumping unsterilized industrial liquid silicone into the bodies of other transgender people.

There are a number of adverse effects of silicone pumping, including the silicone dropping down into the ankles and feet, the immune system's rejection of silicone, and the risk of silicone entering the bloodstream or vital organs.

Fortunately, in recent years, transwomen have become more aware of these issues. There is an increased tendency to resist clandestine medical practices, including hormone treatment without medical supervision and silicone pumping.

Marginalization and Ritualistic Culture

Discrimination leads to marginalization, and Brazilian transgender people until recently tended to live in their own hermetically sealed world with minimal points of contact with mainstream society. The Internet—in particular social media and the ability to research and exchange information—is gradually increasing transgender people's awareness and bringing them into contact with mainstream society.

Transgender people are generally excluded from many religious communities and are warmly welcomed only by the Afro-Brazilian religious orders. In fact, the majority of transgender sex workers are members of one of the three Afro-Brazilian religious orders: Umbanda, Candomblé, and Quimbanda.

Transgender people have their own street vocabulary, *pajuba*, to denote the terms and conditions most common to their lives, such as men, women, sexual organs, good, bad, and so on. Much of this terminology has its origins in Afro-Brazilian religious culture and is shared with Brazilian female street sex workers.

Transgender people have traditionally perceived irrevocable body transformation as a rite of passage. In particular, the pain and risks of silicone pumping resulted in the right to be treated with respect by peers and by those who have not gone through such rites of passage. However, this "silicone dictatorship" is gradually losing ground. Pimps continue to encourage sex workers to undertake silicone pumping.

SEX WORK

General

The formal labor market has been and continues to be largely closed to transgender people. A small minority of transvestites have university educations or professional qualifications. With few exceptions, the only professions open to transwomen have been nursing, domestic service, hairdressing, gay entertainment, and prostitution. In some cases, even those who work as hairdressers, gay nightclub artists, and domestic servants also double as sex workers. This situation is slowly changing.

In the central, north, and northeastern regions of Brazil, transgender people from extremely poor families can begin working as prostitutes as early as 12 years of age, especially if they have been expelled from home by their families. In the south and southeastern regions and in the major capitals of São Paulo and Rio de Janeiro, it is common to find transvestites as young as 16 or 17 working the streets.

Transvestites' clients are generally men who appear "straight" in society. Many, if not most, are married. In the majority of instances, the transvestite sex worker performs the active role in sexual intercourse, the male client assuming the passive, receptive role. AIDS experts believe that a significant hidden route of transmission of AIDS in Brazil is through transgender prostitution: the transvestite passes HIV to the client, and the client in turn passes the virus to his wife or partner.

Street Sex Work

There are two significant differences between transgender and female sex workers in Brazil.

First, a woman has a wider range of career choices. Of course, for a poor person, the choice may be limited. A girl from a low-income background might work in a factory, in a call center, as a shop assistant, or as a domestic servant. Sex work will permit her to earn several times more and give her a certain level of independence that she would not otherwise have. However, the choice exists. For most transwomen, there has, until recently, been no choice.

Second, a girl can choose between several forms of sex work. She can work in a nightclub, in a massage parlor, in a brothel. She can solicit clients in a shopping mall, on the street, in newspapers, and on the Internet. A transgender sex worker had limited choices. At least at the beginning, she had to work on the street. Later, she may be able to solicit clients through newspapers or the Internet. Today, transgender sex workers can work both on the street and through the Internet from the beginning.

Street sex work entails a number of adverse consequences for transgender people, in particular risks to health, drug abuse, STDs, violence, and exploitation.

Risks to Health, Drug Abuse, and STDs

The emotional pressures and fear of violence that accompany sex work, in particular street sex work, lead many sex workers to consume alcohol and drugs in preparation for and during sex work.

The vulnerability of transgender sex workers to STDs, in particular HIV infection, is undeniable. Moreover, it is common for clients to offer an additional payment—which can be more than double the normal price of a trick (*programa*)—for sex without a condom. Transgender sex workers returning from Europe have reported that there are specific streets where it is known that the transvestites work without condoms and where the clients refuse to go with a sex worker who insists on wearing a condom.

Violence

The sex professional working the Brazilian streets lives under the constant threat of violence. The transgender street sex worker lives under the constant fear of being beaten up, run over, stabbed or shot, even of being tortured. Violence can be random. A group of men drive by the street to beat up or shoot a transvestite out of pure malice. Neighbors living on the street where the sex workers ply their trade complain to the authorities and ask them, or pay them, to conduct a cleanup operation. An individual policeman decides to exercise his power and beat a transvestite over the buttocks with his truncheon so that the liquid silicone will spread down her legs, resulting in the silicone becoming lodged in the legs, ankles, and feet. The result is what is known as "elephant feet."

Violence can be premeditated. A client is unable to face himself after a trick and projects his self-revulsion onto the sex worker and beats her up. A client who was robbed by one sex worker wishes to exact revenge. If he cannot find the transvestite who robbed him, he takes his revenge on an innocent person who has done nothing to him. Or he takes out his rage on another sex worker. A motorbike assailant terrorizes and preys on street prostitutes whom he robs and beats up. A drug trafficker punishes nonpayment of drugs. A pimp punishes disobedience or the refusal to pay "protection." One sex worker beats up or stabs a colleague who tries to work on her "patch."

EXPLOITATION AND PIMPING

Cafetinas and Cafetões

Transgender street sex work has traditionally implied exploitation by pimps, at least for new sex workers. In Brazil, there are three kinds of pimp: the male pimp, known as the *cafetão* (plural *cafetões*); and the female and transvestite pimps, known as the *cafetina* (plural *cafetinas*). *Cafetões* are generally low-level drug dealers. *Cafetinas*, both female and transgender, run boardinghouses for transgender people. The majority of those who pimp transgender sex are themselves transgender.

The transgender sex worker's pimp may engage in one or more of a range of activities:

- Managing a group of street sex workers spread out in a city, in a particular neighborhood, or even an entire town

- Distributing drugs to sex workers and other customers

- Supplying basic board and lodging to sex workers: food and a bed. This is normally charged by the day, the payment known as a *diária*

- Money lending and "financing" silicone pumping, plastic surgery, cosmetic treatment, trips to visit family, and international travel

- Charging "protection" for the right to work on the street

- Recruiting, inciting, encouraging, financing, and arranging for the transportation of minor and adult transgender people from one city or state to another within Brazil, generally from the north, northeastern, and central states to São Paulo

- Recruiting, inciting, encouraging, financing, and arranging for the transportation of transgender people from Brazil to Europe.

Pimps and Godmothers

Pimps can be more or less benevolent and more or less malevolent. At the one extreme, there are pimps who charge extortionate daily rates, compelling the transgender sex workers to purchase food and drink at high prices. They encourage the incurring of expenses, which require loans for which high rates of interest are charged, often 100% or more of the amount lent. In particular, they may coerce the sex workers to undergo silicone pumping and cosmetic surgery. Until recently, they encouraged and even coerced their sex workers to be trafficked to Europe. There are pimps who charge a weekly "protection" sum for sex workers who work on the street who are not paying "protection" to another pimp.

Where the pimp provides board and lodging to a transgender sex worker, to the extent that there exists a situation of abuse or power or vulnerability, the pimp is guilty of trafficking.

At the other extreme, there are other pimps, generally transgender *cafetinas*, who do not exploit their sex workers. They provide real protection on the street against violence, especially from other pimps and gangs. They charge justly for board and lodging. They lend money and provide financial assistance without charging interest or at low interest rates. They do not impose fines and do not beat up their sex workers.

The stronger transgender *cafetinas* have a charismatic power over their sex workers. The *cafetina* is called the *madrinha* (godmother), and the sex worker becomes her *filha* (daughter). The *madrinha* fills the role of the family who rejected the *filha*. She gives advice and guidance, creating an emotional bond. She influences behavior and imposes a system of values.

When the *madrinha* is an exploiter, she uses her charismatic hold to impose a Mafia-style respect and discipline rooted in fear, intimidation, and the constant threat of violence. If the *filha* obeys the *madrinha*'s rules, she receives affection. If she disobeys or violates the rules, she will be fined, beaten up, and possibly killed. The exploiting *madrinha* uses her emotional hold to convince her *filha* that it is in her own interests to borrow money for body transformation, to travel to visit her family, and to accept being trafficked to Europe. The *madrinha*'s power is maintained on the basis of the *filha*'s emotional vulnerability, being alone in a big city, far from home. The greater the emotional vulnerability, the stronger the *madrinha*'s hold.

Paradoxically, where the pimp is of a kinder nature and does not exploit or impose a tough regime, the sex workers are left free to use and abuse drugs, to assault clients and passersby, and generally to engage in conduct that is ultimately self-destructive. On the other hand, a strong *madrinha*, one who exploits and mistreats her sex workers, will prohibit assaulting clients and using excessive amounts of hard drugs. She will want her *filhas* to be healthy and to stay clear of trouble to maximize their profit potential. Moreover, these sex workers are better prepared to confront the challenges of being trafficked to Europe. They tend to be tougher, stronger, and more resilient. They also tend to forge stronger, more durable, and mutually supportive bonds with their coworkers and co-trafficking victims.

Charging for Protection

Pimps charge protection in the form of a fixed weekly fee, known as *cobrando rua* ("charging for the street"). This gives the sex worker the right to solicit on the street, free from interference from other pimps. This is extortion in the form of a classic protection racket, based on power, relative disadvantage, and fear. The sex worker is being forced to pay to be protected primarily from her own pimp. Nonpayment results in a fine, which is generally a multiple of the weekly fee. The fine is often accompanied by a beating. The beating serves both as a punishment and as a warning to other potential transgressors. In Brazil, pimps do not generally charge a percentage or proportion of the sex worker's earnings.

In the smaller towns, one transgender *cafetina* can control all the transgender sex workers in the town. The pimp will provide board and lodging to some sex workers. The others will pay the weekly fee.

In the larger towns and cities, several pimps will share the streets, each one controlling a neighborhood or a group of people. In the cities where pimping is not by region, the sex workers can work in any part of the town. When a new sex worker appears on the street, the first pimp to notice her will ask whose "daughter" she is. If she gives a name, the pimp will call that pimp to confirm that the information checks out. If the information is false or if the sex worker is not "protected" by another pimp, the first pimp will claim her. As in all forms of organized crime, violent disputes inevitably arise between pimps.

TRANSGENDER TRAFFICKING

The Central Position of São Paulo in Transgender Trafficking

São Paulo, Brazil's largest city, is the country's largest center of transgender prostitution and transgender trafficking. Some transgender people travel from their home states directly to Europe. Others travel first to São Paulo and other large cities.

Greater São Paulo has the largest concentration of transgender sex workers who have traveled from other states and who intend to travel to Europe. There are no reliable data on how many transgender and other sex workers are in São Paulo, or indeed in Brazil. Some transgender sex workers are born in and around São Paulo and neighboring cities and towns. The majority of transgender sex workers who live and work in São Paulo were born in the poorer north, northeastern, and central regions. São Paulo is seen as a stepping-stone where transgender people transform their bodies in preparation for traveling to Europe. Many transgender sex workers return from Europe and use São Paulo as their base between sojourns in Europe.

Trafficking of Adults and Children within Brazil

Pimps in São Paulo and other cities in Brazil's southeast take transgender sex workers to their houses from the country's north, northeastern, and central regions. Some pimps send recruiters to the poorer regions. Others have arrangements with local pimps to seek out potential candidates. In certain northern states, the pimps seek out effeminate adolescent boys, as well as adults. The candidates are offered the "opportunity" of going to São Paulo and other large cities. Transport is paid for, usually by bus. The bus trip can take up to several days.

In some cases, the candidates do not dress or present themselves as girls in their hometowns. However, as soon as they arrive in the big city, they are made to present themselves as women and are put on the street as sex workers.

The Special Situation of Internal Trafficking of Children

In the case of adults, if there has been no abuse of power or of a situation of vulnerability, there is no human trafficking at this point. In the case of minors, the mere fact of being made to undertake sex work constitutes human trafficking.

Many young effeminate boys and adolescents are rejected by their own families. Many start to feel that they are transgender in their early teens. This is especially the case in Brazil's poorer areas. Many of these children have been abused by their own male relatives, who then reject them. Many are cast out when they are still children.

It is not uncommon for these youths to work as sex professionals in their hometowns from the age of 12. They may even work as drags in local nightclubs. They are thus vulnerable to approaches from pimps and traffickers who offer to take them to the big city. There are cases in which the child's own family encourages the youth to undertake sex work. Some families sell their own children to pimps.

On arrival in the big city, they are put to work on the street. They are forced to have silicone pumped into their bodies. The children are effectively held prisoner in the pimps' houses under a strict debt bondage regime. They are forced to pay for board and lodgings at exorbitant prices and live under the constant threat of beatings.

The children are often encouraged to use drugs. They have to purchase the drugs from the pimps. Thus starts a vicious cycle as the drugs help the children face the life of sex work and violence, creating dependency on the drugs themselves. If, and when, the authorities decide to take action to "rescue" the children, they are sent back to their home states and to the families who rejected them in the first place. In the majority of cases, the children do not want to be "rescued" because they do not consider themselves to be victims. Often, they do not wish to return to their hometowns. They see street sex work as their only chance for a better life.

There are no adequate residential care facilities for transgender minors in São Paulo or in other large Brazilian cities. In boys' care facilities they are subject to abuse and beatings, not to mention the risk of being murdered. They cannot be sent to girls' care facilities because they are not considered female. Some evangelical religious care facilities will accept the children. However, they are seen as "spiritually sick" and in need of being "cured" of their homosexuality and female or transgender gender identity.

Many of the children suffer from serious health problems, and many become infected with STDs, in particular HIV, while still minors. The situation is so serious that even well-intentioned human rights activists regard these children as a lost cause.

International Transgender Trafficking

Transgender sex workers generally choose Italy, France, Spain, Portugal, Switzerland, or Holland for their first sojourn in Europe. With the general recession in Europe and increasing competition for clients, those sex workers who are already established in Europe travel farther afield, moving to and from other European countries.

Transgender sex workers face a number of problems upon arrival in Europe.

First is the need to get through increasingly strict immigration controls. The fortunate ones are granted entry into their chosen destination on the first trip. Those who are refused entry and deported may try again but travel first to a country with slacker immigration controls and then travel within the European Union to their destination of choice. Second, they need to find a place to live. This is difficult in a new country where they have no support system and do not speak the language.

Third, they need to work. In Europe, transgender sex workers work on the streets or through advertisements on the Internet. They need orientation on how to organize themselves and to be able to work on the street without facing problems from other sex workers and local pimps. Fourth, they need to get used to the cold, especially when working on the streets.

There are three ways that a transgender person can finance her first trip to Europe.

1. OWN FUNDS OR LOAN FROM A FRIEND The more mature and independent transgender sex worker will save up to pay for her own travel to Europe. Alternatively, she may obtain a zero-interest or low-interest loan from a friend or from a *cafetina* who does not exploit her *filhas*. She will be aware of the dangers of falling into the hands of exploiters and will have sufficiently strong contacts to enable her to set up in Europe.

A friend might already be established in Europe. She might have been trafficked herself but won her independence. Where there is no exploitation or control by the friend, there is no trafficking.

2. FINANCED BY AN INDIVIDUAL ALREADY ESTABLISHED IN EUROPE It is not uncommon for sex workers who become established in Europe and obtain residence rights to pimp newcomers. There are significant numbers of transgender persons who live and work in Brazil independently, without being controlled by a pimp. Such a person might not have the funds or contacts to enable her to travel to Europe without seeking "financing." The financing would be several times the cost of the airfare. The borrower is tied to the financer until the debt is paid. There is thus both abuse of a position of relative vulnerability and exploitation, which together characterize human trafficking.

3. FINANCED BY A GANG OF PIMPS Powerful pimps have traditionally encouraged and even coerced their transgender sex workers to travel to Europe with financing. There are often networks of such pimps in Brazil with established counterparts in Europe. The latter receive and control the sex workers.

Depending on the country of destination and the strictness of immigration controls at a particular time, the transgender person may be sent directly to the country of destination or to a third country for transit. The third country may be in Eastern Europe. When the third country is far from the country of destination, the transgender person will be met by an intermediary who will assist with entry into the transit country and receive the traveler and take her to the country of destination, where she is then handed over to the receiving pimps.

Upon arrival in the destination country, the sex worker is placed in a house controlled by the Brazilian pimp's local contact. In addition to having to repay the financing, the sex worker is obliged to pay for board and lodging at high prices and to work under the control of the local pimps. She will remain in debt bondage until the financing has been paid in full. Once payment has been made, she is free.

In addition to those sex workers already controlled by pimps in Brazil, independent transgender people seek out these traffickers when they are unable to find alternative sources of financing. The prices will vary depending on the supply and demand of the market at the time and the degree of control that the pimps have over the victims. They might charge a higher fee to sex workers already under their control and a lower fee to independent sex workers who seek them out.

Until recently, financing could have been anywhere from €5,000 to €20,000. In other words, the airfare will cost in the region of €1,000, but the obligation will be to pay back the full amount of the financing. Until the early years of this century, a sex worker could be expected to repay the entire financing within a few months.

Recent Developments
The recession in Europe since 2008, together with increased competition, has meant that it can take many months to pay back a financing of €3,000–€4,000. On the one hand, trafficking has become a low-profit activity for pimps. Consequently, they are no longer encouraging their sex workers to travel to Europe. On the other hand, as transwomen become more independent, they can earn more money in Brazil, where because they are in their own country, they have more security. Alternatively, if they decide to try Europe, they increasingly save up and finance themselves.

A DISTINCT MODEL OF HUMAN TRAFFICKING
There are two differences between transgender trafficking and trafficking of women and men for sexual exploitation. On the one hand, while female and male trafficking victims' consent to travel is obtained through deception, transgender people are fully aware that gangs of pimps will exploit them and that they will live under debt bondage. On the other hand, unlike male and female trafficking victims, transgender sex workers are free once their debt has been paid.

The questions are: Why do transgender sex workers consent to being trafficked? Why are they freed once the debt is paid?

Part of the answer to the first question resides in the second question. No transgender sex worker would consent to a relationship of debt bondage if it were not for a limited time. Whereas male and female trafficking victims are effectively held prisoner without any contact with family and friends, transgender sex workers stay in contact with each other and with their families and friends through telephone and Internet communications networks. Indeed, an intelligence and communications network is a characteristic of underground groups. If a transgender sex worker is murdered in Rome, all her friends and acquaintances in Europe and in Brazil will know within hours through social networks, in particular Facebook. Similarly, if one group of pimps is particularly brutal in Europe and were to try to exert control over its sex workers beyond that which is considered "normal," the information will spread and other potential victims will be warned.

Second, male and female trafficking victims do not imagine they will be become sex workers. Transgender people are fully aware that sex work in Europe offers the only possibility of earning a significant amount of money in a short time.

Third, transgender people need to make their money quickly because they are aware that they have a short "shelf life." They are aware that their female beauty will last into their mid-thirties, or early forties at the absolute maximum. They desire to make the most of their lives while they are still young and able to enjoy their beauty.

Fourth, the international trafficking of women and men is run by large and brutal transnational criminal organizations. Transgender trafficking is run by relatively small gangs of pimps in a small number of countries.

There may be points of contact between transgender traffickers and major organized crime. One example is the acquisition and distribution of drugs. Another example is the arranging of clandestine transport to meet a transgender person who travels from Brazil to an Eastern European country for transport to the country of destination.

Another example is the fact that in Rio de Janeiro, the control of street prostitution is by geographical region. Each region is controlled by a particular organized criminal group that governs all criminal activities in the region, including drug trafficking, pimping, and human trafficking. Thus, all transgender pimps and traffickers are subordinated to the regional criminal organization. Nevertheless, once the transgender people are in Europe, their lives are no longer dominated by the Brazilian organization.

Organized crime, properly so called, cannot dominate, in terms of management, an area of activity where the victims are free and independent once their debts have been paid.

Aspects of International Transgender Trafficking

In some cases, Brazil-based pimps are able to resolve problems and disputes between transgender people and groups in Europe. For example, a newly arrived sex worker on the streets of a European city might draw the attention of clients away from the sex workers who have been there for some time. This can result in a strong and violent reaction against the new arrival. If the Brazilian *cafetina* is powerful and respected, she may be called on to impose order, thereby protecting her *filha*.

There are instances in which, once the trafficking debt has been paid, a powerful *madrinha* will attempt to exploit the fact that an illiterate sex worker will have trouble opening bank accounts and transferring funds. The *cafetina* will put pressure on her illiterate *filha* to send her savings to the *madrinha* so she can "look after" the money for her *filha*. The greater the extent that the *filha* continues to be emotionally dependent on her *madrinha* and is unable to manage her own finances, the greater the control the pimp is able to continue to exert from Brazil.

On the other hand, the greater the charismatic power the *madrinha* has over her *filha* in Brazil, with the resulting belief on the part of the *filha* that the *madrinha* is looking out for her best interests, the greater the *filha*'s deception will be upon her arrival in Europe. She finds herself alone, in a strange country, where she does not speak the language, being forced to work on the street in winter. She discovers that she is being controlled and exploited by a pimp in Europe. She is terrified. She cannot look to her Brazilian *madrinha* for emotional support. To the extent that she becomes aware of the *madrinha*'s dissembling, she tends to become revolted and cynical.

TRANSGENDER TRAFFICKING: LAW ENFORCEMENT OR PREVENTION?

Law enforcement is generally ineffective against transgender trafficking. In the first place, whereas law enforcement is national or possibly regional, criminal activity that involves more than one country is intrinsically transnational.

For example, an investigation into the trafficking of a group of transgender sex workers from São Paulo to Paris will involve at least three police forces: the French police, the Brazilian Federal Police, and the São Paulo State Civil Police. If the same groups are also operating in Spain, the Spanish police will be involved and also possibly INTERPOL and EUROPOL. In each country the prosecutorial and judicial authorities may also be involved. Thus, effective law enforcement will at the very least require:

- National cooperation between the Brazilian Federal Police and the São Paulo State Civil Police.

- Bilateral cooperation between the Brazilian police forces and the French police.

- Bilateral cooperation between the Brazilian police forces and the Spanish police.

- Multilateral cooperation among the Brazilian police, the French police, and the Spanish police.

- Multilateral cooperation among these entities and INTERPOL/EUROPOL.

Organizing such cooperation requires time, resources, and the political will and honesty of all the authorities involved. On the other hand, the criminals act without borders and are able to communicate, travel, and transfer resources instantly. Transnational crime is always several steps ahead of law enforcement.

In the second place, there are intrinsic difficulties involved in obtaining intelligence about the closed and isolated transgender underground. Tracing and following the money—large numbers of small transactions—is extremely costly and effectively impossible. Moreover, to understand the structure and functioning of gangs that operate together in several countries, it is necessary to monitor communications, which is also effectively impossible. Further, the infiltration of undercover agents and the recruitment of informers is not a viable option with transgender gangs.

In the third place, the authorities' relative operational disadvantage compared with the criminals' operational advantage has the practical consequence that law enforcement operations may result in more suffering on the part of the victims while barely affecting the criminals' operations.

Consider the above example of a transgender gang operating among São Paulo, France, and Spain. An initial joint operation between the Brazilian Federal Police and the Spanish police results in the arrest of a Brazilian pimp in Madrid. The Spanish police rescue a Brazilian transgender sex worker, managed by the pimp in question. The rescued sex worker is a victim of human trafficking.

The victim has no direct knowledge of all the key members of the gang. Even if she knew their female names, she would not know their registered birth names. Arresting the entire gang would require a coordinated operation involving the Brazilian federal and state police forces, the Spanish police, and the French police. Each police force would have to involve the prosecutor service and judicial authority of its respective jurisdiction. The processes could take years and might even result in one or more convictions in one of the countries. The chances of obtaining convictions against the entire gang are minuscule.

In the past, the victim might be pressured into providing information against the exploiters under threat of being deported. She would then receive threats from the gang or pimp warning against providing information regarding the traffickers. She or her family may receive messages that she will be killed if she returns to Brazil.

This aspect is improving with the 2007 Council of Europe Convention on Action against Trafficking in Human Beings, which requires that potential victims of trafficking are provided with a period of a minimum of 30 days' reflection and recovery, during which they will receive support, including accommodations, subsistence, and access to relevant medical and legal services, along with potential eligibility for discretionary leave to remain in the country if they are recognized as a victim.

Notwithstanding this improvement, the gang can split up and reconstitute itself in another form quickly and silently without any significant effect on its business.

CONCLUSION: PREVENTION IS THE ONLY SOLUTION

Once the nature of the problem is understood, the solution becomes clear. The distinguishing aspect of transgender trafficking is the fact of consent. Transgender sex workers are aware of and consent to being trafficked, controlled, and exploited. Without this consent there would be no trafficking and no victims. Without the willingness to become a victim, trafficking would not exist.

Of course, the clandestine nature of sexual exploitation and illegal immigration provides the bedrock against which the criminals are able to flourish. However, even transgender people who have no option other than sex work will tend not to fall prey to the exploiters to the extent that they gain self-worth, assume their dignity as human beings, and demand their civil rights. For its part, it is up to Brazil to provide education, care facilities for children and vulnerable adults, health services, and recognition of basic civil rights.

Without victims willing to be exploited, the pimps and traffickers will have to find other sources of income. In recent years, as more and more transgender sex workers have become aware of their worth as human beings, a growing number of transgender pimps have been developing new careers as priestesses in Afro-Brazilian religious orders.

There are those who deny that these changes are taking place. There are a growing number of transgender militants who work in and run NGOs. Many were and continue to be sex workers. Some were and continue to be pimps. Those who refuse to acknowledge these changes have a vested interest in such denial. Their earnings now depend on government and NGO funding. They cannot admit to the situation's improving. They need to accentuate the seriousness of the problem in order to obtain funding. Ironically, the fact that there is a growing number of militants who are former sex workers is itself evidence of the very trend they seek to deny.

LIMITATIONS

The observations and conclusions contained in this chapter are based on my experiences as an international lawyer and years of personal involvement with transgender sex workers in Brazil. Generalizations of these observations and conclusions should be made with caution. They may not apply to individuals whom I did not observe and, in particular, they may not apply to transgender sex workers outside Brazil.

REFERENCES

Cecília Patrício, M. (2008, January 31). *No truque: Transnacionalidade e distinção entre travestis brasileiras*. Tese de Doutorado em Antropologia da UFPE. Retrieved from http://repositorio.ufpe.br/handle/123456789/431.

Couto, E. S. (1999). *Transexualidade: O corpo em mutação*. Salvador, Brazil: GrupoGay da Bahia.

Figueiredo, D. E. (2008). Methodology for attendance of victims of trafficking for sexual exploitation, women, and transgenders that return to Brazil through the international airport of Guarulhos/São Paulo/Brazil. *Revista Interdisciplinar da Mobilidade Humana 16* (31), 468–475. Retrieved from www.csem.org.br/remhu/index.php/remhu/article/view/129/121.

Figueiredo D., & Novaes, M. M. (2002). *Tráfico de seres humanos: Gênero, raça e criança e adolescentes. Guarulhos.* Retrieved from https://xa.yimg.com/kq/groups/26082696/1357650916/name/Texto_semana_7B%5B1%5D.pdf.

Foureaux de Souza, J. L., Jr. (ed.) (2002). *Literatura e homoerotismo: Umaintrodução.* São Paulo: Scortecci.

Garcia, W. (2005). *Corpo, mídia e representação: Estudos contemporâneos.* São Paulo: Thompson.

Graça M., & Gonçalves, M. (2015). Support services for sex workers in Portugal: Ideologies and practices. *Physis: Revista de Saúde Coletiva, 25* (2), 547–570. Retrieved from www.scielo.br/scielo.php?pid=S0103-73312015000200547&script=sci_arttext.

Green, J. N. (1999). *Beyond Carnival: Male homosexuality in twentieth-century Brazil.* Chicago: University of Chicago Press.

Haddad, A. (2015). A nossa igual humanidade e as diferenças entre discriminação de gênero e a discriminação em razão das identidades transgêneros e de orientação sexual. *Revista Jurídica da Universidade de Cuiabá e Escola da Magistratura Mato-Grossense, 3*, 9–32. Retrieved from http://revistaemam.kinghost.net/revista/index.php/unicemam/article/view/269.

Kulick, D. (1998). *Travesti: Sex, gender, and culture among Brazilian transgendered prostitutes.* Chicago: University of Chicago Press.

Kulick, D., & Klein, C. H. (2010). Scandalous acts: The politics of shame among Brazilian *travesti* prostitutes. *In* D. Halperin and V. Traub (eds.), *Gay Shame.* Chicago: University of Chicago Press. Retrieved from http://works.bepress.com/charles_klein/4/.

Lancaster, R. (1998). Transgenderism in Latin America: Some critical introductory remarks on identities and practices. *Sexualities, 1* (3), 261–274.

Lopes, D., Bento, B., Aboud, S., & Garcia, W. (eds.). (2004). *Imagem & diversidade sexual: Estudos da homocultura.* São Paulo: Nojosa Edições.

Lyra, B., & Garcia, W. (eds.). (2001). *Corpo e cultura.* São Paulo: Xamã-ECA/USP.

McCallum, C. (1999). Review of *Travesti: Sex, gender, and culture among Brazilian transgendered prostitutes*, by Don Kulick. *Mana, 5* (1), 165–168.

Moreno, A. (2001). *A personagem homossexual no cinema brasileiro.* Rio de Janeiro: Funarte, Niterói: EdUFF.

Mott, L. R. B. (1996). *Epidemic of hate: Violations of the human rights of gay men, lesbians, and transvestites in Brazil.* San Francisco: Grupo Gay da Bahia/International Gay and Lesbian Human Rights Commission.

Mott, L. R. B., & Cerqueira, M. (1997). *As travestis da Bahia e a AIDS.* Salvador, Brazil: Ministério da Saúde e Grupo Gay da Bahia.

Nederstigt, F., & Almeida, L. C. R. (2007). Brazil. In *Global Alliance against Traffic in Women* (eds.), *Collateral damage: The impact of anti-trafficking measures on human rights around the world.* Bangkok: GAATW. Retrieved from http://gaatw .org/Collateral%20Damage_Final/CollateralDamage_BRAZIL.pdf.

Pelúcio, L. (2007). *Nos nervos, na carne, na pele: Uma etnografia sobre prostituição travesti e o modelo preventivo de AIDS.* Universidade Federal de São Carlos, Programa de Pós-Graduação em Ciências Sociais.

———. (2005). Na noite nem todos os gatos são pardos: Notas sobre a prostituição travesti. *Cadernos Pagu, 25,* 217–248.

Pereira, G. E. A., & Gonçalves, C. F. (2009). Tráfico ou escravidão de pessoas? *ETIC — Encontro de Iniciação Científica, 5,* (5). Retrieved from http://intertemas.tole doprudente.edu.br/revista/index.php/ETIC/article/viewArticle/2134.

Piscitelli, A. (2007). [Confronting corporalities: Brazilian women in the transnational sex industry.] *Ver Bras de Ciênc Sociais, 22* (64), 17–32. Retrieved from www .observatoriodeseguranca.org/files/Brasileiras%20na%20industria%20do% 20sexo.pdf.

Reis, P. (2006). *Mapa da violência e discriminação praticada contra gays, lésbicas, travestis, transexuais, e bissexuais.* São Paulo: Centro de Referência GLTTB da Secretaria da Cidadania Trabalho, Assistência e Inclusão Social da Prefeitura Municipal de Campinas.

Secretaria Nacional de Justiça (SNJ). (2012). *Diagnóstico sobre tráfico de pessoas nas áreas de fronteira.* Brasília: SNJ. Retrieved from www.sinait.org.br/arquivos/arti gos/Artigo_160.PDF.

Silva, H. R. S. (2007). *Travestis: Entre o espelho e a rua.* Rio de Janeiro: Rocco.

Teixeira, F. d. B. (2008). L'Italia dei Divieti: [In between the dream of being European and the "babado" of prostitution]. *Cadernos Pagu, 31,* 275–308. Retrieved from www.justica.sp.gov.br/StaticFiles/SJDC/ArquivosComuns/Programas Projetos/NETP/L%27Italia%20dei%20Divieti.pdf.

TGEU. (2015, May 8). *Transgender Europe.* IDAHOT TMM 2015. Retrieved from http:// transrespect.org/en/transgender-europe-idahot-tmm-2015/.

Trevisan, J. S. (2000). *Devassos no paraíso: A homossexualidade no Brasil, da colônia à atualidade.* São Paulo: Record.

United States Department of State. (2015). Trafficking in persons report (TIP).

CHAPTER 17

Sociocultural Context of Sex Work among Mak Nyah (Transgender Women) in Kuala Lumpur, Malaysia

Tooru Nemoto[1]   Yik Koon Teh[2]   Karen Troki[1]
Rebecca de Guzman[1] Mariko Iwamoto[1]

1 Public Health Institute, Oakland, CA.
2 National Defence University of Malaysia, Kuala Lumpur

SUMMARY

In Malaysia, transgender women (*mak nyah*) are a highly stigmatized and persecuted group. Mak nyah have little to no access to gender-affirming healthcare and are exposed to widespread societal stigma, employment discrimination, persecution by Islamic religious authorities, and police harassment. Violence, HIV risk, and criminalization are further compounded for mak nyah who engage in sex work. This study aimed to explore and describe the health and social needs of mak nyah on the basis of in-depth qualitative interviews with 18 mak nyah sex workers in Kuala Lumpur. We adapted grounded theory and qualitative descriptive methods to analyze the themes that emerged. Narratives of mak nyah illustrated a complex web of mutually reinforcing vulnerabilities. Mak nyah faced hypervisibility in public settings, where they endured routine intimidation and harassment, and near invisibility when seeking access to and information about hormone use and other health needs. Faced with these and other injustices, many mak nyah engaged in a beneficial informal network of support with peers and allies, though the mak nyah's needs extended well beyond the resources available. Study results suggest that public health and advocacy efforts to improve mak nyah's safety and well-being will require the commitment of a broader human rights agenda.

KEY TERMS   *mak nyah;* Malaysia; sex work; transgender women

Nuttbrock, Larry, *Transgender Sex Work and Society*
dx.doi.org/10.17312/harringtonparkpress/2017.11.tsws.017
© 2018 by Harrington Park Press

Amid its national institutions, Malaysia's current HIV/AIDS policies open a small space that counters the invisibility and denigration of mak nyah, including those who engage in sex work. Fears that HIV is moving from its concentration among injection drug users (IDUs) to the generalized population, and that such an epidemic would curtail economic development, have prompted greater attention and resources to prevent transmission (Teh, 2008). The need for public health resources notwithstanding, such a move affirms the trinity of heteronormative patriarchal family, foreign investment, and capitalist growth that characterizes the current Malaysian government policies. Nevertheless, public health fears have opened up opportunities for research on mak nyah, and this small but significant body of work reveals vital insights into the challenges members of this community face.

Yik Koon Teh's book *The Mak Nyahs: Malaysian Male to Female Transsexuals* (2002) offers the most comprehensive scholarly study to date. Based on surveys and qualitative interviews conducted with mak nyah, Teh's book offers a rigorous perspective into the health challenges and social exclusion they face. A recent qualitative study of mak nyah found numerous unmet health needs, including a lack of access to gender-affirming health care, HIV/STI testing, and mental health resources (Gibson et al., 2016). Though the majority of studies of mak nyah were conducted in Kuala Lumpur, Samsul and colleagues' cross-sectional study with 33 mak nyah in Kuantan, Pahang, the majority of whom were sex workers, indicates low levels of knowledge about HIV prevention (2016). High rates of unemployment and employment discrimination were reported in a survey with 20 mak nyah recruited through a drop-in center serving mak nyah in Kuala Lumpur (Wei et al., 2012).

HIV/AIDS was central to the development and execution of our qualitative study of mak nyah sex workers, but our findings revealed that it was not the most pressing or central concern of the women we interviewed, which prompted us to adopt a slightly different approach in this analysis. Following Teh's recommendation that HIV/AIDS interventions be connected to broader efforts that address discrimination, unemployment, and persecution by authorities (Teh, 2008), this chapter explores the processes by which mak nyah sex work practices intersect with and are shaped by contextual factors, such as transphobia, religious regulation, rural-urban migration, and the unrelenting criminalization of both sex work and gender identity. This approach reflects important developments in scholarship about sex work, namely, a departure from a narrow emphasis on individualistic models to focus on the social issues and contextual factors that shape sex workers' experiences (Vanwesenbeeck, 2001).

This chapter is organized as follows. In the next section, we offer a brief summary of some sociocultural factors shaping contemporary life in Malaysia, contextualizing the struggles, challenges, and resiliencies among mak nyah who have engaged in sex work. Next, we describe methodologies of the current study, which consisted of in-depth qualitative interviews with 24 mak nyah. Our findings are organized to highlight the salient themes that emerged in this study: (1) sex work practices; (2) state intervention, criminalization, and persecution; and (3) healthcare access and transgender care. We conclude with some reflections on this study's limitations and discuss how public health researchers might address the unique challenges facing this vulnerable population.

MALAYSIAN NATIONALISM AND CONTEMPORARY CULTURE

Malaysia has seen robust economic growth since its independence from British rule in 1957. In 2015 its GDP reached almost 300 billion USD, a massive leap from its GDP of two billion USD in 1960 (World Bank, 2016). Between 1970 and 2002, rates of poverty fell from 52.4 to 5.1% (Mok, Gan, & Sanyal, 2007). Significant improvements in health since the advent of decolonization are evident in the reductions in infant mortality (a decrease of 75.5 to 5.9 deaths per 1,000 births) and marked increases in life expectancy for both men and women (14.2 and 18.2 years, respectively) (Chee, 2008).

These markers of progress notwithstanding, Malaysia's modernizing nationalist projects have promoted a state with extraordinary authority and broad reach into the everyday lives of its citizens. The issue of race or who counts as Malay is at the heart of Malaysia's postcolonial nationalist projects (Thompson, 2003). At the eve of independence from Britain, the National Front Alliance, a coalition representing the three major political parties (the United Malays National Organisation [UMNO], the Malaysian Chinese Association [MCA], and the Malaysian Indian Congress [MIC]), drafted the Federal Constitution of Malaysia to designate Islam as the religion of the federation, though it was meant to be limited to the sphere of Muslim personal and customary law (Ling-Chien Neo, 2006). In the decade following independence, racial tensions and conflicts erupted amid growing poverty and income inequality, though the physical and social segregation of Malays, Chinese, and Indians had long been entrenched in British colonial policies of labor migration and control over land use (Hirschman, 1986).

Following race riots in 1969, the New Economic Policy (NEP) was introduced, its aim to "pull up the majority Malay demographic to a more prosperous and involved position in the domestic economy" (Charette, 2006, p. 59). This period also saw the rise of what Stivens (2006) calls "dramatic Islamisation" promoted by state-driven modernizing projects (p. 355). During this time, various political factions sought to promote their blueprints for Malay nationalism. In their various bids for power, these groups aimed to establish themselves as "the ultimate Islamic authority" (Goh, 2012a, p. 217), which saw vigorous interventions into Malay life. It was during this time that the policing of sex and gender gained new visibility; in 1983 the Malaysian Conference of Rulers issued a fatwa prohibiting genital-reconstruction surgery and cross-dressing.

Economic globalization has transformed Malaysia on a scale rarely seen in the modern world. The implementation of the New Development Policy (NDP) in 1991 consolidated the aims of the 1970s NEP, facilitating Malaysia's shift from its agricultural economies and roots in *kampung*, or village relations, to a nation of manufacturing, finance, energy, and industry concentrated in expanding urban centers and connected to global networks. At the heart of the NEP, NDP, and Vision 2020, a program of similar proposed reforms, is the image of the "New Malay" (*Melaya Baru*), which is implicitly male, a defender of Islam, urban-based, and successfully poised to compete in the global economy (Thompson, 2003, p. 428).

Malaysia's nationalist programs have given rise to "expansive state projects geared towards cleansing and otherwise 'tidying up'" (Peletz, 2006, p. 322) those who do not conform to heteronormative, patriarchal kinship roles. A spurious call to Malay tradition is often deployed to justify the numerous injustices facing mak nyah (and other people who fall outside heteronormative gendered and sexual arrangements of marriage and male-dominated family structure). But the subjugation and policing of mak nyah are in many ways unique to this historical moment. Mak nyah played important and valued roles in the sanctification and reproduction of local politics in the early modern era

(Peletz, 2006), and empirical research with older mak nyah documents their recollections of the acceptance and tolerance they experienced before the 1980s (Teh, 2002).

Though the intensification of Islamic authority in Malaysia is clearly relevant to understanding the persecution of mak nyah, religious beliefs that are analyzed independently of their sociocultural contexts cannot fully account for the scale and scope of this repression. In his research on Muslim and Christian persecution of mak nyah, the theologian Joseph Goh (2012b) concluded that religious authority must not be analyzed in a vacuum, stating that "many civil and religious authorities understand that having credible moral authority also confers greater political power" (para. 7). The contemporary treatment of mak nyah bears the hallmarks of British colonialism in its civil law (under the Minor Offences Act of 1955, cross-dressing is illegal), as well as postcolonial nation-building projects.

Goh Beng Lan (2008) argues that the trope of Malay tradition as timelessly patriarchal and heteronormative (despite evidence to the contrary) has been valorized through "a long and passionate rhetoric on new expressions of national identity, highlighting new national sensibilities that were responsive to market instrumentalities" (p. 9). How these seemingly divergent goals of global economic participation and the protection of cultural tradition manage not only to coexist, but to thrive, is a topic engaging many scholars of Southeast Asia. According to Shamsul (1997), the *dakwah*, or Islamic resurgence movement most prominent in the new Malay middle classes, is highly in favor of "the continued expansion of the market and the promotion of aggressive individualism, thus making it hostile to tradition. . . . Its political survival depends on the manipulation and persistence of tradition for its legitimacy, hence its attachment to conservatism about the nation, religion, gender, and the family" (p. 255).

It is against this backdrop that mak nyah have become the target of routine abuse and oppression through interrelated social and legal institutions affecting virtually every facet of their lives. This brief summary highlights how Malaysia's social and political-economic processes are deleterious to mak nyah's struggles to experience safety and well-being, and to be treated with dignity and respect, as both transgender women and sex workers.

METHODS

This study was based on 24 in-depth, face-to face interviews with mak nyah who were part of a larger study investigating substance use and HIV risk behaviors among mak nyah and men who have sex with men (MSM) in Kuala Lumpur, Malaysia. The study had two stages. First we completed 48 qualitative interviews (24 MSM and 24 mak nyah), and then 300 survey interviews (150 MSM and 150 mak nyah). We obtained an Institutional Review Board (IRB) approval from the Public Health Institute, as well as from a local collaborating hospital and Malaysian government agencies (Malaysian National Medical Research Register [NMRR]; Institute of Health Behavioral Research [IHBR]; and Medical Research and Ethics Committee [MREC], Ministry of Health, Malaysia).

Staff Training

Research assistants were recruited from the targeted mak nyah communities. Research assistants were also recruited from among university students who had experience in collecting data for research studies conducted by Teh. Nemoto and Trocki (US team) and Teh (Malaysian team) provided intensive training for Malaysian research assistants in terms of the study's theoretical background, protocol, human subjects issues, informed consent process, study design, and data collection and maintenance. In addition, follow-up training was provided for the project staff and research assistants, particularly for the first phase of the qualitative study. The training covered the following topics: (1) study goals and objectives; (2) study protocol for the qualitative interviews; (3) human subjects protection and obtaining informed consent using the informed consent form; (4) community outreach, mapping, and recruitment; (5) qualitative interview guide; and (6) data collection and reporting. The attendees discussed cultural appropriateness and sensitivity toward the target groups regarding the informed consent forms and qualitative interview guide. Revisions were made to the qualitative interview guide with structured open-ended and probing questions.

Recruitment

Recruitment activities for mak nyah were conducted mainly through a local collaborating AIDS service organization, Social and Enabling Environment Development (SEED) Foundation, which provides HIV prevention and treatment services and advocacy for marginalized communities, specifically homeless people affected with HIV and mak nyah in Malaysia. Mak nyah and other research assistants in the Malaysian team frequently visited the SEED Foundation, built a rapport with program staff and clients of the agency, and identified potential participants. The project staff also distributed recruitment fliers at other collaborating agencies in Kuala Lumpur. Word of mouth and personal connections of the Malaysian research team were also effective in recruiting mak nyah. Using snowball and purposive sampling methods, we carefully monitored the demographics of participants to diversify them in terms of age, ethnicity, education, and areas of residence in Kuala Lumpur.

Qualitative Interviews

After obtaining the informed consent, research assistants conducted qualitative interviews using a structured qualitative guide, which included the following sections: (1) background; (2) social support; (3) health in general; (4) concerns about HIV/STIs and testing; (5) gender-affirmation surgeries and hormone use; (6) safe sex with committed and casual partners; (7) sex work; (8) alcohol and illicit drug use; (9) services for mak nyah; (10) religion; and (11) future plans. The interviews took 90 minutes on average and were digitally recorded. Upon completion of the interview, participants were reimbursed RM100 (equivalent to about US $30) and were provided with information about health and social services in Kuala Lumpur that are sensitive to mak nyah. The interviews were conducted in English or Malay and transcribed by research or project assistants. Transcriptions in Malay were translated into English and carefully examined to ensure their validity. All personal identifiers were removed from the transcripts.

Qualitative Analyses

We analyzed these qualitative data in several iterative stages. First, project staff conducted a close reading of each interview transcript. Close reading is a process that adopts an inductive, careful approach to reviewing interview texts, which allowed us to immerse ourselves in each participant's story and grasp its implicit meanings (Ayres, Kavanaugh, & Knafl, 2003, p. 876). This proved to be a critical step to developing awareness of and familiarizing ourselves with the details, subtleties, and nuances in each narrative. As these qualitative interviews were in-depth and lengthy texts, we composed a written summary of each interview to highlight key findings. While the process was time-consuming, we found that close reading and careful summarizing offered insights into the particulars of each participant's story that might have been overlooked had we too quickly tried to establish commonalities across the sample as a whole.

We used these summaries to develop the next stage of our data analysis. We were guided by our a priori research themes, which were the basis of the qualitative interview protocol, which included sex work and other employment, healthcare, partnerships and relationships, substance use, and encounters with religious and criminal authorities. We also included additional themes as they emerged in our close readings and written summaries. In part because so little has been written about mak nyah, our data collection and analysis followed the tenets of an approach called "fundamental qualitative description," which aims for "a comprehensive summary of events in the everyday terms of those events" (Sandelowski, 2000, p. 334).

Our analysis explored the sociocultural contexts of mak nyah engagement in sex work. We discussed the challenges mak nyah encountered in embracing their gender identities; their experiences with and perspectives about sex work; the risks they faced to their health and safety and the strategies they used to manage these risks; and how their marginalized status as mak nyah and sex workers intersected with their religious or spiritual beliefs, class, and migration status.

Participants

We completed a total of 24 qualitative interviews with mak nyah from September to November 2013. Among 24 mak nyah participants, 15 were then engaged in sex work, three had previously engaged in sex work, and the remaining six had never engaged in sex work. For this study, we focused on mak nyahs and their experiences with sex work; therefore, we excluded the six participants who had no experience with sex work from this analysis. Participants ranged in age from 24 to 51; the average age was 37.5 years old. Eleven participants identified themselves as Malay. Two participants described themselves as of mixed background: one as Chinese Melano and the other as Malay Indian.

One participant described herself as Chinese, and another as Iban. Data regarding ethnicity were inadvertently not collected for three participants. Fifteen participants described their religious or spiritual background as Islam. Of the remaining three, one described herself as Catholic, another as Hindu, and the third as a "free thinker." Of the 18 participants, all but one had migrated to Kuala Lumpur from other provinces in Malaysia: five from Sarawak, six from Selangor, two from Johor, and one participant each from Sabah, Kelantan, Serembam, and Perak. Participants had some variation in terms of their educational background: eight had completed Form 3 (equivalent to the ninth grade); three had completed Form 5 (eleventh grade); and four had received their Malaysian Certificate of Education (roughly equivalent to a high school diploma in the United States). One participant could not recall any formal schooling beyond a very young age. One participant held a college degree and the other had earned a culinary diploma. Twelve participants identified their relationship status as single; the remaining were partnered.

RESULTS

Results were thematically organized into the following sections, although there was considerable overlap between these areas. In the first section, we describe mak nyah's pathways to engaging in sex work, exploring what initially drew them to this work, for what reasons, and whether they remained in the sex trade. This section also examines the mak nyah's substance use in relation to managing the emotional stresses and psychological burdens of sex work and discusses how different types of venues—street-based and Internet platforms—shaped mak nyah experiences with sex work, particularly with regard to safety and autonomy in the trade. The second section describes the issue of criminalization and religious persecution, exploring how mak nyah were subjected to various types of moral policing from both civil and religious authorities. The last section examines the effects of mak nyah's limited access to transgender healthcare, such as hormones and gender-affirmation surgeries. The repression of transgender expression proved to be especially salient for the Muslim participants, who constituted the majority of our sample.

Sex Work Engagement among Mak Nyah

PATHWAYS AND PRACTICES OF SEX WORK Mak nyah's pathways into sex work highlighted a convergence of factors, among them economic need (including funds needed to access hormones and gender-affirmation surgeries, and mak nyah–sensitive healthcare), discrimination in the workforce, and peer involvement in sex trades. All but one of the mak nyah in our analysis had migrated to Kuala Lumpur, typically from rural villages. Owing in part to the hostilities many faced from family members in their communities of origin, coupled with a desire to live more independently, many mak nyah sought support and community from peers in Kuala Lumpur. Mak nyah's initial entry into sex work was often tied to both economic need and the longing for friendships and community that affirmed their emergent mak nyah identities. Susan (we used fictional names for all participants), a 41-year-old Malay, stated: "I came to Kuala Lumpur, suddenly I met people like me and I mingled with them. I met them out of sudden, I ask where they stay, how could they turn out like this, as pretty as women, then I went to pharmacy, to ask what medication do they take, I bought them, do what they are doing. They gather every night, I asked, why is that, they said that they are looking for customers, I joined them as well, and finally I turned out to be like them too. I earn RM200–250 every night."

Sex work, which typically brought more income than a job in the service industry, enabled mak nyah to procure hormones, healthcare, and other means to gender expression or transition. Suzie, a 51-year-old Chinese Melano mak nyah, stated: "I was a sex worker quite a long time because you know I need money, and then I want to change myself. Doing sex work at that time was very interesting because you can make a lot of money. And then every week I go and see doctor, I go for hormone injection, I take hormone, definitely I change. At that time, I was young; compare to now; now I am 51 years old."

Win, a 44-year-old Ibanese mak nyah, described a similar situation, whereby sex work became a viable option to secure the costs associated with her gender expression, along with meeting other basic needs, such as food. She stated: "Before sex work, I worked, worked at food stalls, clothes stall, but the pay was not high. At that time in Sarawak, the pay was only RM150, what to eat? Even that amount of money is insufficient for you to look pretty. When I was in sex work, I got a lot of money, I saved up."

The healthcare costs associated with hormone use and other aspects of gender expression and identity were often linked to mak nyah's economic survival to meet basic needs. Most of the mak nyah did not have promising options or alternatives to sex work, and almost all worked in other capacities, such as bridal assistance and providing makeup and hair services. Tania was a 40-year-old Malay mak nyah. Employment discrimination and a lack of formal education and job training are all present in Tania's account, a story that, while unique, was paradigmatic of the subjugation of many mak nyah whose options beyond sex work were limited: "I've tried so hard to apply for a job, perhaps I have no luck. . . . I have to be patient. In the future, I want to help my family, take care of my parents who are old, if possible I want to work like a normal person [having] a decent job; there is no risks with customers, everything, including HIV; beaten [by customers], everything. I don't want all these things, because I have gone through it, I feel sad. People say it's like hopeless. Work like this [is] difficult."

Economic desperation was a regular theme in the mak nyah experiences with sex work, and when these pressures were reduced, they were able to exhibit greater control over their encounters. Rowena, a 40-year-old Malay woman, explained how a secure job, as an outreach health worker at a nonprofit agency, enabled her to achieve greater autonomy as a sex worker: "Maybe the difference for the current situation, now it is different. Last time I think of HIV/AIDS, last time I think about not having enough money. Now I have a full-time job. The mind-set is different, when I have a stable income, if the customer is arrogant and does not want to wear condom, yet at the same time they have a bad odour and look dirty . . . I reject."

SEX WORK VENUE The venues in which participants had engaged in sex work allowed them greater freedom, but in some cases, less control in their encounters. Bella, a 30-year-old of mixed Malay and Indian ancestry, met customers through the Internet, which allowed her certain safeguards, including time to interact with a customer before the sexual encounter. She explained, "You can actually set the ground rules upfront and, normally, before you actually get down to business, you meet up, have some casual talk, dinner, and then only you for business." Having had previous experience with street-based sex work, Bella also liked being able to access a location or other information before an encounter, which she would share with friends as another safeguard. Internet-based sex work also gave Bella greater control over the price of her services: "On the street, there is basically you choosing a spot for yourself, posing there, attracting those who are interested, negotiating price, and then bring them to your place of business. . . . Being a street-based sex worker, you don't really have the negotiation power, you don't have the leverage to negotiate, in the sense that they can only say, well, the person over there is offering RM50."

Like Bella, Lily, who is 46 years old and Chinese, subscribed to a hierarchy of sex work, distancing herself from the kinds of prostitution that are the most vilified. Lily viewed herself as an escort, carving a sharp distinction between her activities and those of sex workers: "I never be a sex worker, I don't do that, I do go out, I meeting up people, I am a type of . . . is just like a working girl. When I went to the bar, sometimes somebody need a companion, I just sit with him, drink with him, I accompany them, like foreigners, they are tourists, they want to go to KL's places, I bring them out, they pay me money, but I don't sleep with them."

Massage work was identified as another form of non-street-based sex work that reduced the stigma involved in sex work. Win, 44 years old and Ibanese, provided makeup and massage services in her home, and she shared her struggle to earn enough money to meet her basic needs. Although massage sometimes involves sexual services, it bears a categorical difference from the sex work she had previously engaged in, which was conducted through discos and hotels. It appeared that Win's primary role of masseur, which might or might not involve sexual services for an additional cost, gave her an identity that yielded some relief from the stigmas associated with sex work. She stated: "I never say I am a sex worker, I don't want others to say I am a prostitute. . . . When I work as a masseuse, sex [becomes] not important, [because] I want to work, my intention is to work, even without sex I still get money, because I massage first."

A few of the mak nyah experiences illustrate the interconnectedness of labor, migration, and other processes of economic globalization that shape the conditions of their labor as sex workers. Though these accounts were not representative of the sample as a whole, they nevertheless deserve our attention, as they reveal the unpredictable conditions of mak nyah's flexible labor in sexual economies. Karen, a 31-year-old of Malay descent, offered insights into the uncertainties that constricted her ability to earn money as a sex worker:

> I am working at a place where it is full of women, female prostitute place, and I am working together with women, what caused me the difficulty now is, many foreign workers are working together, when they are too many, I don't have chance to work. For example, this month I only work for three, four days. I couldn't work for the rest of the days, I have to seek for it on my own, near where I want to work, or at outside, or at Chow Kit, or on the street, or anywhere. There is a pimp [*bapa ayam*], each of us sitting in our rooms, waiting for customers to come, waiting to be chosen. . . . I used to work every day, even if take a leave, I was off for two days in a week. I don't have place for me to work now, I have to wait for calls. If they call saying there is a room for you to work today, then I go to work. [Research assistant asked: Why is there no place for you to work?] Because there are getting more foreigners, so the priority is for the foreign workers, *lah*, whenever they go back to hometown for stamping, or whatever, if there are any rooms vacant, I could work. [RA asked: Do you try to get clients from the streets?] Yes, can get, but I'm scared, I dare not to. [RA asked: Why?] Because when I go down to the street, I got caught, then police ask for money. I don't think so, *lah*.

Since its independence from Britain, Malaysia's dramatic shift from a network of regional agricultural economies to a major center of global finance and manufacturing propelled new desires into its sexual economies. As Karen's discussion illustrates, she was summarily drawn into and expelled from the place where she worked to suit client demand.

ALCOHOL AND DRUG USE Not all mak nyah participants used drugs or alcohol, but for those who did (whether regularly or occasionally), sexual economies figured centrally in the settings in which they consumed.

Erica, a 35-year-old (she did not disclose her ethnic background to her interviewer), described her introduction to heroin and methamphetamines by friends and her subsequent use of these drugs several times a week for approximately six years. "He told us that using the drug could let us always be pretty, thin, and even for the customers who used the drug they would pay more." Erica's drug use gave intimate shape to her experiences as a sex worker, facilitating the kind of self-presentation that was required of her. She described how her drug use was motivated in part by "want[ing] the feelings of fear to be disappear, a sense of lack of self-confidence, and feel like want to have sex. . . . Ah, when we make this sex work, when we go out, we have to look like confident, nor afraid of the competitors, seem like we are the queen of the day."

Like Erica, Alison, a 38-year-old of Malay descent, smoked *shabu* (a street name for methamphetamine), which gave her the energy and affect she needed to engage in sex work: "When I work, I take drugs, when I am on leave, not working, I'm relax. . . . I won't be sleepy, then I will be brave, things like that."

Sabrina, a 43-year-old Malay, described her heroin use in somewhat mechanistic, functional terms, highlighting how she sought to avoid the pain of withdrawal and the way she earned money: "If I am addicted, pain, I look for customers, get one first, earn money, then buy, sniff, then I regain energy, I am fit to earn money. . . . I'm not quite addicted. I'm keen to take it mainly because I want to earn money, not to release tension."

Susan, a 41-year-old Malay, described her use of "Ice" and ecstasy, which helped her deal with stresses of sex work and engendered a certain harmony she shared with customers. Susan became intrigued with these drugs upon seeing their effects on fellow sex workers in the disco:

> Friends in disco . . . sex workers . . . they look very happy, too happy, like us, our face shows as if we are having problems, why are they happy, I asked around, they said each time I go to disco, I take this pills, such colors and with such names, if you take this, you don't scold customers, you talk to customers, you turn to be friendly, your problems will be gone, you are happy, you love the music, so I tried. . . . Feeling was really good, it was good for sex workers like me to take the pills, if not, we feel like, you know disco, boom . . . boom . . . cannot, *lah*, must have that pills, we could forget.

Criminalization and Persecution

One of the dominant themes to emerge in this study of mak nyah sex workers was the persecution, criminalization, and violence they faced. Mak nyah are subjected to Malaysian federal laws that prohibit prostitution and "indecent behavior" that, while not specifically targeting mak nyah, are often used to criminalize them. The Federal Territories Islamic Department, or JAWI, upholds sharia laws on gender identity that criminalize a "male person posing as a woman" (section 28 of the Syariah Criminal Offences [Federal Territories] Act 1997; Human Rights Watch, 2014, p. 82). Our findings illustrate the profound effects of these discriminatory laws on mak nyah, negatively affecting their health and welfare. To highlight the scope and reach of each institution, we present examples first of mak nyah experiences with the civil police, followed by their experiences with JAWI. However, in these instances it is not easy to distinguish between the civil police and JAWI; several examples highlight the relationship between them, which extends their authoritative reach over the mak nyah. Finally, this section concludes with a brief discussion of the physical and sexual violence against mak nyah, for which they had no recourse for the reasons described above.

POLICE HARASSMENT AND ABUSE Identification of a person as mak nyah is often conducted through scrutiny of state-registered identification cards and perceptions of their physical appearance by police or religious authority. This discriminatory process facilitates their entry into criminal justice settings, irrespective of allegations of sex work. Malaysia's National Registration Department forbids anyone, Muslim and non-Muslim, to change the sex category on their identity cards, which contain their biological sex at birth (Human Rights Watch, 2014, p. 3). In the following account, Bianca, a 33-year-old Malay mak nyah, shared how her gender presentation or expression led to harassment by police:

> Normally when police do roadblock, then they block me and ask for IC [ID card], when they see the IC and my face, they show weird face, then they ask my full name, then they ask me to stop at the side, every time like that. So, I stop, I ask them, what is my fault? They usually say nothing; just want to ask for my phone number. They

always like that. Some of them good, some of them ask for phone number, then they call, chitchat and we become friends, some of them they call me and ask me having sex for free. I reject them and scold them.

Mak nyah's lack of social and political power proved to be critical factors in the misconduct and abuse by the police. Ann, a 27-year-old Malay, described the sexual torment she has experienced: "I've never been arrested, only he asked me to come here, show your ID card, I gave it to him, then he asked, do you take drugs? I replied I don't, need a urine test, he brought me there, I wasn't scared, because I don't take drugs. After that he . . . asked me to take off the clothes, he wanted to see my breasts. Because there are ten of them, no matter if I am willing or not, I had to take off the clothes."

Sex work is illegal and criminalized in Malaysia. But for many mak nyah who engage in sex work, it is not the allegation of involvement in sex work but their mak nyah identity that makes them a target for police harassment and violence, especially for Muslim mak nyah, for whom being a mak nyah is considered a wrong against Islam. Muslim mak nyah sex workers suffer double criminalization. Cecilia, a 36-year-old (she did not disclose her ethnic background), shares how her location in Chow Kit, a business area in Kuala Lumpur for sex workers, made her a target for police harassment: "When I walked by Chow Kit even though I was not having sex there at Chow Kit, they just catch every transsexual they see. And I have been caught before . . . they seized our bra, scarf, and everything."

Fines—or bribes—were costly, but mak nyah made every effort to pay them to avoid further harassment, including incarceration, as Win, a 44-year-old Ibanese explained: "Police have all sorts. Some who really do their tasks, some don't do their tasks, that means there are those who don't do their tasks, when they see people like us, they ask for money. If [we] don't give them money, they will bring us back to the police station."

As noted, mak nyah surveillance and harassment by police occurred in tandem with subjugation by religious authorities. Erica, who is 35 years old (she did not disclose her ethnic background), shared her experiences of how the police use the threat of JAWI to harass, intimidate, and extract bribes from her: "Was caught by JAWI for about three times. And was fined about RM800 due to being femininity. [RA asked: Apart from the religious persecution, religious devotees, or religious authorities, have you been harassed by the police too?] Many times with the police, one of the reasons is the police asks for money from us, as long as we have money, they will consistently ask for it, if not, they will send us to the nearby Department of Islamic Religion. In order to avoid for paying higher penalty, we have to give the police whatever amount that they ask."

JAWI HARASSMENT AND ABUSE Sabrina, a 43-year-old Malay, described her experience being disrupted by the religious authority, and the intensification of punishment mak nyah face: "In the past, yes [have been disrupted by religious authority]. Now will be fined for RM1,000. It used to be RM50 only. If refuse to pay, have to go to jail, cut the hair. I used to pay for the fine. Now, even my friends pay for the fine, they [still] have to go to the jail, waste of money."

The growing scope of religious authority to enact fines, promote "reeducation," and incarcerate mak nyah is also described by Suzie, a 51-year-old who described herself as Chinese Melano. Suzie offered a historical perspective that underscores the difficulties and injustices mak nyah face in contemporary Malaysia. She recalled her experience as a sex worker, which began upon her arrival in Kuala Lumpur in 1981 and lasted until she left sex work in the mid-1990s, and the persecution facing mak nyah sex workers today:

> Police, yes, they raided because of prostitution. I was once arrested, then after that they release me out. . . . The harassment they are saying is *lelaki berpakian wanita* [man dressed as a woman] is wrong. Paid fine. At that time, in the 80s, fine is RM25, they catch you today, tomorrow they release you, you pay the fine of RM25. . . . Compare to before, now is very difficult. If you are being caught, it is very difficult for you to get release. Some of them straight away to jail; some of them go two, three months in jail. I heard it now, I said oh my God.

Kelly, a 29-year-old Malay, tells the story of her arrest and incarceration, which illustrates the domino effect that began with, as she described, "being caught by JAWI, guy dress up like a woman." Under sharia law, Kelly's mak nyah expression exposed her to scrutiny, interrogation, and violence. Her narrative captured the multiple levels of fallout she suffered during her arrest, period of incarceration, and subsequent dislocation as she lost her home, clothes, and a modicum of stability she had managed to build before her arrest:

> I called up my mother saying I was caught by JAWI, she cried. My mother asked me what I was doing in KL, I lie about my work, I work in a club, *lah*, I didn't tell her I work as a GRO [guest relation officer], so I was weeping. . . . I got it for three months, I was bald, they didn't know where I have been, I didn't tell them, I don't want to trouble my family. After I was released from JAWI, my head was bald. . . . I used to stay at Sentul, I rent a room at Sentul, my belongings, bed, TV, clothes, my shoes there, the aunty didn't know I was caught, she threw away all my belongings. I was caught in Sg Buloh for three months, I went back there, my head was bald, I showed it to my aunty, telling her that I was caught, she didn't believe, she rent the room to other people. I'm heartbroken, I don't know where I can go. . . . I am okay now, I have a little bit of money, I buy clothes, shoes. . . . [When I was released] I bathed in toilet, washed face in toilet, hanging around, I didn't have clothes, I didn't have money. Oh my God, I start my life, looked for customers, then I managed to get one or two, I earn money, I rent a hotel room, I sleep there. I didn't want to trouble my family.

Given that every one of the mak nyah sex workers had experienced police harassment and abuse at the hands of religious authorities (double jeopardy), it was not surprising that none would report victimization to police. In our interviews, there emerged only one participant who formally filed a police report in response to a client who had stolen personal items from her. When another participant, Erica, was asked if she had ever reported her various experiences of being robbed or beaten by clients, she replied: "Never. Probably because of [my] status as a sex worker, therefore . . . would never be in front for reporting on what had happened." Many mak nyah suffered violence from clients, but they had little recourse to institutions that could support or protect them. The neglect of civil institutions to support mak nyah in reporting crimes is illustrated in the following examples, in which mak nyah shared their experiences of violence:

> Before having sex, he robbed me, all his friends came, I was frightened, gave him money, I said please don't beat me, don't do anything to me, you want money, I have money, but it is not much, it is only this much I have. I gave him the money, he gave me RM10 to get home. (Susan, 41 years old, Malay)

> I was working, there were three guys in a car, the driver came out, my friends had ran away, I was dizzy after exposing myself to the rain, it was six in the morning, I didn't expect he came that way. . . . The moment he came close [to] me, I've stood up, he kicked at me straight away, and I ran, I fall down, he came again, he kept on kicking me, then he ran away. (Jane, 24 years old, Malay)

Healthcare Access, Gender Transitions

Our interviews with mak nyah explored their experiences at clinics, with healthcare providers, and regarding the biomedical management of gender identity. Malaysian citizens are able to receive healthcare provided by the state, but mak nyah face multiple barriers to receiving quality healthcare. The majority of mak nyah encountered discrimination in clinic settings when attempting to receive medical treatments or advice for their health concerns. The absence of established standards of transgender healthcare was part of this pattern of discrimination and neglect that mak nyah faced in meeting their health needs.

CLINICAL ENCOUNTERS Many mak nyah shared their experiences of discrimination in healthcare settings. Some of their encounters with medical staff left them feeling that they were an object of revulsion, which was especially devastating because they were suffering and in desperate need of care. Sabrina, a 43-year-old Malay, described her experience needing care at a hospital, which was met with disgust by hospital staff: "The treatment at _____, when we want to check, they ask loudly: 'What sickness do you have?' The way they talk is rude, saucy, [and] they don't say in a nice way, polite way. The way they talk showed they are disgusted that we are a *Pondans* [gay]. There was once, I wanted to do dressing for the wounds, the doctor felt disgusting to do it, I told the doctor, it is ok, never mind if you don't want to do it. I went back and told PT (Pink Triangle Foundation) staff that the doctor there was rude."

Not all discrimination toward mak nyah was overtly hostile but, rather, fostered an uncomfortable and even intimidating environment for mak nyah who sought care. Bianca, a 33-year-old Malay, described the microaggression of the staff toward her gender presentation: "I been to a hospital, I don't [know] whether the staff there [are] well trained or not. When they saw people like me, they something like show face. There is something lack of respect."

When asked how she felt about the healthcare services she received at the hospital, Erica, a 35-year-old, replied: "At hospital, definitely quite difficult, one of those was if we took the STI or HIV/AIDS test, when reached the hospital, when he/she knew exactly what our status, they will begin, one said this, one said that, one would look as if we're like animals."

However, not all mak nyah had universally negative experiences with public healthcare. Susan, a 41-year-old Malay, describes the support and encouragement she received to adhere to her HIV medications and return for her follow-up appointments: "Good, the doctors and nurses don't insult, they really are helpful, supportive so that I could get well. They told me, you want to be healthy, you take medicine. They are really helpful, really are helping us. They said, remember, when the medication finished, when the doctor asks you to come on certain dates, you don't refuse to come, and you must come. I follow his instruction, I have never missed it."

Many mak nyah reported their preferences for private clinics over governmental ones, despite the costs these health visits incurred. A shared understanding emerged among several mak nyah participants who expressed their beliefs that private medical clinics were not as hostile to them. Ann, a 27-year-old Malay, compared the care she received at a publicly funded clinic with visits to a private clinic, which she paid for: "Although people have been saying there is no discrimination (at public hospitals), actually there was, they stared at me, then whispering, but I just don't care at that time, because I thought of getting well soon. . . . At private clinic, we pay, so they really treat us well. It is a bit different from government-owned clinic."

TRANSGENDER HEALTHCARE Since the fatwa banning gender-reassignment surgery was enacted in 1982, there have been no settings in Kuala Lumpur where these services are available. Overall, mak nyah healthcare services, particularly for cross-gender hormone therapy and gender-affirmation surgeries, are virtually nonexistent. The state does not provide cross-gender hormone therapy and other medical treatments for gender transition; therefore, mak nyah seek hormones and related care elsewhere, usually at high costs and without medical follow-up or clinical monitoring. All mak nyah participants in our study had used hormones to enhance their gender identity and expression and described obtaining hormones outside medical settings. The unpredictability of accessing hormones presented difficulties in adhering to any hormone regimen. Bella's discussion of her hormone use illustrates the irregularities of her access to and intake of hormones:

> For the injection is every two weeks, but sometimes it becomes every three weeks, sometimes becomes one month, depending on my time. Normally I try to keep it within two weeks, twice a month. For the anti-androgen, I would take one tablet per day, fifty milligrams, normally after I finish fifty tablets, I would take a break, and I will stop for a while, normally about a month. [RA asked: Is it the advice from the doctor?] No, unfortunately in Malaysia we don't have doctors who officially prescribe any hormone therapy regimen, none, in my case is more like you have to Google, you do a bit of research, you look at Internet, you have to trial and error as well. . . . Most of my information I get it from Internet. Not many clinics are willing to provide the information. The only clinic I can remember provide this kind of information although you have to pay for it is _____. There is lack of expertise within this field and that's why

we look at the transsexual community in Malaysia, a lot of them are doing things on trials and errors basis and unfortunately it also lead to a lot of medical complications as well.

In the following exchange, Rowena, a 40-year-old Malay, and a research assistant discussed how she obtained hormones from friends. In the absence of medical care and clinical monitoring of her hormone use, Rowena used her peers as a gauge to assess that her hormone intake was relatively safe, noting that she did not know anyone who died because of her hormone use.

RA: Where do you buy [hormones]?
Rowena: Buy from friends, don't know friends got from where.
RA: How much they charge for the pill?
Rowena: One box, three pills for RM40 to 50, I just found out.
RA: But no doctor's advice; are you worried?
Rowena: No, *lah.* Last time, I almost 100 percent be mak nyah I never worry. But the risk is low, never heart, at age 40, those whom I know, never heard they died because of eating hormone, because of this. Maybe it is mind-set, *lah,* thinking, never really thought.

Lily, 46 years old and Chinese, was one of only two mak nyah in our study who had undergone genital reconstruction surgery. She had recently started using hormones again following her surgery, after a period of discontinuation:

RA: Currently are you still taking hormone?
Lily: Hormone injection is Proluton Depot [hydroxyprogesterone hexanoate].
RA: How often do you have the injection?
Lily: One month once, one time two doses.
RA: Where do you get the injection?
Lily: Is in the clinic,———.
RA: How much they charge?
Lily: RM80.
RA: Did the doctor advise you before the injection?
Lily: No.

RA: So you just go there and the nurse will give you the injection?
Lily: Yes.

Some participants recalled surgical procedures they had wanted in the past or were hoping to undergo in the future. Until 1983, when the fatwa outlawed gender-reassignment surgery for all Muslims (the language of the fatwa offers an exception for "hermaphrodites"), mak nyah did not have to travel to Thailand (the destination for most mak nayh to obtain surgeries). Even if mak nyah could afford and arrange for such a surgery, they would face barriers in receiving medical monitoring and follow-up, especially because knowledge and expertise in gender-affirmation surgeries are not required or monitored by medical service providers licensed by the Malaysian government. The absence of care and support by the government for mak nyah who seek gender-affirmation surgeries and hormone therapy presented clear risks to their overall health and well-being.

DISCUSSION

To date, there have been only a few research studies that illustrate the range of health, social, and economic challenges that mak nyah sex workers face in Malaysia (Teh, 2002; Teh, 2008; Gibson et al., 2016). On the basis of in-depth qualitative interviews, we further described the lives of mak nyah sex workers in contemporary Kuala Lumpur and explored the interwoven contexts of their unmet health needs for mak nyah—specific healthcare, fear and vulnerability as sex workers, criminalization and persecution that is based on civil and sharia law, harassment and abuse by police and religious authorities, and substance use to cope with stress and discrimination. Though facing a number of challenges in their everyday lives, mak nyah participants showed their resiliency to protect themselves from violence at the hands of customers and police and adjustment skills to get healthcare (e.g., going to private clinics).

Findings from our interviews with mak nyah illustrated the relevance of theories of intersectionality to understand the interactive effects of the various social categories they inhabit. The concept of intersectionality, and its application to public health, posits that social categories are "multiple, interdependent, and mutually constitutive" (Bowleg, 2012, p. 1268). Data from this study underscore the idea that mak nyah's engagement in sex work and their lived experiences as mak nyah had synergistic effects. The ongoing threats of criminalization and religious persecution exacerbated mak nyah's health risks and barriers to accessing care. Similarly, poverty and employment discrimination magnified the vulnerabilities they encountered as sex workers, and substance use further entrenched them in the sex trade.

Our findings illustrate that the majority of mak nyah lacked access to education and training that would have enabled them to find employment other than sex work. And even those mak nyah with trade school or some university education faced significant barriers to regular employment. Employment discrimination against transgender persons is widely practiced, and consequently many become involved in commercial sex (Wong, 2005). This study clearly shows that discrimination in the workplace was a salient factor that structured mak nyah involvement with sex work.

A few mak nyah reported some satisfaction with sex work, most often citing their participation in a community of other mak nyah and quick money to sustain their survival needs. However, these accounts were more often eclipsed by the uncertainties and vulnerabilities they faced in the sex trade. Mak nyah who exercised the most control over their conditions of sex work—namely, those who conducted sex work outside street settings—seemed to experience the least amount of stigma and harm. It was in street settings that the mak nyah seemed most vulnerable to risk from civil police and JAWI. A study of *kathoey* (transwomen) sex workers in Bangkok, Thailand, revealed that street-based settings had exposed kathoey sex workers to riskier situations than controlled commercial venues, such as bars and clubs, in terms of possible infection with HIV/STIs and exposure to violence (Nemoto et al., 2016). The authors recommended venue-specific HIV prevention and health promotion programs for kathoey sex workers. There is a significant difference between mak nyah and kathoey sex workers; specifically, the number of controlled work environments, such as massage parlors and bars or clubs where mak nyah can solicit customers, is limited because mak nyah cannot reveal their identities at any workplaces, and businesses cannot openly hire mak nyah. One mak nyah participant mentioned using the Internet for soliciting and screening customers to increase her safety and negotiation power.

This study's findings demonstrate the effects of a lack of access to resources, such as hormone therapy, gender-affirming surgeries, and interventions that follow biomedical and psychosocial standards of care as outlined by the World Professional Association for Transgender Health (2016). Mak nyah cannot get access to hormones through legitimate medical service providers, and no participant had enrolled in hormone therapy through the state hospitals. They obtained hormones from a variety of sources, such as friends and the Internet. They often relied on knowledge gained from friends or websites. Because they had neither prescriptions nor monitoring by medical professionals, their hormone intake varied in dosage and frequency. One participant revealed her idea about the safety of her hormone use: none of her friends died of hormone overdose. Two of the eighteen mak nyah had undergone gender reconstruction surgeries. Three participants had undergone vaginoplasty and breast augmentation and five had completed surgeries to enlarge their hips or breasts (or both). The majority of the mak nyah underwent surgeries in Thailand, a popular destination for gender-affirmation surgeries (Aizura, 2010). None of the mak nyah participants reported whether she had received follow-up care upon her return to Malaysia. Widespread underground hormone use and gender-affirming surgeries in Thailand among mak nyah highlight their disparate needs for access to mak nyah–specific medical care.

Mak nyah have persisted in carving out meanings and practices that support their experiences as women, but the denial by medicolegal regulation of gender-affirming surgeries and care for mak nyah is unjust and needs to be corrected through political and community movements as part of country-level policy changes to increase and ensure human rights for mak nyah and other gender and sexual minorities. Suzie's remarks illustrate how mak nyah develop and enact a robust ontology of what being a woman means to them that both challenges the primacy of biomedicine in defining mak nyah and defies the force of the 1983 fatwa banning gender-affirmation surgeries. Like Suzie, many mak nyah locate their gender identities and expressions through a series of social roles and responsibilities that affirm their status as women. Suzie, 51 years old and Chinese Melano, replied to a question about her desire to undergo gender-affirmation surgery: "Darling, I don't need it. I am comfortable [with] what I am. You know what, transgender is not about sexuality; it's about our brain. It's your mind, my mind says oh, I am a woman, so I am a woman. Even though

I am transsexual, but to me, I am a woman. I am living my life as a woman. Because of my partner, I am a woman. From the way I treated him, I do housework, I do everything, laundry, cooking, everything. That makes me feel like I am a woman."

Suzie clearly presented her idea of women that conforms to traditional roles. Future research needs to further investigate the development of gender identity among mak nyah, particularly in relation to normative gender roles defined by Malaysian society, religion, and ethnic culture.

According to the activist and scholar Khartini Slamah, the term *mak nyah*, which derives from *mother*, was coined in 1987 as members of this group sought "to define ourselves from a vantage point of dignity rather than from the position of derogation" (Slamah, 2006, p. 99). We believe that mak nyah's willingness to take part in this study and share their everyday lived experiences provides a necessary counterpoint to the routinely negative beliefs about and mischaracterizations of them, and yields insights about their lives that are salient for public health, civil police, JAWI, and other institutions. The SEED Foundation, where we recruited the study participants, has been providing health promotion, legal, and other services to mak nyah in Kuala Lumpur. Researchers, including us, must collaborate with them to advocate for ensuring basic human rights for mak nyah through presenting compelling scientific data.

In addition to its strengths, this study also has several limitations that may be addressed by further research. Mak nyah are generally a hidden population, and purposive and snowball sampling was deemed to be the most culturally appropriate recruitment and sampling strategy for this study, although these findings may not be representative of general mak nyah populations who engage in sex work in Kuala Lumpur. The consistency of this research with previous studies supports the validity of our findings.

ACKNOWLEDGMENT

This study was supported by the National Institute on Drug Abuse (principal investigator, Tooru Nemoto, grant no. R21DA033869). The opinions and recommendations expressed in this study are solely those of the authors and do not necessarily represent the views of the National Institute on Drug Abuse.

REFERENCES

Aizura, A. Z. (2010). Feminine transformations: Gender reassignment surgical tourism in Thailand. *Medical Anthropology, 29* (4), 424–443.

Ayres, L., Kavanaugh, K., & Knafl, K. A. (2003). Within-case and across-case approaches to qualitative data analysis. *Qualitative Health Research, 13* (6), 871–883.

Baral, S., Poteat, T., Strömdahl, S., Wirtz, A. W., Guadamuz, T. E., & Beyrer, C. (2013). Worldwide burden of HIV in transgender women: A systematic review and meta-analysis. *Lancet Infectious Diseases, 13,* 214–222.

Bowleg, L. (2012). The problem with the phrase *women and minorities*: Intersectionality—an important theoretical framework for public health. *American Journal of Public Health, 102* (7), 1267–1273.

Charette, D. E. (2006). Malaysia in the global economy: Crisis, recovery, and the road ahead. *New England Journal of Public Policy, 21* (1), 55–78.

Chee, H. L. (2008). Ownership, control, and contention: Challenges for the future of healthcare in Malaysia. *Social Science & Medicine, 66,* 2145–2156.

Gibson, B. A., Brown, S., Rutledge, R., Jeffrey, A., Wickersham, A. K., & Altice, F. L. (2016). Gender identity, healthcare access, and risk reduction among Malaysia's mak nyah community. *Global Public Health, 11* (7), 1010–1025.

Goh, B. L. (2008). Globalization and postcolonial nation in Malaysia: Theoretical challenges and historical possibilities. *Kasarinlan: Philippine Journal of Third World Studies, 23* (2), 4–19.

Goh, J. N. (2012a). Mary and the mak nyahs: Queer theological imaginings of Malaysian male-to-female transsexuals. *Theology & Sexuality, 18* (3), 215–233.

———. (2012b). Abuse of gender-variant people and religious justifications for trans-persecution. *Queer Asian Spirit E-Zine, 1.* Retrieved from www.queerasianspirit.org/qas-e-zine-volume-1.html.

Hirschman, C. (1986). The making of race in colonial Malaya: Political economy and racial ideology. *Sociological Forum, 1* (2), 328–361.

Human Rights Watch. (2014, September 24). "I'm scared to be a woman": Human rights abuses against transgender people in Malaysia. Retrieved from https://www.hrw.org/report/2014/09/24/im-scared-be-woman/human-rights-abuses-against-transgender-people-malaysia.

Ling-Chien Neo, J. (2006). Malay nationalism, Islamic supremacy and the constitutional bargain in the multi-ethnic composition of Malaysia. *International Journal on Minority and Group Rights, 13,* 95–118.

Ministry of Health Malaysia, HIV/STI Section. (2016). *Global AIDS response progress report.* Retrieved from www.moh.gov.my.

———. (2015). *Global AIDS response progress report.* Retrieved from www.moh.gov.my.

Mok, T. Y., Gan, C., & Sanyal, A. (2007). The determinants of urban household poverty in Malaysia. *Journal of Social Sciences, 3* (4), 190–196.

Nemoto, T., Cruz, T., Iwamoto, M., Trocki, K., Perngparn, U., Areesantichai, C., . . . & Robert, C. (2016). Examining the sociocultural context of HIV-related risk behaviors among kathoey (male-to-female transgender women) sex workers in Bangkok, Thailand. *Journal of the Association of Nurses in AIDS Care, 27* (2), 153–165. doi:10.1016/j.jana.2015.11.003.

Peletz, M. G. (2006). Transgenderism and gender pluralism in Southeast Asia since early modern times. *Current Anthropology, 47* (2), 309–340.

Samsul, D., Razman, M. R., Ramli, M., Mohd Aznan, M. A., Maliya, S., Muhamad Shaiful Lizam, M. A., . . . & Mohamad Faquihuddin, H. (2016). Knowledge and attitude towards HIV/AIDS among transsexuals in Kuantan, Pahang. *International Medical Journal Malaysia, 15* (1), 45–50.

Sandelowski, M. (2000). Whatever happened to qualitative description? *Research in Nursing & Health, 23* (4), 334–340.

Shamsul, A. B. (1997). The economic dimension of Malay nationalism: The socio-historic roots of the new economic policy and its contemporary implications. *Developing Economies, 35* (3), 240–261.

Slamah, K. (2006). The struggle to be ourselves, neither men nor women: Mak nyahs in Malaysia. *In* R. Chandiramani & G. Misra (eds.), *Sexuality, gender, and rights: Exploring theory and practice in South and South East Asia* (pp. 98–112). Thousand Oaks, CA: Sage Publications.

Stivens, M. (2006). "Family values" and Islamic revival: Gender, rights, and state moral projects in Malaysia. *Women's Studies International Forum, 29,* 354–367.

Teh, Y. K. (2008). HIV-related needs for safety among male-to-female transsexuals (mak nyah) in Malaysia. *SAHARA-J: Journal of Social Aspects of HIV/AIDS, 5* (4), 178–185.

———. (2002). *The mak nyahs: Malaysian male to female transsexuals.* Singapore: Eastern Universities Press.

———. (1998). Understanding the problems of mak nyah (male transsexuals) in Malaysia. *South East Asia Research, 6,* 165–180.

Thompson, E. (2003). Malay male migrants: Negotiated contested identities in Malaysia. *American Ethnologist, 30* (3), 418–438.

Vanwesenbeeck, I. (2001). Another decade of social scientific work on sex work: A review of research, 1990–2000. *Annual Review of Sex Research, 12,* 242–289.

Wei, C. L., Baharuddin, A., Abdullah, R., Abdullah, Z., & Por Chhe Ern, K. (2012). Transgenderism in Malaysia. *Journal of Dharma, 37* (1), 79–96.

Wong, E. L. (2005, February 1). Neither here nor there: The legal dilemma of the transsexual community in Malaysia. *Malaysian Bar.* Retrieved from www.malaysianbar.org.my/gender_issues/neither_here_nor_there_the_legal_dilemma_of_the_transsexual_community_in_malaysia.html.

World Bank. (2016). *World development indicators: GDP* [Data file]. Retrieved from http://data.worldbank.org/data-catalog/world-development-indicators.

World Professional Association for Transgender Health. (2016). *Standards of Care for the Health of Transsexual, Transgender, and Gender Non-Conforming People* (7th ed.). Retrieved from www.wpath.org.

CHAPTER 18

Sociocultural Context of Health among Kathoey (Transwomen) and Female Sex Workers in Bangkok, Thailand

Tooru Nemoto[1]
Usaneya Perngparn[2]
Chitlada Areesantichai[2]
Charlene Bumanglag[3]
Mariko Iwamoto[1]
Julia Moore[1]

1 Public Health Institute, Oakland, CA.
2 College of Public Health Sciences, Chulalongkorn University, Bangkok.
3 John A. Burns School of Medicine, University of Hawaii, Manoa.

SUMMARY

Although prostitution is illegal in Thailand, a number of *kathoey* (male-to-female transgender women) and women engage in sex work mainly for economic reasons. Both kathoey sex workers (KSW) and female sex workers (FSWs) face health risks, such as sexually transmitted infections (STIs), substance abuse, and violence; however, risk behaviors and surrounding environmental and sociocultural contexts significantly differ.

KEY TERMS

female sex worker; kathoey; sex work; Thailand; transwomen

Nuttbrock, Larry, *Transgender Sex Work and Society*
dx.doi.org/10.17312/harringtonparkpress/2017.11.tsws.018
© 2018 by Harrington Park Press

The HIV epidemic in Thailand began in the mid-1980s (Family Health International and Ministry of Public Health, Thailand, 2008). The number of reported HIV cases in Thailand is particularly high compared to that in other Asian countries (Dokubo et al., 2013; Park et al., 2010). Prostitution (sex work) has been illegal in Thailand since 1960. Rather than eliminating prostitution, however, the Thai government has moved toward controlling sex work (Hannenberg & Rojanapithayakorn, 1998). These controls are made possible because sex work occurs mainly at commercial sex establishments, performed by a few sex workers who freelance their services. Reports document female sex workers (FSWs) and more recently male sex workers, though national reports for sex work involvement among transgender women (kathoey) are unclear.

Sex work has historically been perceived and documented as "female" work and not "male" work. Further, even if shifts to move away from classifying kathoey in the category of men who have sex with men (MSM), governmental practices and reporting still consider kathoey as MSM. A national campaign for HIV prevention has encouraged the general Thai population to increase condom use (e.g., 100% condom use among FSWs) and drastically lowered HIV prevalence in heterosexual populations (Park et al., 2010; Punpanich, Ungchusak, & Detels, 2004). However, HIV prevalence has not declined among MSM, including kathoey, but has remained stable, near 30% (Centers for Disease Control and Prevention, 2013; van Griensven et al., 2010). Despite a lack of government data on HIV prevalence among kathoey, recent studies have focused on kathoey or kathoey sex workers (KSWs) in terms of HIV prevention, health promotion, and human rights advocacy.

There is a growing body of literature about HIV prevalence among sex workers, including men and transwomen sex workers. A special issue of the *Lancet* in 2015 addressed structural determinants of HIV, community empowerment, human rights violations, and an action agenda among FSWs and transgender sex workers (TGSWs). Biomedical, behavioral, and structural interventions tailored to the cultural context have been shown to be effective for FSWs (Bekker et al., 2015). The five levels of intervention include biological (level 1) (e.g., pre-exposure prophylaxis [PrEP]), network (level 2), community-based advocacy (level 3), environmental or policy factors (level 4) (e.g., locations of sex exchange or transactions), and the epidemic context (level 5). Existing prevention strategies, which include condom provision, control of STIs, HIV testing and counseling, and gender-based violence prevention interventions, have been scaled up as the HIV epidemic expands. New prevention strategies have been advocated, including PrEP, post-exposure prophylaxis (PEP), and earlier treatment of HIV for FSWs.

In the context of human rights, violations place sex workers at risk for HIV infections (Decker et al., 2015), as has been documented in Russia, Serbia, Mexico City, Nepal, Slovakia, Namibia, the United States, Kenya, and Uganda. Not only are sex workers vulnerable to HIV infections, but they also suffer risks of homicide; police repression, extortion, and physical and sexual abuse; police interference in possession of condoms and syringes; discrimination in access to justice; forced rehabilitation and detention; violence; unsafe working conditions and an absence of labor protection; institutional discrimination (e.g., discrimination in access to health and welfare services); mandatory and forced HIV testing and health examinations; and criminalization of sex work through punitive law. Therefore, the human rights framework for policy change, such as decriminalization of sex work, was recommended by the United Nations High Commissioner for Human Rights and UNAIDS (Decker et al., 2015). Community empowerment and health promotion interventions (e.g., HIV/STI testing and treatment, free condom distribution, and PrEP) are strongly advocated, as are increasing human rights for sex workers.

The World Health Organization (WHO) advises that persons diagnosed with HIV initiate antiretroviral therapy (ART) regardless of their CD4 count (World Health Organization, 2015). In October 2014 Thailand implemented this guideline for ART (National AIDS Committee, 2015). While the UNAIDS GAP Report indicates that HIV testing among FSWs in Thailand was 50% to 75% in 2010–2015, HIV testing among KSWs was unreported (UNAIDS, 2016a). There are an estimated 445,000 people living with HIV/AIDS (PLHIV) in Thailand; 84% knew their status, 76% were on ART, and 34% were virally suppressed (UNAIDS, 2016a).

A meta-analysis reported a higher HIV prevalence for transwomen engaging in sex work (27.3%) compared with those not engaging in sex work (14.7%) (Operario, Soma, & Underhill, 2008). Another meta-analysis reported that transwomen were 48.8 times more likely to be infected with HIV than all adults of reproductive age (Baral et al., 2013). High HIV prevalence was attributed to their engagement in sex work and substance use, exposure to transphobia, and lack of access to transgender-sensitive healthcare services (Nemoto et al., 2005; Nemoto et al., 2006; Sugano, Nemoto, & Operario, 2006). Transwomen sex workers face structural, interpersonal, and individual levels of vulnerability to HIV (van Griensven, Na Ayutthaya, & Wilson, 2013; Poteat et al., 2014). Most preoperative transwomen engage in receptive and insertive anal sex that elevates their vulnerability to HIV, much as it does MSM's; however, their gender identification and expression and social marginalization further elevate their risks of HIV (Baral et al., 2013; Herbst et al., 2008; van Griensven et al., 2013). Socioeconomic factors also contribute to their HIV risk (e.g., housing instability, discrimination in the job market, poverty, and a lack of access to health services) (De Santis, 2009; Poteat, German, & Kerrigan, 2013).

Risk behaviors and high HIV seroprevalence among kathoey in Thailand were reported (12% in Bangkok, 18% in Chiang Mai, and 12% in Phuket), and particularly among those engaged in sex work (17%) (Wimonsate et al., 2006). Furthermore, kathoey reported coerced sex more often than MSM (Guadamuz et al., 2011), and only 29% of kathoey reported using a condom during their last anal sex encounter (Chemnasiri et al., 2006). Our recent study showed that kathoey sex workers had engaged in unsafe sex with customers, as well as sex under the influence of substances (Nemoto et al., 2012). Though high HIV prevalence and risk behaviors have been identified among KSWs who tend to work side by side with FSWs in Bangkok, little research has sought to differentiate the sociocultural context of risk behaviors among KSWs compared with FSWs. HIV prevention and health promotion programs have to be tailored to the target groups in intersecting individual and structural factors (e.g., health outcomes, risk behaviors, and sociocultural context). The current study aims to illustrate risk behaviors in relation to sociocultural factors among KSWs in comparison to FSWs and provide scientific evidence for future intervention programs specific to KSWs and FSWs in Thailand.

METHODS

The current study used two data sets that were collected from a study targeting KSWs in 2006 and another study targeting FSWs in 2005. These two studies used a similar survey questionnaire and recruitment methods. During the preparation period, we trained Thai female and kathoey interviewers regarding recruitment and data collection procedures, as well as obtaining informed consent. First, female and kathoey interviewers conducted mapping in the targeted areas in Bangkok; they first identified the location of commercial venues and areas where FSWs and KSWs solicited customers, and they then collected information about those work environments using an environmental checklist. We described the environment using the following factors: location or area, approximate numbers of FSWs and KSWs per business venue, solicitation methods, age groups, types of customers (e.g., local Thai and foreigner or tourist), and hours of operation. Also, street corners where FSWs and KSWs solicited customers were identified. Locations were categorized into three types: (1) the street, (2) bars and clubs (e.g., go-go bars and karaoke bars), and (3) massage parlors (only for FSWs). Using the mapping data, the trained Thai interviewers approached potential participants and screened them for eligibility: (1) age of 18 years or older, (2) self-identification as female or kathoey, (3) engaged in sex work in Bangkok at that time, and (4) ability to communicate in Thai. After obtaining informed consent, the interviewers administered a survey in person in a place where participants' privacy was ensured. A total of 112 KSWs and 205 FSWs completed the survey. A survey interview took about one hour, on average. Participants received financial compensation after completing the survey and were provided with information about HIV/STI testing and given health promotion pamphlets. The study protocols were approved by the Committee on Human Research, University of California – San Francisco and the Ethical Committee for Research Involving Human Subjects and/or Use of Animals in Research, Health Science Group of Faculties, College and Institute, Chulalongkorn University, Thailand.

MEASURES

The survey questions about HIV-related sexual and drug use behaviors and demographics were modified from those used for our previous studies among Asian FSWs who worked at massage parlors in San Francisco (Nemoto et al., 2003) and Vietnamese FSWs in Ho Chi Minh City, Vietnam (Nemoto et al., 2008). The questionnaire consisted of anchored questions and Likert-type measurements, asking about drug use and HIV-related sexual behaviors with customers and nonpaying private partners, access to HIV/STI testing and healthcare services, history of STIs, and demographic information. The psychosocial measurements included (1) AIDS knowledge (ten true-or-false questions about HIV transmission), (2) subjective norms toward practicing safe sex (α =.72), (3) perceived economic pressure (α = .64), and (4) self-esteem (Rosenberg, 1965) (α = .79). Other than the true-or-false questions used to gauge AIDS transmission knowledge, other measurements used a five-point Likert scale (1 = strongly disagree to 5 = strongly agree). The measurements of AIDS knowledge, norms toward practicing safe sex, and economic pressure were taken from our previous studies (Nemoto et al., 2003; Nemoto et al., 2006). The survey questionnaire and informed consent form were translated into Thai and carefully examined for their validity and cultural compatibility by Thai researchers associated with this study. Statistical analyses were conducted to compare two groups (KSWs and FSWs) on the basis of chi-square or t-test and linear regression analyses on risk behaviors.

PARTICIPANT CHARACTERISTICS

Participants had a mean age of 27 years (SD = 6.9), ranging from 18 to 58 years. KSWs (m = 25 years) were younger than FSWs (m = 28 years) ($p < .01$) (Table 18.1). KSWs were more likely to be single (87.5%), and FSWs were more likely to be married (28.3%) or divorced (52.2%). More FSWs (71.1%) reported an education level of less than high school, compared with KSWs (38.4%) ($p < .01$). However, 33% of FSWs reported a monthly income of more than 40,000 baht (about $1,207), compared with 11.9% of KSWs ($p < .01$).

RESULTS

Work Environment

There was a significant difference in work venues where KSWs and FSWs were recruited: KSWs—29% from the street and 71% from bars or clubs; and FSWs—13% from the street, 48% from bars or clubs, 10% from brothels, and 29% from massage parlors. There were significant differences in working conditions between KSWs and FSWs. Both groups worked about six days a week, but KSWs (m = 6 hours) worked fewer hours per day than FSWs (m = 8 hours) (see Table 18.1). On average, FSWs had had sex with three times more customers per week (m = 12 customers) than KSWs (m = 4). Also, more FSWs reported having had jobs other than sex work (16%) than KSWs (8%) ($p < .05$). In gen-

TABLE 18.1

Demographic Characteristics

	KSWs (N = 112) %	FSWs (N = 205) %	Total (N = 317) %	χ^2	t
Age (years)	25.0	27.9	26.9		3.66***
Marital status				139.44***	
Single	87.5	19.5	43.5		
Married	9.8	28.3	21.8		
Divorced/separated/widowed	2.7	52.2	34.7		
Educational attainment				34.29***	
Less than high school	38.4	71.1	59.6		
High school/vocational school graduate	54.5	27.3	36.9		
College graduate	7.1	1.5	3.5		
Monthly income (baht)				44.49***	
Less than 12,000 (< $362)	0.9	7.3	5.0		
12,001–24,000 (≈ $362–$724)	18.8	18.0	18.3		
24,001–40,000 (≈ $724–$1,207)	67.9	35.1	46.7		
40,001–60,000 (≈ $1,207–$1,811)	11.6	21.0	17.7		
More than 60,001 (> $1,811)	0.3	12.0	12.3		
Seen healthcare provider (past 12 months)	0.9	98.0	63.7	295.75***	
Received HIV prevention information (past 12 months)	89.3	100.0	96.1	21.74***	

	KSWs (N = 112) %	FSWs (N = 205) %	Total (N = 317) %	χ^2	t
Ever been tested for HIV	52.7	99.5	83.0	112.41***	
Work conditions					
Work hours per day	6.1	8.2	7.5		8.97***
Number of work days per week	6.1	5.8	5.9		ns
Number of customers per week	4.0	11.8	9.0		8.31***
Send money to family	75.0	87.3	83.0	7.78**	
Have job other than sex work	8.0	16.0	13.0	4.16*	
Psychosocial measures					
AIDS knowledge[a]	7.3	6.4	6.8		ns
Subjective norms toward practicing safe sex[b]	4.0	3.6	3.8		–5.41***
Self-esteem[b]	3.8	3.8	3.8		ns
Economic pressure[b]	2.8	3.0	2.9		ns

NOTE: *ns* = not significant.
[a] Mean score out of 10 items.
[b] Five-point Likert scale (1 = strongly disagree to 5 = strongly agree).
*$p < .05$. **$p < .01$. ***$p < .001$.

eral, the major reason for engaging in sex work was economic necessity or survival; however, significantly more FSWs (87%) sent money to their families at home than KSWs (75%). And, a significantly higher number of FSWs (86%) reported their willingness to engage in unsafe sex for extra money than KSWs (35%).

HIV/STI Testing

Only one KSW reported having seen doctors in the previous 12 months, compared with 98% of FSWs. Nearly all FSWs reported having being tested for HIV (99.5%), compared with only 53% of KSWs. Only one FSW reported living with HIV. As only one KSW reported having seen a doctor, no KSWs reported having been tested for STIs, whereas a high percentage of FSWs reported being infected with STIs in the preceding 12 months (91% for chlamydia; 22% for gonorrhea; 20% for genital herpes).

Hormone Use among KSWs

Almost all KSWs (97%) reported having ever used hormones, and 79% reported current use. Injecting hormones was common (86% of participants in their lifetime); however, no participant reported having ever shared needles or syringes with others for hormone injection. In addition, 58% reported having ever injected silicone.

Substance Use Behaviors

Significantly higher percentages of KSWs reported using substances in their lifetimes and over the previous 12 months (Table 18.2). In the preceding 12 months, significantly more KSWs reported drinking alcohol and using marijuana and ecstasy than FSWs (99% vs. 94%, 32% vs. 22%, and 36% vs. 11%, respectively). There was no significant difference in amphetamine use in the previous 12 months between the two groups (9.8% in each group). In their lifetimes, there was no significant difference on alcohol use between the two groups; however, more KSWs reported use of illicit drugs than did FSWs (marijuana: 51% vs. 32%; amphetamines: 32% vs. 22%; ecstasy: 51% vs. 12%, respectively). Only KSWs reported using ketamine in the previous 12 months and in their lifetimes.

Sexual Behaviors

In the previous six months, a significantly higher number of FSWs (79.0%) reported not always using condoms with customers for anal or vaginal sex than KSWs did (26.4%). Similarly, a significantly higher number of FSWs (79.0%) reported not always using condoms with nonpaying partners than did KSWs (26.9%). Significantly higher numbers of KSWs had engaged in sex with customers under the influence of alcohol in the preceding six months than had FSWs: 98.2% vs. 79.5%.

We conducted two multiple linear regression analyses on the frequency of condom use for vaginal or anal sex with customers and of

TABLE 18.2

HIV-Related Risk Behaviors

	KSWs (N = 112)	FSWs (N = 204)	Total (N = 316)	χ^2
	%	%	%	
Inconsistent condom use for anal/vaginal sex with customers in past 6 months	26.4	79.0	60.6	83.17*
Inconsistent condom use for anal/vaginal sex with non-paying partners	26.9	79.0	61.5	79.09*
Willing to have unprotected sex with customers for extra money	34.8	85.9	67.08	86.43*
Substance use behaviors				
Substance use in the past 12 months				
Alcohol	99.1	94.1	95.9	4.56*
Marijuana	32.1	22.1	25.6	3.86*
Amphetamines (yaba)	9.8	9.8	9.8	a
Ketamine	19.6	a	19.6	a
Ecstasy	35.7	10.9	19.7	28.02*
Substance use in lifetime				
Alcohol	99.1	99.0	99.1	ns
Marijuana	50.9	31.9	38.6	11.05*
Amphetamines (yaba)	32.1	22.1	25.6	3.86*
Ketamine	28.6	a	28.6	a
Ecstasy	50.9	11.8	25.6	58.07*
Having sex under the influence of substances in the past six months				
Alcohol use with customers	98.2	79.5	21.47*	
Drug use with customers Number of customers	26.9	83.1	79.8	0.72

NOTE: *ns* = not significant.
a No statistics are computed.
*p < .05.

having sex under the influence of drugs in the previous six months by entering the following variables: FSWs versus KSWs, age, the levels of education and income, subjective norms toward practicing safe sex, perceived economic pressure, and self-esteem (Tables 18.3a and 18.3b). Sex worker group and perceived economic pressure were independently and significantly correlated with the frequency of condom use with customers in the previous six months ($R^2 = .42$, F [7, 297] = 8.82); that is, KSWs compared with FSWs and those who felt a lesser degree of economic pressure were more likely to have used condoms with customers for vaginal or anal sex. Sex worker group and subjective norms toward practicing safe sex were independently and significantly correlated with the frequency of having sex under the influence of drugs in the preceding six months ($R^2 = .30$, F [7, 273] = 3.92); that is, KSWs compared with FSWs and those who had lower levels of subjective norms toward practicing safe sex were more likely to have engaged in sex under the influence of drugs in the previous months.

TABLE 18.3a

Multiple Linear Regression Analysis on Frequency of Condom Use for Vaginal or Anal Sex with Customers in the Previous Six Months

Variables	Beta	t
FSWs vs. KSWs[a]	5.42	5.42**
Age	-.06	-.98
Education level	-.02	-.36
Income	-.06	-.98
Norms toward practicing safe sex[b]	.03	.61
Economic pressure[b]	-.14	-2.40*
Self-esteem[b]	.09	1.69
$R^2 = .42$, F (7, 297) = 8.823, $p < .01$		

[a] Group 1 = FSW, 2 = KSW.
[b] Five-point scale (1 = "strongly disagree" to 5 = "strongly agree").
*$p < .05$. **$p < .01$.

TABLE 18.3b

Multiple Linear Regression Analysis on Frequency of Sex under the Influence of Drugs in the Previous Six Months

Variables	Beta	t
FSWs vs. KSWs[a]	.28	4.19**
Age	-.11	-1.78
Education level	-.12	-1.82
Income	.05	.78
Norms toward practicing safe sex[b]	-.13	-2.07*
Economic pressure[b]	-.03	-.49
Self-esteem[b]	-.02	-.33
R^2 = .30, F (7, 273) = 3.916, $p < .01$		

[a] Group 1 = FSW, 2 = KSW.
[b] Five-point scale (1 = "strongly disagree" to 5 = "strongly agree").
*$p < .05$. **$p < .01$.

DISCUSSION

KSWs and FSWs work closely with one another at venues and on the street in Bangkok, though very few KSWs work at massage parlors. Kathoey who completed gender-reassignment surgery (vaginoplasty) may engage in sex work as kathoey or women at various venues. A study showed 15.5% of kathoey sex worker participants reported vaginoplasty (Nemoto et al., 2012). However, there are no data on the numbers and description of postoperative kathoey who engage in sex work as women. Both KSWs and FSWs face health risks, such as sexually transmitted diseases (STDs) and HIV/AIDS, substance abuse, and violence; however, risk behaviors and surrounding environmental and sociocultural contexts significantly differ. Multivariate analyses of our current study clearly revealed that the type of sex workers (KSWs or FSWs) was strongly correlated with the frequency of condom use with customers and of sex under the influence of drugs in the previous six months. These analyses also revealed that study participants, regardless of whether they were KSWs or FSWs, who felt strong economic pressure less frequently used condoms with customers, and those who did not have strong norms to practice safe sex were more likely to engage in sex under the influence of drugs. The results confirmed the theory of reasoned action (Fishbein, Middelstadt, & Hitchcock, 1994); that is, behaviors or intended behaviors (e.g., practicing safe sex) are strongly influenced by the actor's perceived norms and attitudes toward the behaviors. Therefore, future HIV prevention programs for KSWs and FSWs must increase norms toward practicing safer sex and address issues of economic pressure among sex workers. Results of this study further pinpoint the sources of or reasons for economic pressure specific to KSWs and FSWs; most of all, distinctive factors that separate these two groups must be addressed for future HIV prevention and health promotion programs that are specific to KSWs or FSWs.

This study revealed that KSWs were younger, single, and better educated, worked fewer hours a day, and had a smaller number of customers than FSWs. Compared with KSWs, FSWs earned more money and were more likely to have jobs other than sex work. These background factors significantly differentiate KSWs from FSWs; however, our previous studies showed that within each group, these factors differed depending on the types of venues they worked (Nemoto et al., 2012, 2013). Female street sex workers were exposed to higher risk of HIV/STIs and violence than venue-based FSWs working at bars or clubs and massage parlors because sexual transactions among street FSWs occur at hotels, apartments, or cars that are chosen by customers, whereas venue-based FSWs are protected by managers of the venues, and the price for sexual transaction is often set by managers (Nemoto et al., 2013). Street-based FSWs tended to use illicit drugs (15% used *yaba*—amphetamines—or ecstasy) and have sex under the influence of drugs. In contrast, FSWs at massage parlors and bars or clubs tended to engage in sex with customers under the influence of alcohol. There were no significant differences on substance use and having had sex under the influence of substances between street and bar or club KSWs (Nemoto et al., 2012). The current study showed that KSWs were more likely to use illicit drugs and to have had sex with customers under the influence of substances than FSWs, though it should be noted that a high proportion of FSWs reported alcohol use (94.1%) in the previous 12 months and having had sex under the influence of alcohol with customers in the preceding six months (79.5%).

The work environment at bars or clubs puts KSWs and FSWs in a vulnerable situation for possible alcohol abuse or sex under the influence of alcohol with customers. Sex workers at bars and clubs receive a commission from those venues when their customers purchase drinks, and they tend to think that they can entertain customers through drinking with them for extra tips, or they can gain potential "regular" customers for the future. However, drinking influences judgment and elevates risk for HIV/STIs (Reisner et al., 2010). KSWs at bars and clubs stated the following (Nemoto et al., 2016): "I drink every day because I'll get money—a drinking commission from having customers drink with me. I won't be embarrassed to have sex after drinking. I can do whatever the customer tells me to. . . . I think drinking is part of my work and it's very much necessary" (p. 160); "I admit that I don't use condoms every time. For instance, I tend to forget when I'm drunk, or when I really like the customers" (p. 160). It would be very difficult to change the work environment at bars and clubs, where drinking is part of business and entertainment; however, it is possible to educate KSWs and FSWs that drinking alcohol will elevate their risks for exposure to HIV/STIs and violence, as well as to educate owners and managers of these venues that drinking can distract their employees' performance and lead to alcohol addiction and possibly diseases (e.g., HIV/STIs and sclerosis). Also, owners and managers could make the commission for consuming alcoholic and nonalcoholic beverages the same, which should discourage workers from drinking with customers.

In addition to alcohol use, illicit drug use among KSWs must be addressed: 35.7% ecstasy; 32.1% marijuana; 19.6% ketamine; 9.8% amphetamines (Nemoto et al., 2012). Kathoey are accepted in Thai society and receive some support from family members (Totman, 2003). However, our studies revealed that kathoey have been abused by family members (typically father and brothers), discriminated against in the job market, and exposed to transphobia (Nemoto et al., 2012, 2016). To avoid abuse and transphobia and pursue gender transition through medical interventions, many kathoey leave home and look for a better environment in Bangkok. Many kathoey engage in sex work because of limited job opportunities and to save money for gender-affirmation surgeries. More than 60% of KSWs in this study were high school or vocational school graduates or had a college degree, compared with 28.8% of FSWs. Stress that is due to the exposure to transphobia and limited job opportunities may trigger them to initiate or continue use of illicit drugs. Future research must address illicit drug use among KSWs and kathoey in general in relation to transphobia and gender transition issues.

As we previously described, economic pressure is a key factor in whether KSWs and FSWs engage in safe sex. The current study showed that both KSWs (75%) and FSWs (87%) sent money home to support their families, but a higher number of FSWs (86%) expressed their willingness to engage in unsafe sex with customers for extra money than KSWs (35%), even though FSWs earned more money than KSWs. In addition, the levels of economic pressure were higher among FSWs than KSWs. The majority of FSWs and KSWs had migrated from rural areas in Thailand and engaged in sex work for economic reasons; however, the passageway to sex work and current economic situation may differ between KSWs and FSWs. Many FSWs first work at factories or service sectors in Bangkok and surrounding areas. They are introduced to sex work by friends and often start working through business venues, not on the street. To earn higher incomes, FSWs often work at various business venues and on the street, where they can engage in freelance work, but where they get minimum protection from physical abuse, rape, and robbery. Our previous study showed an extremely demanding work environment among FSWs (Nemoto et al., 2013). For example, FSWs working at brothels reported working 11 hours a day, six days a week, and having 31 customers a week, on average. Future HIV prevention and health promotion programs need to address economic pressure on FSWs who are compelled to work hard and subjugate their bodies to male customers so that they can send money home. Our previous study showed that FSWs who had higher levels of self-esteem were more likely to use condoms with customers (Nemoto et al., 2013); this result showed strong resiliency and protection of their own bodies among some FSWs. It is important that future HIV prevention and health promotion programs for FSWs address their strengths and provide skills for managing income from sex work while maintaining good health and sending money home.

Like FSWs, KSWs who felt strong economic pressure were more likely to engage in unsafe sex; however, their sources of economic pressure might differ from those of FSWs. Three-quarters of KSW participants in the study reported sending money home, despite the fact that many of them escaped from transphobia and abuse at home. Our recent qualitative study revealed that the majority of KSWs thought that their gender identity or transition from male to female was fate, but engaging in sex work was their choice, not fate (Nemoto et al., 2016). Even though many have a college or high school degree, their opportunities in the job market are limited; typically, many work as hairdressers or in the entertainment business. Establishing economic independence through sex work provided them with strong sense of self as kathoey. This also showed strong resiliency. From adolescence to their current lives, they have been exposed to individual and system-level transphobia, abuse, and harassment, but they try to establish economic independence through sex work, save money for gender-affirmation surgeries and hormone use, and still send money to reestablish a supportive relationship with family members at home. Future HIV prevention and health promotion programs for KSWs must recognize their strength and resiliency and address their substance use behaviors. Few mental health and substance use prevention programs specifically designed for kathoey are available in Bangkok and elsewhere. It is alarming that only one KSW participant in this study reported having seen health service providers in the previous 12 months, and only about half reported having being tested for HIV. Health centers especially for kathoey, where they can obtain medical and mental health and social services, as well as participate in peer-led support groups, are desperately needed. These are ideal and long-term goals for community advocates and public health service providers and researchers, but at least this study clearly indicates that comprehensive HIV/STI prevention and health promotion programs must be implemented that are specific to KSWs (e.g., reducing substance abuse) and FSWs (e.g., addressing economic pressure).

ACKNOWLEDGMENTS
This study was supported by the National Institutes of Health (principal investigator: Tooru Nemoto, grant no. R01DA013896; Center for AIDS Prevention Study, University of California–San Francisco, grant no. P30MH062246). Part of the study results were presented at the Joint International Conference on Alcohol, Drug, and Addiction Research in Commemoration of H.M. the King's 84th Birthday Anniversary, Bangkok, Thailand. The opinions and recommendations expressed in this study are solely those of the authors and do not necessarily represent the views of the National Institutes of Health.

REFERENCES

Baral, S. D., Poteat, T., Strömdahl, S., Wirtz, A. L., Guadamuz, T. E., & Beyrer, C. (2013). Worldwide burden of HIV in transgender women: A systematic review and meta-analysis. *Lancet Infectious Disease, 13* (3), 214–222. doi:10.1016/S1473-3099(12)70315-8.

Bekker, L., Johnson, L., Cowan, F., Overs, C., Besada, D., Hillier, S., & Cates, W. (2015). Combination HIV prevention for female sex workers: What is the evidence? *Lancet, 385* (9962), 72–87. doi:10.1016/S0140-6736(14)60974-0. PubMed PMID: 25059942.

Centers for Disease Control and Prevention. (2013, June 28). *HIV and syphilis infection among men who have sex with men — Bangkok, Thailand, 2005–2011.* Retrieved from www.cdc.gov/mmwr/preview/mmwrhtml/mm6225a2.htm.

Chemnasiri, T., Guadamuz, T. E., Naorat, S., Utokasenee, P., Visarutratana, S., Varangrat, A., . . . & van Griensven, F. (2006). Predictors of condom use during most recent anal intercourse among populations of young men who have sex with men in Thailand. Paper presented at the XVI International AIDS Conference, Toronto, Canada.

Decker, M., Crago, A., Chu, S., Sherman, S. G., Seshu, M. S., Buthelezi, K., Dhaliwal, M., & Beyrer, C. (2015). Human rights violations against sex workers: Burden and effect on HIV. *Lancet, 385* (9963), 186–199. doi:10.1016/S0140-6736(14)60800-X.

De Santis, J. P. (2009). HIV infection risk factors among male-to-female transgender persons: A review of the literature. *Journal of the Association of Nurses in AIDS Care, 20* (5), 362–372. doi:10.1016/j.jana.2009.06.005.

Dokubo, E. K., Kim, A. A., Le, L. V., Nadol, P. J., Prybylski, D., & Wolfe, M. I. (2013). HIV incidence in Asia: A review of available data and assessment of the epidemic. *AIDS Reviews, 15* (2), 67–76.

Family Health International (FHI) and Bureau of AIDS, TB and STIs, Department of Disease Control, Ministry of Public Health, Thailand. (2008). *The Asian Epidemic Model (AEM) projections for HIV/ AIDS in Thailand.* Retrieved from http://www.aidsdatahub.org/sites/default/files/documents/The_Asian_Epidemic_Model_Projections_for_HIVAIDS_in_Thailand_2005_2025.pdf.

Fishbein, M., Middlestadt, S. E., & Hitchcock, P. J. (1994). Using information to change sexually transmitted disease–related behaviors: An analysis based on the theory of reasoned action. *In* R. J. DiClemente & J. L. Peterson (eds.), *Preventing AIDS: Theories and methods of behavioral interventions* (pp. 61–78). New York: Plenum Press.

Guadamuz, T. E., Wimonsate, W., Varangrat, A., Phanuphak, P., Jommaroeng, R., Mock, P. A., . . . & van Griensven, F. (2011). Correlates of forced sex among populations of men who have sex with men in Thailand. *Archives of Sexual Behavior, 40* (2), 256–266. doi:10.1007/s10508-009-9557-8.

Hannenberg, R., & Rojanapithayakorn, W. (1998). Changes in prostitution and the AIDS epidemic in Thailand. *AIDS Care, 10* (1), 69–79.

Herbst, J. H., Jacobs, E. D., Finlayson, T. J., McKleroy, V. S., Neumann, M. S., & Crepaz, N. (2008). Estimating HIV prevalence and risk behaviors of transgender persons in the United States: A systematic review. *AIDS and Behavior, 12* (1), 1–17. doi:10.1007/s10461-007-9299-3.

National AIDS Committee. (2015). *Thailand AIDS response progress report, 2015: Thailand ending AIDS*. Retrieved from www.unaids.org/sites/default/files/country/documents/THA_narrative_report_.pdf.

Nemoto, T., Cruz, T., Iwamoto, M., Trocki, K., Perngparn, U., Areesantichai, C., Suzuki, S., & Robert, C. (2016). Examining the sociocultural context of HIV-related risk behaviors among kathoey (male-to-female transgender women) sex workers in Bangkok, Thailand. *Journal of the Association of Nurses in AIDS Care, 27* (2), 153–165. doi:10.1016/j.jana.2015.11.003.

Nemoto, T., Iwamoto, M., Colby, D., Witt, S., Pishori, A., Le, M. N., . . . & Giang, L. T. (2008). HIV-related risk behaviors among female sex workers in Ho Chi Minh City, Vietnam. *AIDS Education & Prevention, 20* (5), 435–453.

Nemoto, T., Iwamoto, M., Perngparn, U., Areesantichai, C., Kamitani, E., & Sakata, M. (2012). HIV-related risk behaviors among kathoey (male-to-female transgender) sex workers in Bangkok, Thailand. *AIDS Care, 24* (2), 210–219. doi:10.1080/09540121.2011.597709.

Nemoto, T., Iwamoto, M., Sakata, S., Perngparn, U., & Areesantichai, C. (2013). Social and cultural contexts of HIV risk behaviors among female sex workers in Bangkok, Thailand. *AIDS Care, 25* (5), 613–618.

Nemoto, T., Operario, D., Keatley, J., Nguyen, H., & Sugano, E. (2005). Promoting health for transgender women: Transgender Resources and Neighborhood Space (TRANS) program in San Francisco. *American Journal of Public Health, 95* (3), 382–384. doi:10.2105/AJPH.2004.040501.

Nemoto, T., Operario, D., Soma, T., Bao, D., Vajrabukka, A., & Crisostomo, V. (2003). HIV risk and prevention among Asian/Pacific Islander men who have sex with men: Listen to our stories. *AIDS Education and Prevention, 15* (Suppl. 1), 7–20.

Nemoto, T., Sausa, L. A., Operario, D., & Keatley, J. (2006). Need for HIV/AIDS education and intervention for MTF transgenders: Responding to the challenge. *Journal of Homosexuality, 51* (1), 183–202. doi:10.1300/J082v51n01_09.

Operario, D., Soma, T., & Underhill, K. (2008). Sex work and HIV status among transgender women: Systematic review and meta-analysis. *Journal of Acquired Immune Deficiency Syndrome, 48* (1), 97–103. doi:10.1097/QAI.0b013e31816e3971.

Park, L. S., Siraprapasiri, T., Peerapatanapokin, W., Manne, J., Niccolai, L., & Kunanusont, C. (2010). HIV transmission rates in Thailand: Evidence of HIV prevention and transmission decline. *Journal of Acquired Immune Deficiency Syndrome, 54* (4), 430–436. doi:10.1097/QAI.0b013e3181dc5dad.

Poteat, T., German, D., & Kerrigan, D. (2013). Managing uncertainty: A grounded theory of stigma in transgender health care encounters. *Social Science and Medicine, 84*, 22–29. doi:10.1016/j.socscimed.2013.02.019.

Poteat, T., Wirtz, A. L., Radix, A., Borquez, A., Silva-Santisteban, A., Deutsch, M. B., . . . & Operario, D. (2014). HIV risk and preventative interventions in transgender women sex workers. *Lancet, 385* (9964), 274–286. doi:10.1016/S0140-6736(14)60833-3.

Punpanich, W., Ungchusak, K., & Detels, R. (2004). Thailand's response to the HIV epidemic: Yesterday, today, and tomorrow. *AIDS Education and Prevention, 16* (3 Suppl. A), 119–136. doi:10.1521/aeap.16.3.5.119.35520.

Reisner, S. L., Mimiaga, M. J., Bland, S., Skeer, M., Cranston, K., Isenberg, D., et al. (2010). Problematic alcohol use and HIV risk among black men who have sex with men in Massachusetts. *AIDS Care, 22* (5), 577–587.

Rosenberg, M. (1965). *Society and the adolescent self-image.* Princeton: Princeton University Press.

Sugano, E., Nemoto, T., & Operario, D. (2006). The impact of exposure to transphobia on HIV risk behavior in a sample of transgendered women of color in San Francisco. *AIDS and Behavior, 10* (2), 217–225. doi:10.1007/s10461-005-9040-z.

Totman, R. (2003). *The third sex: Kathoey—Thailand's ladyboys.* Chian Mai, Thailand: Silkworm Books.

UNAIDS. (2016a). *Prevention gap report.* Retrieved from www.unaids.org/sites/default/files/media_asset/2016-prevention-gap-report_en.pdf.

———. (2016b). *90-90-90: On the right track towards the global target.* Retrieved from http://reliefweb.int/sites/reliefweb.int/files/resources/90_90_90_Progress_ReportFINAL.pdf.

van Griensven, F. (2010). Inconsistent condom use among young men who have sex with men, male sex workers, and transgenders in Thailand. *AIDS Education and Prevention, 22* (2), 100–109. doi:10.1521/aeap.2010.22.2.100.

———. (2006). Predictors of condom use during most recent anal intercourse among populations of young men who have sex with men in Thailand. Paper presented at the XVI International AIDS Conference, Toronto, Canada.

van Griensven, F., Na Ayutthaya, P. P., & Wilson, E. (2013). HIV surveillance and prevention in transgender women. *Lancet Infectious Disease, 13* (3), 185–186. doi:10.1016/S1473-3099(12)70326-2.

van Griensven, F., Varangrat, A., Wimonsate, W., Tanpradech, S., Kladsawad, K., Chemnasiri, T., . . . & Plipat, T. (2010). Trends in HIV prevalence, estimated HIV incidence, and risk behavior among men who have sex with men in Bangkok, Thailand, 2003–2007. *Journal of Acquired Immune Deficiency Syndrome, 53* (2), 234–239. doi:10.1097/QAI.0b013e3181c2fc86.

Wimonsate, W., Naorat, S., Varangrat, A., Phanuphak, P., Kanggarnrua, K., & McNicholl, J. (2006). Risk behavior, hormone use, surgical history and HIV infection among transgendered persons (TG) in Thailand, 2005. Paper presented at the XVI International AIDS Conference, Toronto, Canada.

World Health Organization. (2015). *Guideline on when to start antiretroviral therapy and on pre-exposure prophylaxis for HIV.* Retrieved from http://apps.who.int/iris/bitstream/10665/186275/1/9789241509565_eng.pdf?ua=1.

CHAPTER 19

Transgender Sex Work in the Andean Region

Between Vulnerability and Resilience

Ximena Salazar[1]
Aron Núnez-Curto[1]
Angélica Motta[2]
Carlos F. Cáceres[3]

1 Anthropologist who graduated from Universidad Nacional Mayor de San Marcos at Lima (Peru).
2 Doctor of collective health from the Institute of Social Medicine (Rio de Janeiro State University).
3 Completed medical training at Universidad Peruana Cayetano Heredia (Lima, Peru).

SUMMARY

This chapter describes transgender sex work in the Andean region in South America (formed by Peru, Ecuador, Colombia, and Bolivia). The history and current situation of transgender sex work in this region are presented in conjunction with the workers' legal status, HIV risks, and other characteristics. Some unique features of conducting transgender sex work in this area are summarized briefly.

KEY TERMS

Andean region; HIV risks; transgender sex workers

Nuttbrock, Larry, *Transgender Sex Work and Society*
dx.doi.org/10.17312/harringtonparkpress/2017.11.tsws.019
© 2018 by Harrington Park Press

Transgender is a term widely used to describe people whose gender identity and gender expression do not correspond to the norms and expectations traditionally associated with the sex assigned at birth. Transgender people's behavior and presentation transcend culturally defined parameters of gender (i.e., male vs. female) (Operario et al., 2008; Baral et al., 2013; Bianchi et al., 2014; Poteat et al., 2014).

Transwomen have often been incorrectly included in research related to HIV from an epidemiological perspective as men who have sex with men (MSM) (Silva-Santisteban et al., 2012; Beyrer et al., 2015). Sex work is defined as the "provision of sexual services for money or its equivalent" (Harcourt & Donovan, 2005). UNAIDS (2002) defines sex workers as "female, male and transgender adults and young people who receive money or goods in exchange for sexual services, either regularly or occasionally, and who may or may not consciously define these activities as income-generating" (p. 3). Sex work is extremely widespread and practiced in major urban centers, as well as in small towns and rural areas. The diversity of ways in which sex work is performed makes defining its boundaries problematic. This vagueness results in a spectrum of implications for public health and health service provisions (Harcourt & Donovan, 2005). Commonly, two contrasting approaches to sex work are identified. One approach emphasizes the constraints and oppression experienced by sex workers (e.g., Farley, 2004; Raphael & Shapiro, 2004). The other emphasizes agency and empowerment as the main issues (e.g., Bernstein, 2007; Burnes, Long, & Schept, 2012). Regardless, sex work varies depending on the context and circumstances (Bianchi et al., 2014).

The proportion of transwomen who perform sex work is uncertain owing to nonprobability sampling methods' estimates and different definitions of sex work (Poteat et al., 2014). However, it is known that many of them engage in sex work because of employment discrimination and lack of other income opportunities (Garber, 1992; Clements-Nolle et al., 2001; Baral et al., 2013; Poteat et al., 2014).

Discrimination against transgender sex workers (TSWs) stems from many forms of stigma relating to gender identity, gender expression, perceived sexual orientation, and involvement in sex work (Poteat et al., 2014). In addition, legal and psychological protection of any kind remains scarce (Poteat et al., 2014). Transwomen's well-being is strongly compromised in countries where their gender identity is not legally recognized, which leads, for instance, to limited access to HIV services and other forms of healthcare (Cáceres et al., 2010; Silva-Santisteban et al., 2012).

Some studies have explored the relationship between sex work and body modification. A more feminine appearance in sex work increases earning capacity (Poteat et al., 2014). It was also found that through sex work, TSWs could obtain some sense of gender validation from male clients seeking TSW sexual services (Bockting, Robinson, and Rosser, 1998; Sevelius, 2013).

In the Andean region (formed by Peru, Ecuador, Colombia, and Bolivia), common sense, laws, and policies have traditionally assumed sex work to be an activity performed mainly by women. Therefore, the reality of transgender sex work has remained invisible and neglected (Poteat et al., 2014). Fifteen years ago, transwomen, and among them those who engage in sex work, began to make themselves visible in public documents and academic studies in Latin America. The reason for that was the relationship established between sex work and HIV (Salazar, 2009) and probably also the misclassification of transwomen as men who have sex with men (MSM) (Beyrer et al., 2015). This invisibility did not allow for an understanding of their life conditions and deep vulnerabilities, which limited regional and national information on this issue (UNAIDS, 2002; Salazar, 2009).

Because of structural, interpersonal, individual, and biological factors (Poteat et al., 2014), transwomen doing sex work are known to be at high risk for HIV acquisition (Kenagy, 2002; Baral et al., 2013; Beyrer et al., 2015; Poteat et al., 2014, Clements-Nolle et al., 2001; Melendez & Pinto, 2007; Silva-Santisteban et al., 2012). TSWs are four times more likely to be living with HIV than female sex workers are (Baral et al., 2013). Worldwide, HIV prevalence is about 19.1% in transwomen, with an odds ratio of 48.8 (95% CI 21.2–76.3), compared with the general adult populations (Poteat et al., 2014). Nonetheless, results stratified by transgender status are rarely available, which reduces the understanding of HIV epidemiology and the possibility of intervention effects.

TRANSGENDER SEX WORKERS IN THE ANDEAN REGION

Key Features of Transgender Sex Work

In the Andean region, sex work has been assumed to be performed only by women and has been considered a "necessary evil" in society since the early twentieth century. Even though sex work is not a crime in Peru, Ecuador, Colombia, and Bolivia, its regulation by the state and cities remains ambiguous because it is considered immoral and thus socially criminalized, especially when carried out on the streets and in unauthorized settings. The regulation also implies sanitary control for sex workers, as well as restrictions on spaces where and conditions under which sex work can be performed (Salazar, 2009).

TSWs often experience two levels of discrimination: against their gender identity and against the work they perform (Salazar & Villayzán, 2009; Rodríguez, 2010). These situations of discrimination and resulting violence are rooted in the societies of the Andean region and have become naturalized. In our society, where greater importance and value are given to men, many people cannot tolerate an individual assigned at birth as a male identifying with the female gender (Salazar, 2010). Many TSWs in the Andean region are expelled from their homes at a very young age and as a result engage in sex work sometimes from childhood (International HIV/AIDS Alliance, 2008; Salazar, 2010). For many of them, sex work is their main livelihood (Estrada-Montoya & García-Becerra, 2010; Bianchi et al., 2014).

Legislation relating to sex work does not take into account TSWs and the twofold stigma related to them: specifically, their human rights are regularly violated, and they are frequently exposed to different kinds of aggressions perpetrated by security officials (Salazar & Villayzán, 2009; Rodríguez, 2010). Additionally, TSWs in the Andean region often experience not only physical but also psychological violence from clients, pimps, and gangs. Pimps and gangs charge TSWs money in exchange for allowing them to work on specific streets or avenues, or force them to use certain hotels. Social stigma and criminalization, together with the shortcomings of the justice system, are critical barriers to reporting these events and accessing health services for the TSW population.

TSWs in the Andean region play a significant role in the sexual labor market (Salazar, 2010). However, as is true in other parts of the world, they are invisible to public policy. Moreover, this invisibility has generated a lack of knowledge about their vulnerabilities and the conditions in which they perform this activity.

In some countries in the region, such as Peru, tourism has created a demand for TSWs (Nureña et al., 2011), who migrate from the hinterland not only to the capital but also abroad. An example of this migration is the movement of TSWs from the Peruvian rainforest region to the capital city (Silva-Santisteban et al., 2012). Additionally, Europe is a very common destination for migration abroad for many TSW (Kulick, 2008; Loehr, 2007; Rodríguez, 2010; Nureña et al., 2011). Temporary migration may also occur, in search of new sex work markets (Nureña et al., 2011). In any case, immigration creates loneliness, alienation from family and friends, and breakdown of social networks. It also results in an unawareness of the rules and regulations in a new location and further limits access to health services (UNAIDS, 2002).

Transgender sex work in Peru, Ecuador, and Bolivia occurs in many different venues, but mainly on the streets, which can become highly violent settings (Silva-Santisteban et al., 2012; Rodríguez, 2010) with very competitive dynamics (Nureña et al., 2011). It also takes place in bars and discos, saunas, video clubs, hotels, houses and apartments, nightclubs, brothels, prisons, riverboats, and highways (Nureña et al., 2011). Studies have shown that transgender sex work is associated with substance use (Nemoto et al., 2004; Silva-Santisteban et al., 2012). Transgender sex work performed in the conditions mentioned is, in fact, a dangerous and socially marginalized practice. In contrast, in Colombia, sex work is allowed in areas designated by the government as "tolerance zones." TSWs are required to carry identification and a health card and are expected to undergo training sessions at least once a year on sexual health and human rights. Owners of commercial establishments involved in the sex work industry within the tolerance zones are required to provide condoms and promote their use, participate in health training, and prevent minors from working as sex workers in their establishments (Bianchi et al., 2014).

Regarding sexual roles performed in sex work, TSWs are asked not only to be penetrated but also to penetrate clients, which is usually a sexual service with a higher rate (Nureña et al., 2011; Urrea & La Furcia, 2014). In Peru, for example, receptive sexual roles (passive) are most frequent, but about a fifth of the TSWs assume both roles (penetrative and receptive) (Cáceres et al., 2012). This sexual versatility with their male clients is not performed with their close partners, with whom they tend to take the receptive role during sex (PAHO/WHO, 2011). In Latin America, TSWs often have male clients of different social classes, ages, and sexual preferences. Usually, clients are men whose sexual fantasies involve women with male genitalia who penetrate them. Therefore, the anatomy of the "woman with a penis" has a determining effect on the demand and success of TSWs (Urrea & La Furcia, 2014).

In Colombia, Urrea & La Furcia (2014) have found a racialization of TSWs. Black TSWs are overvalued because of an alleged "hypersexuality." In that sense, clients see a "woman with a penis and dark skin color" as exotic and highly sexual. Transgender sex work is diverse, multifaceted, and polymorphous (Bianchi et al., 2014; Nureña et al., 2011; Weitzer, 2009). At the individual level, some transwomen may get involved in this practice as a way to exteriorize and affirm their identity (Silva-Santisteban et al., 2012; Rodríguez, 2010; Salazar & Villayzán, 2009). Therefore, in spite of the dangers and marginality associated with it, transgender sex work is a space for personal fulfillment and appropriation of public space (Urrea & La Furcia, 2014). According to recent studies, it seems that leaving sex work is considered a difficult option to consider for TSWs in Ecuador (Rodríguez, 2010). In Lima, Peru, 40% of TSWs have reported trying to leave sex work at least once.

Who, Where, and How Many?

It is unclear how many TSWs are in each country of the Andean region, as there are no estimates of population size of transwomen, including those engaged in sex work. In Peru, Segura and colleagues (2010) have estimated 22,456 transgender women using the technique of Network Scale Up.

Transwomen who finish school often do not pursue higher education, or they leave higher education owing to the stigma and discrimination they are subject to (less than 9% of the participants had obtained a university degree) (Cáceres et al., 2012). Transwomen often pursue occupations regarded as "feminine," including hairdressing, makeup, or decoration (Rodríguez, 2010; Silva-Santisteban et al., 2012; MCP Colombia, 2012), or they opt for sex work (Salazar & Villayzán, 2009). This situation reflects their lack of employment opportunities.

According to available data for some countries in the Andean region, the percentage of transwomen engaged in sex work is high: in Medellín (Colombia) 44.4% of transgender women are involved in sex work, whereas in Bogotá (Colombia), 25% are engaged in sex work (MCP Colombia, 2012). In the city of Lima, 64% of transgender women are engaged in sex work (Silva-Santisteban et al., 2012), and the average age at which they begin working is 18.

TABLE 19.1

HIV Prevalence in the Andean Region

	Transwomen	TSWs
Peru	29.0% (Silva-Santisteban et al., 2012)	20.8% (Dirección General de Epidemiología—IMPACTA, 2011)
Ecuador	31.9% (Ministerio de Salud Pública del Ecuador, 2012)	—
Colombia	—	15.1% (MCP Colombia, 2012)
Bolivia	19.7% (Ministerio de Salud de Bolivia, 2012) 21.80% (Ministerio de Salud de Bolivia, 2014)	—

In Lima 61.6% of TSWs work every day and have between three and seven clients per day. In Colombia the average number of customers per TSW in the preceding month was 20 (MCP Colombia, 2012).

HIV Prevalence, Health Needs, and Access to Care

TSWs are, as a group, most profoundly affected by HIV. It has been shown that the denial of fundamental rights often has adverse effects on the health of affected groups; for example, isolation hinders access to preventive information and healthcare systems. Therefore, in the case of TSWs, there is a close connection among stigma, discrimination, violence, and vulnerability to HIV (Salazar & Villayzán, 2009). The social and psychological damage caused by stigma can be a barrier to accessing health services, both for prevention and treatment of HIV, and for healing the physical and psychological wounds caused by violence. Isolation forces TSWs to face many serious problems and leaves them feeling abandoned, devalued, and guilty. The resulting low self-esteem affects their capacity to take care of their health, leading them to believe that they are not worthy of protecting themselves from HIV.

Studies among transwomen in different countries in Latin America reveal that between 33% and 75% of all transwomen are involved in sex work. Condom use varies according to the type of partner. The rates of condom use with clients range from 40% to 98%, whereas among TSWs' stable partners, rates are between 22% and 46% (Sotelo, 2008; Silva-Santisteban et al., 2012; Hernández, Guardado, & Paz-Bailey, 2010;

Morales-Miranda et al., 2010). A high rate of substance use among TSWs in Peru has also been found. In Lima, for instance, a study shows that TSWs have a high consumption of cocaine powder and cocaine base paste (Cáceres et al., 2012). The criminalization of sex work generates a series of vulnerabilities among people who perform it, which directly affects their health. UNAIDS (2002) states that the legal status of sex work is directly related to the effectiveness of HIV programs. Therefore, decriminalization constitutes a platform for preventing HIV.

A survey of people living with HIV found that transwomen were associated with lower access to HIV services, including the provision of antiretrovirals (Cáceres et al., 2010; Cáceres et al., 2012). Similarly, there are no specialized providers to prescribe hormone therapy or perform complicated surgeries to reduce the damage caused by the informal application of liquid silicone in different body parts (Cáceres et al., 2010). The lack of comprehensive health services for TSWs is a barrier to acquiring new skills, especially about issues related to gender and body modification strategies according to their gender identity. Table 19.1 summarizes HIV prevalence in the Andean region.

Recent reviews comparing HIV prevalence among TSWs and transwomen not involved in sex work illustrate how sex work can significantly increase the risk of HIV for many transwomen (Estrada-Montoya & García-Becerra, 2010).

Studies focusing on transwomen involved in sex work reveal HIV infection prevalence of 28–63% in Latin America and the Caribbean, confirming sex work as a significant risk factor (Grandi et al., 2000; Sotelo, 2008; dos Ramos Farías et al., 2011; Toibaro et al., 2009; Lobato et al., 2007; Salazar & Villayzán, 2010; PAHO/WHO, 2011). Unfortunately, there are limited data on the prevalence of hepatitis B, human papillomavirus (HPV), and herpes simplex (HS) (PAHO/WHO, 2011) among this population.

In Peru, the prevalence of HIV among TSW is 20.8% (104/500), with an incidence of 9.07 per 100 people/year (Dirección General de Epidemiología, 2011). In Colombia, HIV prevalence among transgender sex workers was 10% in Medellín, 13.1% in Barranquilla, 17.1% in Bogotá, and 18.8% in Cali (MCP Colombia, 2012).

In Colombia, TSWs report a less frequent use of condoms with their stable partners than with casual partners and when they are under the influence of alcohol or drugs (MCP Colombia, 2012). Less than 40% of respondents reported having had an HIV test in the previous 12 months (MCP Colombia, 2012). The limited data that exist show that TSWs remain the population most affected by HIV.

In conclusion, in the context of stigma and marginalization, the many difficulties that TSWs must endure, their lack of access to healthcare, and their self-administration of hormones and silicone can lead to multiple health risks (PAHO/WHO, 2011). Additionally, TSWs may have other health problems that are not covered by health services.

Meanings of Sex Work for Andean TSWs: Identity, Vulnerability, and Agency

In recent years, the concept of vulnerability has been incorporated and applied to sex work. Moser (1997) postulated that this concept should be understood as a dynamic one that captures the many dimensions of the life of particular social groups. This vulnerability is ascribed not only at the individual level, but also at family and community levels, and it involves existing disadvantages in addressing social problems. Affected groups are exposed to situations that hinder their well-being and their ability to exercise their rights, and they are confronted with processes of decomposition of the social tissue. Toro-Alfonso (1997) suggests that social vulnerability results from the experience of social isolation, lack of support, and the limited existence of organization and empowerment. Vulnerability produces the inability to confront health problems. Risk context is an important factor to consider when processes of vulnerability are analyzed.

Populations that suffer social exclusion, such as TSWs, often face multiple forms of vulnerability. Sexual risk among TSWs, usually the most evident factor of unprotected sexual intercourse, should be analyzed in the context of vulnerability. In that sense, possible actions to change risk situations that can lead to HIV/STI are connected with educational, economic, and empowerment issues, as well as with public policies for this population (Salazar, 2009).

While poverty, stigma, and criminalization have an important role in the condition and meanings related to sex work among TSWs in the Andean region, it is also necessary to take into account the forms of agency that they develop in these contexts (Urrea & La Furcia, 2014). For example, it was found that sex work, besides its economic benefits, is an activity that produces a sense of gender validation and reaffirmation of femininity (Bianchi et al., 2014) and thus strengthens self-esteem (Salazar & Villayzán, 2010; Bianchi et al., 2014). Sex work also enables TSWs to afford the products, clothes, and treatments that enhance their femininity (Prada et al., 2012), which at the same time increases their ability to attract clients (Bianchi et al., 2014). Sex work may be a rational choice in pursuit of new income (Calhoun, 1996), but also pleasure and fun (Nureña et al., 2011).

It is common in the Andean region to find TSWs who are introduced to sex work by another transwoman with longtime experience in the field, who is usually called "mother" by the initiates, and who teaches them all the tricks of sex work (Urrea & La Furcia, 2014). In return, the "mother" is usually rewarded with money, domestic labor, and care work. Accordingly, Bianchi and colleagues (2014) found in Bogotá that TSWs with experience in sex work are relevant models and mentors for other young TSWs, integrating them into the transgender community. What Bianchi and colleagues (2014) pointed out in the case of Colombia could be extended to the Andean region.

CONCLUSIONS

The role of sex work in the spread of HIV depends on local conditions and structural factors. However, in spite of local variations, it is possible to conclude that decriminalization of sex work with a human rights perspective can allow for better living situations for TSWs in the region. For example, the establishment of legal tolerance zones for sex work in Colombia has helped to promote HIV knowledge and condom use (Bianchi et al., 2014), but also to protect TSWs against violence. Although governments and security entities, most notably the police, have crucial roles in helping establish environments that support human rights and public health goals, they are often impediments to achieving protection.

In the Andean region, transgender sex work continues to be invisible within the legal framework. Change, then, should operate at two levels: first at the cultural level, through changes in the mentality and sensitivity of the general population, and second at the policy level. It is not easy, nor can it be done overnight, but it is clear that both levels are needed to achieve a real improvement in the conditions of vulnerability and exclusion of TSWs (Salazar & Villayzán, 2010).

The diversity and varied patterns of sex work practices emerge from the confluence of individual, social, historical, and structural factors (and not only by focusing on discrete "determinants" or isolated psychological traits) (Nureña et al., 2011).

Finally, because the burden of HIV among TSWs is very high, HIV prevention and care need to be addressed while considering significant structural and social barriers. TSW community engagement in HIV prevention and social empowerment requires political will, structural and policy reform, and innovative programs (Beyrer et al., 2015). Few evidence-based HIV prevention interventions have been assessed among TSWs, and none addresses structural drivers. Evidence suggests that prevention interventions among TSWs should include activities such as education on rights and self-esteem, and strengthening the awareness of authorities to reduce systematic violence (Salazar & Villayzán, 2010; Silva-Santisteban et al., 2011). Better-quality research and surveillance are needed to differentiate TSWs from other trans-

REFERENCES

Baral S. D., Poteat, T., Strömdahl, S., Wirtz, A. L., Guadamuz, T. E., & Beyrer, C. (2013). Worldwide burden of HIV in transgender women: A systematic review and meta-analysis. *Lancet, 13* (3), 214–222.

Bernstein, E. (2007). *Temporarily yours: Intimacy, authenticity, and the commerce of sex.* Chicago: University of Chicago Press.

Beyrer, C., Crago, A. L., Bekker, L. G., Butler, J., Shannon, K., Kerrigan, D., Decker, M., . . . & Strathdee, S. (2015). An action agenda for HIV and sex workers. *Lancet, 385,* 287–301.

Bianchi, F. T., Reisen, C. A., Zea, M. C., Vidal-Ortiz, S., Gonzalez, F. A., Betancourt, F., Aguilar, M., & Poppen, P. J. (2014). Sex work among men who have sex with men and transgender women in Bogotá. *Archives of Sexual Behavior, 43,* 1637–1650.

Bockting, W. O., Robinson, B. E., & Rosser B. R. S. (1998). Transgender HIV prevention: A qualitative needs assessment. *AIDS Care, 10,* 505–525.

Burnes, T. R., Long, S. L., & Schept, R. A. (2012). A resilience-based lens of sex work: Implications for professional psychologists. *Professional Psychology: Research and Practice, 43,* 137–144.

Cáceres, C., Salazar, X., Silva-Santisteban, A., & Villayzán, J. (2012). Estudio sobre los factores que incrementan la vulnerabilidad al VIH, riesgos de la Feminización Corporal, necesidades de educación y laborales de la Población Trans en las regiones intervenidas (not published). USSDH-UPCH, Fondo Mundial de Lucha contra el Sida, la Tuberculosis y la Malaria.

Cáceres, C. F., Segura E., Silva-Santisteban A., et al. (2010). Non-conforming gender identification as the determinant of lower HIV care access among people living with HIV in Peru: The HIV, economic flows and globalization study. Presented at AIDS 2010—XVIII International AIDS Conference.

Calhoun, T. C. (1996). Rational decision-making among male street prostitutes. *Deviant Behavior*, *17*, 209–227.

Clements-Nolle, K., Marx, R., Guzman, R., & Katz, M. (2001). HIV prevalence, risk behaviors, health-care use, and mental health status of transgender persons: Implications for public health intervention. *American Journal of Public Health*, *91*, 915–921.

Dirección General de Epidemiología—IMPACTA. (2011). *Vigilancia epidemiológica en VIH en Población HSH 2011*. Lima: Ministerio de Salud del Perú.

Dos Ramos Farías, M. S., Garcia, M. N., Reynaga, E., Romero, R., Vaulet, M. L., Fermepín, M. R., . . . & Avila, M. M. (2011). First report on sexually transmitted infections among trans (male to female transvestites, transsexuals, or transgender) and male sex workers in Argentina: High HIV, HPV, HBV, and syphilis prevalence. *International Journal of Infectious Diseases*, *15*, 634–640.

Estrada-Montoya, H., & García-Becerra, A. (2010). Reconfiguraciones de género y vulnerabilidad al VIH/Sida en mujeres transgénero en Colombia. *Revista Gerencia Políticas de Salud*, *9* (18), 90–102.

Farley, M. (2004). Bad for the body, bad for the heart: Prostitution harms women even if legalized or decriminalized. *Violence against Women*, *10*, 1087–1125.

Garber, M. (1992). *Vested interests: Cross-dressing and cultural anxiety.* New York: Routledge.

Grandi, J. L., Goihman, S., Ueda, M., & Rutherford, G. (2000). HIV infection, syphilis, and behavioral risks in Brazilian male sex workers. *AIDS and Behavior*, *4* (1), 129–135.

Harcourt, C., & Donovan, B, (2005). The many faces of sex work. *Sexually Transmitted Infections*, *81*, 201–206.

Hernández, F. M., Guardado, M. E., & Paz-Bailey, G. (2010). *Encuesta centroamericana de vigilancia de comportamiento sexual y prevalencia de VIH/ITS en poblaciones vulnerables (ECVC): Subpoblación transsexual, travesty y transgénero.* San Salvador: Ministerio de Salud El Salvador.

International HIV/AIDS Alliance. (2008). The hidden HIV epidemic: A new response to the HIV crisis among transgender people. Presentation at the 2008 International AIDS Conference.

Kenagy, G. (2002). HIV among transgender people. *AIDS Care, 14,* 127–134.

Kulick, D. (2008). *Travesti: Prostituição, sexo, gênero e cultura no Brasil.* Brasil: Editora Fiocruz.

Lobato, M. I., Koff, W. J., Schestatsky, S. S., Pedrollo de Vasconcellos, C., Petry, M., Crestana, T., . . . & Annes, A. (2007). Clinical characteristics, psychiatric comorbidities and sociodemographic profile of transsexual patients from an outpatient clinic in Brazil. *International Journal of Transgenderism*, *10* (2), 69–77.

Loehr, K. (2007). *Transvestites in Buenos Aires: Prostitution, poverty, and policy.* Master's thesis, Georgetown University and Universidad Nacional de San Martín, Argentina.

Mecanismo de Coordinación de País—MCP Colombia. (2012). *Resultados del estudio comportamiento sexual y prevalencia de infección por VIH en mujeres trans en cuatro ciudades de Colombia.* CHF International—Colombia. MCP Colombia.

Melendez, R. M., & Pinto, R. (2007). "It is really a hard life": Love, gender, and HIV risk among male-to-female transgender persons. *Culture, Health & Sexuality, 9* (3), 233–245.

Ministerio de Salud de Bolivia. (2014). *Informe nacional de progresos en la respuesta al VIH/SIDA, 2014.* Seguimiento a la Declaración Política sobre el VIH/SIDA 2011.

———. (2012). *Vigilancia epidemiológica, 2012.*

Ministerio de Salud Pública del Ecuador. (2012). *Estudio de vigilancia de comportamientos y prevalencia del VIH y otras infecciones de transmisión sexual en personas trans en Quito.*

Morales-Miranda, S., Álvarez-Rodríguez, B. E., Arambú, N., Aguilar-Martínez, M., Huamán, B., . . . & Castillo, A. (2010). *Encuesta centroamericana de vigilancia de comportamiento sexual y prevalencia de VIH e ITS en poblaciones vulnerables y en poblaciones clave* (ECVC). Capítulo Guatemala. Guatemala: Ministerio de Salud Pública y Asistencia Social de Guatemala, Universidad del Valle de Guatemala.

Moser, C. (1997). *Household responses to poverty and vulnerability,* vol. 1, *Confronting crisis in Cisne Dos, Guayaquil, Ecuador.* Urban Management Programme Policy Paper no 21. Washington, DC: World Bank.

Nemoto, T., Operario, D., Keatley, J., & Villegas, D. (2004). The social context of HIV risk behaviors among male-to-female transgenders of color. *AIDS Care, 16* (6), 724–735.

Nureña, C. R., Zúñiga, M., Zunt, J., Mejia, C., Montano, S., & Sánchez, J. L. (2011). The diversity of commercial sex among men and male-born trans people in three Peruvian cities. *Culture, Health & Sexuality, 13* (10), 1207–1221.

Operario, D., Burton, J., Underhill, K., & Sevelius, J. (2008). Men who have sex with transgender women: Challenges to category-based HIV prevention. *AIDS Behavior, 12* (1), 18–26.

PAHO/WHO. (2011). *Por la salud de las personas trans: Elementos para el desarrollo de la atención integral de personas trans y sus comunidades en Latinoamérica y el Caribe.* Retrieved from www.paho.org/arg/images/gallery/Blueprint%20Trans%20Espa%C3%83%C2%B1ol.pdf.

Poteat, T., Wirtz, A. L., Radix, A., Borquez, A., Silva-Santisteban, A., Deutsch, M. B., . . . & Operario, D. (2014). HIV risk and preventive interventions in transgender women sex workers. *Lancet, 385* (9964), 274–286.

Prada, N., Herrera, S., Lozano, L. T., & Ortiz, A. M. (2012). *"¡A mí me sacaron volada de allá!" Relatos de vida de mujeres trans desplazadas forzosamente hacia Bogotá.* Bogotá: Universidad Nacional de Colombia.

Raphael, J., & Shapiro, D. L. (2004). Violence in indoor and outdoor prostitution venues. *Violence against Women, 10,* 126–139.

Rodríguez, D. (2010). *Estudio psico-social sobre el trabajo sexual en jóvenes transexuales y transgéneras de 15 a 29 años de edad de Guayaquil, durante el año 2010.* Guayaquil: Silueta X.

Salazar, X. (2010). *Estudio sobre la efectiva participación de mujeres y personas transgénero en los procesos del Fondo Mundial Perú.* Lima: AID for AIDS.

———. (2009). *Diagnóstico de la violencia contra los y las trabajadores/assexuales, mujeres, transgénero y varones y su vulnerabilidad frente a las ITS y el VIH.* Lima: CARE—Peru, Global Fund.

Salazar, X., & Villayzán, J. (2010). *La situación de la población trans el Perú en el contexto del acceso universal a tratamiento, atención y apoyo en VIH/SIDA.* Lima: IESS-DEH, UNAIDS.

———. (2009). *Guidelines for multisector work with transgender populations, human rights, sex work, and HIV/AIDS.* Lima: IESSDEH, UNFPA, Red Lac Trans.

Segura E. R., Cáceres, C. F., Mahy, M., Ghyos, P., Leyrla, R., & Salganik, M. (2010). *Estimating the size of populations of men who have sex with men, transgender women, and people living with HIV/Aids in Lima, Peru: A study using the Network Scale-Up Method.* USSDH-UPCH. Policy Brief distributed at the International AIDS Conference in Vienna.

Sevelius, J. M. (2013). Gender affirmation: A framework for conceptualizing risk behavior among transgender women of color. *Sex Roles, 68,* 675–689.

Silva-Santisteban, A., Raymond, H. F., Salazar, X., Villayzán, J., Leon, S., McFarland, W., & Cáceres, C. F. (2012). Understanding the HIV/AIDS epidemic in transgender women of Lima, Peru: Results from a seroepidemiologic study using respondent-driven sampling. *AIDS and Behavior, 16* (4), 872–881.

Sotelo, J. (2008). Estudio de seroprevalencia de VIH en personas trans. *In* Ministerio de Salud de Argentina, *Salud, VIH-Sida y sexualidad trans* (pp. 49–56). Buenos Aires: Organización Panamericana de la Salud.

Toibaro, J. J., Ebensrtejin, J. F., Parlante, A., Burgoa, P., Freyre, A., Romero, M., & Losso, M. H. (2009). Infecciones de transmisión sexual en personas transgénero y otras identidades sexuales. *Medicina, 69,* 327–330.

Toro-Alfonso, J. (1997). Vulnerabilidad de hombres gays y hombres que tienen sexo con hombres (HSH) frente a la epidemia del VIH/SIDA en América Latina: La otra historia de la masculinidad. *In* C. Cáceres, M. Pecheny, & J. Terto (eds.), *Sida y sexo entre hombres en América Latina: Vulnerabilidades, fortalezas y propuestas para la acción* (pp. 57–81). Lima: Universidad Peruana Cayetano Heredia/ONUSIDA/Red de investigación en sexualidades y VIH/Sida en América Latina.

UNAIDS (2002). *Sex work and HIV/AIDS: Technical update.* Geneva: UNAIDS.

Urrea, F., & La Furcia, A. (2014). Pigmentocracia del deseo en el mercado sexual trans de Cali, Colombia. *Sexualidad, Salud y Sociedad—Revista Latinoamericana, 16,* 121–152.

Weitzer, R. (2009). Sociology of sex work. *Annual Review of Sociology, 35,* 213–234.

CHAPTER 20

Transgender Sex Work in Spain

Psychosocial Profile and Mental Health

Rafael Ballester-Arnal[1]
Maria Dolores Gil-Llario[2]
Jesús Castro-Calvo[3]

Trinidad Bergero-Miguel[4]
José Guzmán-Parra[5]

[1] Associate professor of clinical health psychology at the Universitat Jaume I, Castellón de la Plana, Spain.
[2] Associate professor at the University of Valencia, Spain.
[3] Clinical health psychologist at the Universitat Jaume I, Castellón de la Plana, Spain.
[4] Clinical psychologist at the Regional University Hospital, Málaga, Spain.
[5] Clinical psychologist at the Mental Health Research Unit of the Hospital Carlos Haya, Málaga, Spain.

SUMMARY

This study compared sex workers and non–sex workers among transwomen seeking services at the Transsexual and Gender Identity Clinic in Málaga, Spain. Compared to those with no history of sex work, those with such a history reported more family issues (e.g., having a mother with psychological problems and having been thrown out of the house), a history of having been arrested, sexual abuse, and substance use. The sex workers were also more likely to report behavior consistent with an antisocial personality disorder based on SCID-II. These findings are consistent with studies from other parts of the world and point to transwomen sex workers as a population with distinctive issues and concerns.

KEY TERMS

antisocial personality disorder; sexual abuse; sex work; Spain; substance use

Nuttbrock, Larry, *Transgender Sex Work and Society*
dx.doi.org/10.17312/harringtonparkpress/2017.11.tsws.020
© 2018 by Harrington Park Press

Research on sex work in Spain has focused primarily on females who engage in this activity. Some studies have examined male sex workers (Ballester, Salmerón, Gil, & Gómez, 2012; Ballester, Salmerón, Gil, & Giménez, 2012, 2014; Ballester-Arnal et al., 2014; Ballester-Arnal et al., 2016; Belza et al., 2001; Zaro, Peláez, & Chacón, 2007). Only a few studies have examined transgender sex work.

Perhaps the first published report on transgender sex work in Spain was by Belza and colleagues (2000). They examined 132 transgender sex workers who attended a mobile harm-reduction program in Madrid. Condom use was almost 100% with paying partners; systematic condom use with steady partners was only 49%. Seventy three percent had been tested for HIV, and 22% of those tested indicated a positive seroconversion status.

Meneses and colleagues (2003) later evaluated 176 transgender street sex workers in conjunction with an organization working with victims of sexual exploitation and human trafficking. A significant percentage of these sex workers were from Latin America. They had come to Spain in search of a more tolerant and permissive society while also seeking the funds they needed to pay for sex-reassignment surgery. These transgender sex workers were apparently more stigmatized and ridiculed than men or women who worked in the sex trade (Meneses, 2016). Most of their paying partners were heterosexual or bisexual. Some of their regular clients were heterosexuals in search of new experiences.

An important study of sex work in Madrid, Spain, was the Transmadrid Report sponsored by the Lesbian, Gay, Transgender, and Bisexual Collective Organization (Martín-Pérez & Navas, 2008). This study obtained information on 206 transwomen sex workers. A high percentage of these women (88.2%) were originally from abroad, mainly Latin America. They came from countries where transwomen were frequently abused. They were between 26 and 35 years old, which is older than most male sex workers. Most (82%) indicated that sex work was their only means of subsistence. Almost half had been in the sex trade for more than ten years, suggesting that sex work was not a sporadic activity. Most of them worked independently; very few indicated any type of involvement with a pimp. Only a small number were actively looking for alternative work. Three-quarters of those taking hormones were doing so without a medical prescription.

A later study was sponsored by the Fundación Triángulo (Zaro, Rojas, & Navazo, 2009). The average age of the 58 female transgender sex workers was 30 years. Most of them (91%) were also from Latin America. Most of them entered the sex trade around the age of 20 and had been involved in the trade for about ten years. Only 3.5% engaged in sex work against their will, although 56.9% were looking for alternatives to sex work. Almost all (96.4%) were taking hormones, but only 20.4% were doing so as a prescribed treatment. Condom use with paying partners was almost 100%, but this percentage dropped to 30% for steady partners. Among the 84.5% who had been tested for HIV, 24.5% indicated being seropositive.

These reports have allowed us to better understand the issues and difficulties associated with sex work among transgender persons in Spain. They have also allowed us to develop prevention programs aimed at this population, such as the program Preventrans, developed by the Federación Estatal de Lesbianas, Gais, Transexuales, y Bisexuales (FELGTB) (Martín-Pérez & Redondo, 2014). Additional studies are clearly needed.

We know very little about variables like family background, victimization, stressful life events, and mental health. A few studies (Gómez-Gil et al., 2009; Guzmán-Parra et al., 2016) have assessed mental disorders and other psychological problems among transgenders, but none of them has done so in relation to sex work. No study has directly compared transgender persons who engage in sex work with those who do not. That is what we proposed to do in the current study.

METHOD

Participants

The original sample consisted of 210 male-to-female (MTF) and female-to-male (FTM) transgender persons. Sixteen of them had engaged in sex work at some time in their lives. All 16 sex workers were biologically males (see Chapters 1–3 in this book). To better compare those who engaged in sex work (SWs) with those who had not done so (NSWs), we excluded FTM transgender (N = 101) and also those who did not answer the item about sex work (N = 28). Our final sample is composed of 81 participants, 16 of whom (19.8%) reported a history of sex work.

Instruments

The following instruments were used to evaluate the participants:

- A sociodemographic and mental health questionnaire for transgender patients created for evaluation purposes at the Transsexual and Gender Identity Unit of the University General Hospital of Málaga (Spain). This questionnaire assesses age, sex, nationality, educational level, marital status, sexual orientation, employment status, mental health history, parental psychiatric history, violence suffered in life, use of different illegal substances such as cocaine, and traumatic events during life.

- Beck Depression Inventory II (BDI-II) by Beck, Steer, and Brown (1996). This is a 21-item self-report instrument intended to assess the existence and severity of symptoms of depression as listed in the DSM. There is a four-point scale for each item ranging from 0 to 3, sorted from lowest to highest severity. The Spanish version used by Sanz, Navarro, and Vázquez (2003) has a high alpha coefficient (.89).

- SCID-II (Structured Clinical Interview for DSM-IV Axis II Personality Disorders) (First et al., 1997).

Procedure

All the participants were recruited from among visitors to the Transsexuality and Gender Identity Unit, at the University General Hospital of Málaga. These people came to this unit seeking hormonal or surgical treatment or psychological aid. All of them met the diagnostic criteria established by the ICD-10 (World Health Organization, 2010) and DSM-IV-TR (APA, 2000) for transsexualism. Participants were informed about the study, and those who decided to participate gave their informed consent after the discussion. The study was conducted in accordance with the Declaration of Helsinki and approved by the Hospital Ethics Committee. The evaluations were conducted by clinical psychologists trained in patient diagnosis and evaluation.

Statistical Analyses

With the aim of comparing the profiles of transgenders who had engaged in sex work and those who had not, we conducted Student's t-tests to compare the means for the continuous variables (basically for the total scores on the questionnaires), and chi-square tests for the comparison of the categorical variables.

RESULTS

Our results will be presented in different blocks of content.

Sociodemographic and Sexual Orientation Profile

The sixteen SW transgenders were between 22 and 50 years of age (mean = 34.56, SD = 8.24). A total of 75% were single; 12.5% lived with their partners; the remaining 12.5% were married. Regarding education, 43.8% had finished higher secondary education (high school or vocational training), 18.8% had completed eighth grade (middle school), 25% had completed primary education (elementary school), 6.3% had not finished their primary school studies, and the remaining 6.3% had no formal education. A total of 56.3% were born in Spain, and the rest were born in other countries, mainly Latin American countries. With regard to sexual orientation, the percentage of the SWs who considered themselves to be heterosexuals, that is, sexually attracted to men, was 93.8%; only 6.3% defined themselves as homosexuals, that is, attracted to women.

As Table 20.1 shows, for most of these variables, there was equivalence between SWs and NSWs, except for country of origin. The number of transgender people from other countries was much higher in the SW group (43.7%) compared to the NSW group (6.2%).

Labor Aspects and Discrimination at Work

A second block of results pertains to aspects of discrimination in conjunction with work (Table 20.2). The SW and NSW groups indicate a similar frequency of work and income. The mean number of jobs for SW was 4.7 compared to 3.0 for the NSW group. The mean monthly income of SW was 480 euros versus 560 euros for the NSW group. One noteworthy finding was that 37.5% of the SW group earned less than 300 euros a month, and none of them received more than 1,200 euros. Finally, 81.3% of the SW had suffered discrimination at work

TABLE 20.1

Sociodemographic and Sexual Orientation Characteristics of the Sample for Comparison between Groups (N = 81)

	Sex Worker (N = 16)	Non–Sex Worker (N = 65)	Contrast	p
	% or Mean (SD)	% or Mean (SD)		
Age	Mean = 34.56 (SD = 8.24)	Mean = 31.11 (SD = 11.70)	t = –1.371	.180
Marital status				
Married	12.5%	4.6%	Chi square = 1.471	.479
Living with partner	12.5%	10.8%		
No partner	75%	84.6%		
Level of education				
None	6.3%	1.5%	Chi square = 3.609	.823
Unfinished primary ed.	6.3%	4.6%		
Elementary school	25.0%	21.5%		
Middle school	18.8%	20.0%		
High school	43.8%	52.4%		
Country				
Spain	56.3%	93.8%	Chi square = 15.464	.000*
Other countries	43.7%	6.2%		
Sexual orientation				
Heterosexual	93.8%	81.5%	Chi square = 1.984	.745
Bisexual	0%	4.6%		
Homosexual	6.3%	12.3%		
Asexual	0%	1.5%		

*$p < .001$.

TABLE 20.2

Labor Aspects and Discrimination at Work

	Sex Worker (N = 16)	Non-Sex Worker (N = 65)	Contrast	p
	% or Mean (SD)	% or Mean (SD)		
Has worked in the past	100%	95.4%	Chi square = 0.719	.396
No. of jobs since they started	Mean = 4.7 (SD = 2.36)	Mean = 3.0 (SD = 2.79)	t = -1.794	.078
Income level				
Less than 300 euros/month	37.5%	21.6%	Chi square = 5.396	.494
300-420	12.5%	18.9%		
420-540	0%	10.8%		
540-900	12.5%	16.2%		
900-1,200	37.5%	13.5%		
More than 1,200	0%	13.5%		
Mean income	Mean = 480 euros/month	Mean = 560 euros/month	t = 0.936	.467
Discrimination at work	81.3%	33.8%	Chi square = 11.758	.001*

*$p < 0.001$.

versus 33.8% of the NSW. These differences were statistically significant (chi square = 11.758, $p < .001$).

Family Background and Parents' Mental Health

Perceptions of the mother as having a psychological problem were more likely among the SW group (37.5%) as compared to the NSW group (15.4%) (chi square = 3.962; $p = .047$). A greater number of the SW group reported events that could have been traumatic or stressing (Table 20.3), such as separation of the parents (43.8%), having been thrown out of their homes (37.5%), or having been under pressure from their parents because of their transsexuality (75% of the SW stated

TABLE 20.3

Family Background and Parents' Mental Health

	Sex Worker (N = 16)	Non-Sex Worker (N = 65)	Contrast	p
	%	%		
Parents with psychological problems	50	32.3	Chi square = 1.749	.186
Father's psychiatric history	25	30.8	Chi square = 0.205	.651
Mother's psychiatric history	37.5	15.4	Chi square = 3.962	.047*
Separation of parents	43.8	23.1	Chi square = 2.774	.096
Thrown out of home	37.5	7.7	Chi square = 9.720	.002**
Pressure from parents				
None	12.5	31.2	Chi square = 8.494	.131
Very little	6.3	1.6		
Some	6.3	7.8		
A lot	0	17.2		
Very strong	75	42.2		

*$p < .05$. **$p < 0.01$.

that they were under "very strong" pressure), compared to the NSW (23.1%, 7.7%, and 42.2%, respectively). The differences were statistically significant in the case of "thrown out of home" (chi square = 9.720, $p < .002$) and almost significant in "separation of parents" (chi square = 2.774, $p < .096$).

Mental Health History and Problems with the Law

A fourth block of results is related to the transgenders' own mental health history and having been in trouble with the law (Table 20.4). The frequency of having visited mental health professionals, having been diagnosed with a mental health problem, and having been treated by

TABLE 20.4

Mental Health History and Problems with the Law

	Sex Worker (N = 16)	Non–Sex Worker (N = 65)	Contrast	p
	%	%		
Visit to mental health professional	64.3	72.6	Chi square = 0.382	.536
Diagnosed with mental health problems at some time	46.2	49.2	Chi square = 0.152	.749
Treated by more than one professional	30.8	44.1	Chi square = 1.093	.579
In treatment for mental health at some time	58.3	62.7	Chi square = 0.335	.846
Has been arrested	25.0	7.7	Chi square = 3.894	.048*

*$p < .05$.

one or more mental health professionals was high (46%–73%) but very similar; differences between SW and NSW transgenders were not significant. We found significant differences (chi square = 3.894, $p < .048$) only in the experience of having been arrested: 25.0% of SW versus only 7.7% of NSW had been arrested.

Victimization and Abuse

A high percentage of the respondents reported suffering some form of abuse at some time in their life: 81.3% in the SW group and 80.0% in the NSW group (Table 20.5). The abuse was mostly verbal or emotional (76.9% in the SW and 75.4% in the NSW), although 15.4% of the SW group and 17.4% of the NSW group reported physical abuse. Statistically significant group differences were observed for sexual abuse. This was found for such experiences in childhood (30.8% vs. 12.7%), adolescence (23.1% vs. 11.1%), and adulthood (30.8% vs. 4.8%). Similar findings were observed for experiences of being raped.

TABLE 20.5

Victimization: Abuse Recieved

	Sex Worker (N = 16)	Non–Sex Worker (N = 65)	Contrast	p
	%	%		
Has suffered abuse	81.3	80.0	Chi square = 0.013	.910
Type of abuse				
Verbal/ emotional	76.9	75.4	Chi square = 6.823	.270
Physical	15.4	17.4		
All	7.7	7.2		
Sexual abuse				
In childhood	30.8	12.7	Chi square = 2.647	.104
In adolescence	23.1	11.1	Chi square = 1.350	.245
In adulthood	30.8	4.8	Chi square = 8.716	.003**
Rape				
In childhood	23.1	4.8	Chi square = 4.971	.026*
In adolescence	0	6.3	Chi square = 0.871	.351
In adulthood	15.4	4.8	Chi square = 1.979	.160
Told someone about being raped				
In childhood	15.4	3.2	Chi square = 3.222	.073
In adolescence	0	4.8	Chi square = 0.644	.422
In adulthood	15.4	0	Chi square = 9.954	.002**

(continued)

(Table 20.5 cont.)

	Sex Worker (N = 16)	Non-Sex Worker (N = 65)	Contrast	p
	%	%		
Reported rape to police				
In childhood	0	0	—	—
In adolescence	0	0	—	—
In adulthood	7.7	0	Chi square = 4.911	.027*

*p < .05. **p < .01

Mental Health

The last block of results (Table 20.6) concerns mental health. Differences between the groups with regard to SCID-II (personality disorders) were not statistically significant, with one exception: antisocial personality disorder was higher in the SW group ($t = -2.550$, $p < .013$). High levels of suicidal ideation (46.7% in SW and 49.2% in NSW), attempted suicide (37.5% in SW and 23.1% in NSW), thoughts of self-mutilation (12.5% in SW and 29.2% in NSW), and intentional self-harm (6.3% in SW and 15.9% in NSW) were observed, but differences between the SW and NSW groups were not found.

Earlier substance use was extremely high in both groups, but SWs reported higher levels for most of the drugs: cocaine (90% of SW versus 50%), marijuana (63.6% versus 59.0%), designer drugs (43.8% versus 13.8%), amphetamines (6.3% versus 4.6%), hallucinogens (31.3% versus 6.2%), heroin (12.5% versus 4.6%), and alcohol abuse (6.3% versus 3.1%).

TABLE 20.6

Mental Health

	Sex Worker (N = 16)	Non–Sex Worker (N = 65)	Contrast	p
	% or Mean (SD)	% or Mean (SD)		
BDI	Mean = 7.56 (SD = 9.79)	Mean = 12.12 (SD = 9.65)	t = 1.688	.095
Total SCID II	Mean = 38.06 (SD = 16.92)	Mean = 32.41 (SD = 14.60)	t = –1.338	.185
SCID-II				
Avoidance disorder	Mean = 2.88 (SD = 1.45)	Mean = 2.09 (SD = 1.91)	t = –1.527	.131
Dependence disorder	Mean = 2.44 (SD = 1.63)	Mean = 1.89 (SD = 1.51)	t = –1.273	.207
Obsessive disorder	Mean = 5.00 (SD = 1.83)	Mean = 4.56 (SD = 1.91)	t = –0.827	.411
Passive disorder	Mean = 3.00 (SD = 1.83)	Mean = 2.77 (SD = 1.99)	t = –0.428	.670
Depressive disorder	Mean = 2.31 (SD = 1.81)	Mean = 2.94 (SD = 2.14)	t = 1.072	.287
Paranoid disorder	Mean = 3.69 (SD = 2.02)	Mean = 3.28 (SD = 2.20)	t = –0.671	.504
Schizotypal disorder	Mean = 4.25 (SD = 1.98)	Mean = 3.66 (SD = 2.32)	t = –0.941	.350
Schizoid disorder	Mean = 2.13 (SD = 1.09)	Mean = 1.97 (SD = 1.30)	t = –0.444	.658
Histrionic disorder	Mean = 3.19 (SD = 1.72)	Mean = 2.56 (SD = 1.75)	t = –1.280	.240
Narcissistic disorder	Mean = 5.38 (SD = 3.22)	Mean = 4.72 (SD = 2.52)	t= –0.880	.381
Borderline disorder	Mean = 4.13 (SD = 3.24)	Mean = 3.78 (SD = 2.75)	t = –0.432	.667
Antisocial disorder	Mean = 2.06 (SD = 2.20)	Mean = 0.97 (SD = 1.32)	t = –2.550	.013*

(continued)

(Table 20.6 cont.)

	Sex Worker (N = 16)	Non-Sex Worker (N = 65)	Contrast	p
	% or Mean (SD)	% or Mean (SD)		
Suicidal ideation	46.7%	49.2%	Chi square = 0.032	.858
Age at first thought of suicide	Mean = 20.71 (SD = 4.82)	Mean = 14.82 (SD = 8.58)	t = -1.749	.088
Attempted suicide	37.5%	23.1%	Chi square = 1.391	.238
Number of attempts	Mean = 1.50 (SD = 1.22)	Mean = 2.08 (SD = 1.04)	t = 1.066	.301
Age at first attempt	Mean = 22 (SD = 6.13)	Mean = 18.33 (SD = 9.73)	t = -0.851	.406
Thoughts of self-mutilation	12.5%	29.2%	Chi square = 1.871	.171
Intentional self-harm	6.3%	15.9%	Chi square = 1.292	.524
Substance use (past)				
Cocaine	90.0%	50.0%a	Chi square = 4.480	.034*
Marijuana	63.6%	59.0%	Chi square = 0.078	.780
Designer drugs (ecstasy etc.)	43.8%	13.8%	Chi square = 7.243	.007**
Amphetamines	6.3%	4.6%	Chi square = 0.073	.787
Hallucinogens	31.3%	6.2%	Chi square = 8.188	.004**
Heroin	12.5%	4.6%	Chi square = 1.378	.240
Alcohol	6.3%	3.1%	Chi square = 0.362	.547
Tobacco	31.3%	60.0%	Chi square = 4.277	.039*

$*p < .05.$ $**p < .01.$

DISCUSSION

Transgender persons clearly experience an array of difficulties in contemporary society, including Spain (Bergero et al., 2012). In addition to the dysphoria associated with a gender identity at odds with sexual anatomy at birth, these individuals are often socially marginalized in a society that misunderstands and often rejects them. Difficulties associated with finding legitimate employment prompt many of these individuals to enter the sex trade, but this type of work may lead to additional issues and difficulties. Comparisons between transgender persons who engage in sex work and those who do not have been made in some studies in different parts of the world (see other chapters in this book), but these comparisons have typically been limited in scope, and there have been no such studies in Spain.

The first result of our study, which attempted to make such comparisons, is that in a sample of 210 transgender people, all of those who engaged in sex work were male-to-female transgender persons. This is an important issue (addressed in other chapters in this book) that obviously needs additional scrutiny (Guzmán-Parra et al., 2016). It could be argued that transgender persons with a female sexual anatomy may be more successful in the sex trade. Some paying partners of sex workers may have a fascination with biological males who appear as females. Nadal and colleagues (2012) have suggested that transwomen engage in sex work because it allows them to feel more sexually attractive and accepted as "real" women, a notion proposed in other chapters in this volume (see Chapters 1–3).

We found that significant numbers of transwomen sex workers in Spain emigrated from other countries, where they may have suffered abuse and discrimination. Spanish transgender persons born outside Spain may have additional problems finding employment, which may further their motivation to engage in sex work. Immigrants coming from cultural contexts with a tradition of sex work among transwomen may practice sex work regardless of economic factors (see Chapters 2 and 7).

Whether in the sex trade or not, significant numbers of transgender persons clearly experience mental health challenges. Our study in Spain, which is consistent with this literature (see especially Chapters 3 and 4 of this book), highlights issues with parental figures during adolescence in particular. Compared to those with no history of sex work, the sex workers in our study recalled a greater likelihood of being separated from their parents and having been thrown out of their homes. Apart from the emotional turmoil involved, financial issues stemming from a disruptive early family life may be a factor leading to the decision to enter the sex trade (Belza et al., 2000; see Chapter 2 of this book).

As Beth Hoffman thoroughly reviewed in Chapter 8, substance use is prevalent among transwomen, and it is even more prevalent among transwomen in the sex trade. Similarly, we observed extremely high levels of substance use among transwomen sex workers in Spain.

This study points to transgender sex workers in Spain, as elsewhere in the world, as a distinct population with a range of behavioral and mental health issues that need to be better understood and addressed.

REFERENCES

American Psychiatric Association (APA). (2000). *Diagnostic and statistical manual of mental disorders DSM-IV-TR* (rev. ed.). Arlington, VA: American Psychiatric Association.

Ballester, R., Salmerón, P., Gil, M. D., & Giménez, C. (2014). Sexual behaviors in male sex workers in Spain: Modulating factors. *Journal of Health Psychology, 2* (19), 207–217.

———. (2012). The influence of drug consumption on condom use and other aspects related to HIV infection among male sex workers in Spain. *AIDS and Behavior, 17* (2), 536–542.

Ballester, R., Salmerón, P., Gil, M. D., & Gómez, S. (2012). Sexual risk behaviors for HIV infection in Spanish male sex workers: Differences according to educational level, country of origin and sexual orientation. *AIDS and Behavior, 16* (4), 960–968.

Ballester-Arnal, R., Gil-Llario, M. D., Salmerón-Sánchez, P., & Giménez-García, C. (2014). HIV prevention interventions for young male commercial sex workers. *Current HIV/AIDS Reports, 1* (11), 72–80.

Ballester-Arnal, R., Salmerón-Sánchez, P., Gil-Llario, M. D., & Castro-Calvo, J. (2016). Male sex workers in Spain: What has changed in the last lustrum? A comparison of sociodemographic data and HIV sexual risk behaviors (2010–2015). *AIDS and Behavior.* Advance online publication. doi:10.1007/s10461-016-1494-7.

Beck, A. T., Steer, R. A., & Brown, G. K. (1996). *Manual for the Beck Depression Inventory-II.* San Antonio, TX: Psychological Corporation.

Belza, M. J., Llácer, A., Mora, R., de La Fuente, L., Castilla, J., Noguer, I., & Cañellas, S. (2000). Características sociales y conductas de riesgo para el VIH en un grupo de travestis y transexuales masculinos que ejercen la prostitución en la calle. *Gaceta Sanitaria, 14* (5), 330–337.

Belza, M. J., Llácer, A., Mora, R., Morales, M., Castilla, J., & de la Fuente, L. (2001). Sociodemographic characteristics and HIV risk behavior patterns of male sex workers in Madrid, Spain. *AIDS Care, 13* (5), 677–682.

Bergero, T., Ballester, R., Gornemann, I., Cano, G., & Asiain, S. (2012). Desarrollo y validación de un instrumento para la evaluación del comportamiento sexual de los transexuales: El CSTM. *Revista de Psicopatología y Psicología Clínica, 17* (1), 11–30.

Clements-Nolle, K., Marx, R., Guzman, R., & Katz, M. (2001). HIV prevalence, risk behaviors, health care use, and mental health status of transgender persons: Implications for public health intervention. *American Journal of Public Health, 91* (6), 915–921.

First, M. B., Gibbon, M., Spitzer, R. L., Williams, J. B. W., & Benjamin, L. S. (1997). *Structured clinical interview for DSM-IV Axis II personality disorders (SCID-II).* Washington, DC: American Psychiatric Press.

Garofalo, R., Deleon, J., Osmer, E., Doll, M., & Harper, G. (2006). Overlooked, misunderstood and at-risk: Exploring the lives and HIV risk of ethnic minority male-to-female transgender youth. *Journal of Adolescent Health, 38,* 230–236.

Gómez-Gil, E., Trilla, A., Salamero, M., Godás, T., & Valdés, M. (2009). Sociodemographic, clinical, and psychiatric characteristics of transsexuals from Spain. *Archives of Sexual Behavior, 38* (3), 378–392. doi:10.1007/s10508-007-9307-8.

Guzmán-Parra, J., Sánchez-Álvarez, N., de Diego-Otero, Y., Pérez-Costillas, L., Esteva de Antonio, I., Navais-Barranco, M., & Bergero-Miguel, T. (2016). Sociodemographic characteristics and psychological adjustment among transsexuals in Spain. *Archives of Sexual Behavior, 45* (3), 587–596.

Keuroghlian, A., Reisner, S., White, J., & Weiss, R. (2015). Substance use and treatment of substance use disorders in a community sample of transgender adults. *Drug and Alcohol Dependence, 152,* 139–146.

Mardomingo López, C. (1999). Prevalencia de infección por VIH y factores de riesgo asociados entre los trabajadores del sexo de cuatro áreas españolas. [Prevalence of HIV infection and associated risk factors among sex workers from four Spanish regions]. Master's thesis, Centro Universitario de Salud Pública, Universidad Autónoma de Madrid.

Martín-Pérez, A., & Navas, M. (2008). Informe Transmadrid: Descripción de una población de mujeres trabajadoras del sexo en Madrid. [Transmadrid report: Description of a population of female sex workers in Madrid]. Madrid: COGAM.

Martín-Pérez, A., & Redondo, S. (2014). *No le pongas precio a tu salud: Programa Preventrans.* [Do not put price on your health: Preventrans program]. Madrid: FELGTB.

Meneses, C. (2016). *Riesgo, vulnerabilidad, y prostitución.* [Risk, vulnerability, and prostitution]. Madrid: Universidad P. Comillas.

Meneses, C., Rubio, E., Labrador, J., Huesca, A., & Charro, B. (2003). *Perfil de la prostitución callejera: Análisis de una muestra de personas atendidas por APRAMP.* [Profile of street prostitution: Analysis of a sample of people attended by APRAMP]. Madrid: Universidad P. Comillas.

Nadal, K., Vargas, V., Meterko, V., Hamit, S., & Mclean, K. (2012). Transgender female sex workers in New York City: Personal perspectives, gender identity development, and psychological processes. In M. A. Paludi (ed.), *Managing diversity in today's workplace: Strategies for employees and employers* (pp. 123–153). Santa Barbara, CA: Praeger/ABC–CLIO.

Nemoto, T., Bödeker, B., & Iwamoto, M. (2011). Social support, exposure to violence and transphobia, and correlates of depression among male-to-female transgender women with a history of sex work. *American Journal of Public Health, 101,* 1980–1988.

Nuttbrock, L., Bockting, W., Rosenblum, A., Hwahng, S., Mason, M., Macri, M., & Becker, J. (2014). Gender abuse and major depression among transgender women: A prospective study of vulnerability and resilience. *American Journal of Public Health, 104* (11), 2191–2198.

Nuttbrock, L., Hwahng, S., Bockting, W., Rosenblum, A., Mason, M., Macri, M., & Becker, J. (2010). Psychiatric impact of gender-related abuse across the life course of male-to-female transgender persons. *Journal of Sex Research, 47* (1), 12–23.

Sanz, J., Navarro, M. E., & Vázquez, C. (2003). Adaptación española del Inventario para la Depresión de Beck II (BDI-II): Propiedades psicométricas en estudiantes universitarios. [Spanish adaptation of the Beck Depression Inventory-II (BDI-II): Psychometric properties with university students]. *Análisis y Modificación de Conducta, 29* (124), 239–288.

Wilson, E. C., Garofalo, R., Harris, R., Herrick, A., Martínez, M., Martínez, J., . . . & the Adolescent Medicine Trials Network for HIV/AIDS Interventions. (2009). Transgender female youth and sex work: HIV risk and a comparison of life factors related to engagement in sex work. *AIDS and Behavior, 13,* 902–913.

World Health Organization. (2010). *WHO International Classification of Diseases (ICD).* Retrieved from www.who.int/classifications/icd/en/.

Zaro, I., Peláez, M., & Chacón, A. (2007). *Trabajadores masculinos del sexo: Aproximación a la prostitución masculina en Madrid.* [Male sex workers: Approach to male prostitution in Madrid]. Madrid: Fundación Triángulo.

Zaro, I., Rojas, D., & Navazo, T. (2009). *Trabajadoras transexuales del sexo: El doble estigma.* [Transgender sex workers: The double stigma]. Madrid: Fundación Triángulo.

CHAPTER 21

Prevalence and Associated Factors of Condomless Receptive Anal Intercourse with Male Clients among Transwomen Sex Workers in Shenyang, China

Zixin Wang[1]
Joseph T. F. Lau[2]
Yong Cai[3]
Jinghua Li[4]
Tiecheng Ma[5]
Yan Liu[6]

[1] Research assistant professor in the JC School of Public Health and Primary Care, Faculty of Medicine, Chinese University of Hong Kong.

[2] Professor and associate director of the JC School of Public Health and Primary Care, Faculty of Medicine, Chinese University of Hong Kong.

[3] Associate professor in the School of Public Health, Shanghai Jiaotong University, Shanghai, China.

[4] Associate professor in the School of Public Health, Sun Yat-sen University, Guangzhou, China.

[5] Chief executive of Shenyang Consultation Centre of AIDS Aid and Health Service, Shenyang, China.

[6] On the staff at Shenyang Consultation Centre of AIDS Aid and Health Service.

SUMMARY

Globally, transwomen sex workers have a high prevalence of HIV and condomless receptive anal intercourse with male clients (CRAIMC). We investigated the prevalence of CRAIMC and factors associated with CRAIMC among transwomen sex workers in China. HIV prevalence among transwomen sex workers was high but probably underestimated.

Nuttbrock, Larry, *Transgender Sex Work and Society*
dx.doi.org/10.17312/harringtonparkpress/2017.11.tsws.021
© 2018 by Harrington Park Press

The high prevalence of condomless anal intercourse with male nonclients and high mobility in sex work among this population in China are
causes for concern. Risk factors for CRAIMC were multidimensional
and should be considered when designing interventions targeting transwomen sex workers. Such interventions are urgently needed.

KEY TERMS
China; condomless anal intercourse; HIV prevalence; transwomen
sex workers

Transwomen are assigned male at birth but currently identify as female,
transgender, or transsexual women (Nemoto et al., 2012; Keatley &
Clements-Nolle, 2001; Poteat et al., 2015). They may express their gender identity by means of interventions (e.g., cosmetic surgery, hormone
treatment, and sex-reassignment surgery) or specific behaviors (e.g.,
wearing feminine attire) (Nemoto et al., 2012). In most countries, it is
difficult or impossible for transwomen to change their legal gender
identification, which creates difficulties for them in accessing healthcare, education, and employment (Poteat et al., 2015; Roche & Keith,
2014). The percentage of transwomen engaged in sex work has been
estimated at 24–75% in the United States (Herbst et al., 2008); 9% in
Singapore (Chew, Tham, & Ratnam, 1997); 58.8% in Brazil (Sutmoller
at al., 2002); 61.3% in Thailand (Centers for Disease Control and
Prevention, 2006); 66.7% in Uruguay (Vinoles et al., 2005); and
54–80% in Asia (Poteat et al., 2015).

Transwomen form a key population that requires focused attention
for HIV prevention (Operario, Soma, & Underhill, 2008). Meta-analyses
have reported HIV prevalence of 19.1% among transwomen (49 times
higher than that of the general adult population) and 27.3% among
transwomen sex workers (Vinoles et al., 2005; Operario et al., 2008).
Other studies of transwomen sex workers reported HIV prevalence of
66.7% in India and 67.9% in the United States, which was higher than
that of male (15.1%) and female (4.3%) sex workers as reported by a
meta-analysis covering 14 countries (Operario et al., 2008). Despite the
large size of the population of transgender men and women in mainland
China, estimated at 400,000, only one survey (N = 52) has recorded
self-reported HIV prevalence (11.1%) (Jiang et al., 2014), and no data
are available for transwomen sex workers.

Previous studies have reported high prevalence of condomless receptive anal intercourse with male clients (CRAIMC) among transwomen sex workers: 12.0–77.0% in the United States (Herbst et al., 2008); 25.0% in South Africa (Richter et al., 2013); 26.9% in Thailand (Nemoto et al., 2012); 29.8% in Italy (Spizzichino et al., 2001); and 92% in Pakistan (Hawkes et al., 2009). We found only two quantitative studies that reported risk factors (e.g., financial pressure) and protective factors (e.g., subjective norms) associated with CRAIMC (Nemoto et al., 2012; Lau et al., 2007), and three qualitative studies that described reasons for practicing CRAIMC (Nemoto, Operario, Keatley, & Villegas, 2004; Bockting, Robinson, & Rosser, 1998; Bianchi et al., 2014). These studies were conducted outside China.

Perceptions related to condom use have been associated with condomless sex with clients among male and female sex workers (Lau, Cai, et al., 2012; Lau et al., 2007). Although theory-based interventions have been found to be more effective than non-theory-based ones (Michie et al., 2008), behavioral health theories have not been used to study factors associated with CRAIMC among transwomen sex workers. The Health Belief Model (HBM) (Janz & Becker, 1984) has been used to explain risk behaviors among sex workers more generally (Lau, Cai, et al., 2012; Lau, Gu, et al., 2012) and was used in this study. The HBM postulates that perceived susceptibility, perceived severity, perceived benefit, perceived barrier, cue to action, and perceived self-efficacy are determinants of health-related behaviors.

We investigated four types of factors that may be associated with CRAIMC: (1) background variables (sociodemographics, HIV serostatus, and anal intercourse with noncommercial male sex partners), (2) feminizing medical interventions (cosmetic surgery, hormone treatment, and sex-reassignment surgery), (3) variables related to sex work (e.g., venue, charge, and sex work in other cities), and (4) perceptions related to condom use (both perceived transgender identity's effect on condomless sex and perceptions related to condom use derived from HBM). We further tested two hypotheses: (1) self-efficacy for condom use with male clients would mediate the association between feminizing medical interventions and CRAIMC, and (2) self-efficacy for condom use with male clients would mediate the association between perceived transgender identity's effect on condomless sex and CRAIMC.

METHODS

Study Design

A cross-sectional study was conducted in Shenyang, China, from April to July 2014. Inclusion criteria were: (1) age ≥ 18 years, (2) self- identification as a transwoman, (3) anal intercourse with ≥ 1 male client (within previous three months), and (4) wearing feminine attire and makeup during sexual contact with men. In the absence of a sampling frame, it was not feasible to perform probability sampling. Instead, staff of a nongovernmental organization (NGO), who provided services to transwomen sex workers, contacted all their clients and performed outreach for recruitment. Referrals were also made by some participants. Prospective participants were assured that refusing to participate in the study would not affect their right to receive any services and that they could quit at any time without being questioned. A total of 282 eligible transwomen sex workers were approached for the study; 62 declined to participate in the study, and 220 (78%) provided written informed consent and completed an anonymous face-to-face interview in settings in which privacy was ensured.

In the survey, 37 participants self-reported being HIV-positive. The 183 who self-reported being HIV-negative or having an unknown HIV serostatus were invited to take a finger-prick HIV rapid test (Alere Determine HIV-1/2 rapid HIV screening test; sensitivity = 99.75%; specificity = 100%); 49.2% (90/183) agreed. Those who tested HIV-negative were given counseling. Those who showed HIV-positive test results received psychological support and underwent confirmatory testing at the local Center for Disease Control and Prevention (CDC). All were subsequently confirmed as HIV-positive and referred to appropriate services. Eight of them subsequently started antiretroviral treatment. Monetary compensation (50 RMB, or 8.1 USD) was given to participants upon completion of the procedures. Ethics approval was obtained from the Survey and Behavioral Research Ethics Committee of the Chinese University of Hong Kong.

Measures

PARTICIPANTS' PROFILES Information collected included sociodemographics (age, education level, monthly personal income, city of residence [*hukou*], and duration of stay in Shenyang), use of any HIV prevention services in the preceding six months, any CRAIMC in the previous month, and any anal intercourse with male sex partners who were non-clients in the previous month, and if affirmative, whether condomless anal intercourse was involved. HIV status (self-reported as HIV-positive, tested HIV-positive, tested HIV-negative, and self-reported as HIV-negative or unknown HIV status but refused testing) was recorded (Table 21.1).

FEMINIZING MEDICAL INTERVENTIONS Participants were asked whether they had undergone cosmetic surgery, hormone treatment, or sex-reassignment surgeries (removal of testes, penis, and scrotum, and/or surgeries for reconstruction of female genitalia) (Table 21.2).

VARIABLES RELATED TO SEXUAL PRACTICES WITH CLIENTS Participants were asked about the channel that was most frequently used to recruit sex clients, venues where sexual intercourse with clients took place, the average charge per episode of sex with male clients, the number of male and female clients in the previous week, drug or alcohol use before or during sex with male clients, any performance of sex work in other Chinese cities or other countries, and the proportion of their male clients that might be aware of their identity as a transwoman (see Table 21.2).

PERCEPTIONS RELATED TO HIV AND CONDOM USE Three scales were constructed for this study and were based on the HBM: (1) the four-item Perceived Susceptibility for HIV Scale, (2) the six-item Perceived Barrier against Condom Use Scale, and (3) the three-item Perceived Self-Efficacy of Consistent Condom Use Scale (response categories: 1 = strongly disagree, 5 = strongly agree). In addition, participants were asked to assess their transgender identity's influence on condomless sex (i.e., whether wearing feminine attire during sexual practice with clients, worrying about clients discovering their gender identity, avoiding exposing their genitals to male clients, and avoiding talking to male clients would increase risk of CRAIMC). The four-item Transgender Identity's Impact on Condomless Sex Scale was then constructed by summing up responses to these four items. Another item, "reminders for condom use were displayed in the venues where sexual practice with clients took place," was asked to assess cue to action. All the scale items are listed in Table 21.3.

TABLE 21.1

Background Characteristics of Transgender Sex Workers (N = 220)

	%
Sociodemographics	
Age Group	
25 or less	23.6
25 to 30	27.3
30 to 40	39.1
> 40	10.0
Education Level	
Primary or below	11.8
Junior secondary	35.9
Senior secondary	41.4
Tertiary	10.9
Monthly income (in RMB)[1]	
3,000 or less	25.9
3,001 to 5,000	32.3
5,001 to 8,000	18.2
>8,000	23.6
Residents of Shenyang ("*hukou*")	
Yes	12.7
No	87.3
Duration of stay in Shenyang	
< 1 year	18.2
1–5 years	37.7
>5 years	44.1

(continued)

(Table 21.1 cont.)

	%
HIV prevention services utilization in the previous six months	
No	8.2
Yes	91.8
HIV serostatus	
Self-reported as being HIV-positive	16.8
Tested as positive in rapid HIV testing	9.1
Tested as negative in rapid HIV testing	31.8
Self-reported HIV-negative or unknown HIV serostatus but refused to undergo HIV testing	42.3
Sexual behavior in the previous month	
Had condomless receptive anal intercourse with any male clients (CRAIMC)	
No	73.2
Yes	26.8
Had anal intercourse with noncommercial male sex partner(s)	
No	11.4
Yes	88.6
Had condomless anal intercourse with noncommercial male sex partner(s) (among those having noncommercial male sex partners, N = 195)	
No	73.8
Yes	26.2
Variables related to feminizing medical interventios (% yes)	
Cosmetic surgery	13.2
Hormone treatment	2.3
Sex reassignment surgery to remove testes, penis, and scrotum	0.5
Sex reassignment surgery to reconstruct female genitals	0.5
Any of above	15.0

[1] 1 USD = 6.2 RMB at the time of the survey.

TABLE 21.2

Sexual Practices with Clients (N = 220)

	%
Channels most often used to recruit clients	
Hotel	14.5
Park	44.1
Internet	41.1
Venues where sexual practices with clients took place	
Hotel	24.6
Rented room	45.0
Client's home	2.7
Park	27.7
Engaged in sexual practices with clients in other Chinese cities in the last year	
No	54.5
Yes	45.5
Engaged in sexual practices with clients in other countries in the last year	
No	96.8
Yes	3.2
Number of male sex clients in the last week	
1–10	65.4
11–20	19.1
21–30	6.4
> 30	9.1
Number of female sex clients in the last week	
0	95.5
1–10	4.5

(continued)

(Table 21.2 cont.)

	%
Average charge per episode of sex with clients (in RMB)[1]	
≤ 100 RMB	35.0
101–200 RMB	15.0
201–400 RMB	19.1
≥ 401 RMB	20.9
Ever used alcohol before or during sex with clients in the last month	
No	77.7
Yes	22.3
Ever used drugs before or during sex with clients in the last month	
No	79.1
Yes	20.9
Estimated proportion of male clients who might be aware of one's transwoman status during sex with clients	
All/majority	28.6
Minority/none	47.7
Uncertain	23.6

[1] 1 USD = 6.2 RMB at the time of the survey.

Statistical Analysis

Using CRAIMC in the previous month as the dependent variable, bivariate odds ratios (OR) of the background independent variables were estimated. Those background variables that showed $p < .1$ in the bivariate analysis were adjusted for in subsequent multiple logistic regression analyses to derive the adjusted odds ratios (AOR) and respective 95% confidence intervals (CI).

Following Baron and Kenny's (1986) method, the first mediation hypothesis was tested by inspecting the association between feminizing medical interventions and self-efficacy in condom use. Multiple logistic regression models, including the variables of feminizing med-

TABLE 21.3

Scales Related to HIV and Condom Use

	%	Mean Scale Score (SD)[1]
Perceived susceptibility of HIV transmission (% high/very high)		
Perceived risk of HIV infection via sexual intercourse with male sex partners	24.5	
Perceived risk of HIV infection via sexual intercourse with clients	39.5	
Perceived risk of transmitting HIV to noncommercial male sex partners	26.9	
Perceived risk of transmitting HIV to male clients	22.8	
Perceived Susceptibility for HIV Scale		*8.8 (2.8)*
Perceived barriers to condom use (% agree/strongly agree)		
Condom was not available in venues for sexual practice with clients	27.3	
It is inconvenient for me to use condoms with clients	5.5	
I worry about police arrest when carrying condoms with me	30.9	
Many male clients would not want to use condoms	39.1	
Condom use with male clients would reduce income	39.1	
Condom use with male clients would shorten the duration of sexual intercourse	39.4	
Perceived Barriers against Condom Use Scale		*15.6 (4.2)*
Perceived cue to action for condom use (% agree/strongly agree)		
Reminders for condom use were displayed in the venues where sexual practices with clients took place	50.0	

(continued)

(Table 21.3 cont.)

	%	Mean Scale Score (SD)[1]
Perceived self-efficacy of consistent condom use (% agree/strongly agree)		
I can suggest to clients that they use condoms	98.2	
I can persuade clients who do not want to use condoms to use condoms	71.8	
I am confident in using condoms during all episodes of sexual practices with clients	78.1	
Perceived Self-Efficacy of Consistent Condom Use Scale		11.3 (2.1)
Transgender identity's impact on condomless sex (% agree/strongly agree that circumstance would increase risk of CRAIMC)		
Wearing feminine attire during sexual practice with male clients	18.7	
Worry that male sex clients might know about your identity as a transgender woman	10.0	
Attempts to avoid exposing your genitalia to male clients	13.2	
Avoidance of talking to male clients	11.8	
Transgender Identity's Impact on Condomless Sex Scale		8.5 (3.4)

[1] SD: standard deviation.

ical interventions and self-efficacy, were then fitted. A weakened association between the variable of feminizing medical intervention and CRAIMC would suggest the presence of a mediation effect (Baron & Kenny, 1986). To test the second mediation hypothesis, the same procedure was repeated, but the variable of feminizing medical interventions was replaced by the Transgender Identity's Impact on Condomless Sex Scale. We used SPSS version 16.0; p values < .05 were considered statistically significant.

RESULTS

Background Characteristics

Over half of the participants were under 30 years of age (50.9%), not permanent Shenyang residents (87.3%), and had stayed in Shenyang for less than five years (55.9%). Only 10.9% had attended college or university, and 41.8% had a monthly personal income greater than 5,000 RMB (806.5 USD). About 90% (91.8%) had used HIV prevention services in the previous six months (see Table 21.1).

Over one-quarter (26.8%) had had CRAIMC in the previous month, and the prevalence was 32.4% among those who self-reported being HIV positive. The majority (88.6%) had had anal intercourse with a noncommercial male sex partner(s) in the preceding month, and among these, 26.2% had had condomless anal intercourse with their male sex partners (23.2% among all participants). Only 15.0% had undergone one of the following interventions: cosmetic surgery (13.2%), hormone treatment (2.3%), or sex-reassignment surgery (.5%) (see Table 21.1).

HIV Serostatus

Prevalence of self-reported HIV-positive status was 16.8% (N = 37). The 183 participants who self-reported HIV-negative or unknown HIV serostatus were invited to undergo free HIV testing, and 90 accepted the offer. The testing identified 20 HIV-positive cases (22.2% among the 90 testers and 9.1% among all participants). The HIV serostatus of the 93 participants who refused to be HIV tested remained unknown. Overall, 25.9% of all the participants either self-reported or were tested and confirmed as HIV-positive (see Table 21.1).

Sexual Practices with Male Clients

Almost half of the participants most often recruited their male clients at parks (44.1%), and 45.0% had provided sex services to male clients in a rented room. About one-third (35%) charged 100 RMB or less (16.1 USD or less) per episode of sexual practice. About two-thirds (65.4%) had had 1–10 male clients (9.1% had had more than 30) in the previous week, and 4.5% had also had female clients in that time; 22.3% and 20.9% reported having used alcohol or drugs, respectively, before or during sex with male clients in the preceding month. Almost half

(45.5%) had performed sex work in other Chinese cities, and 3.2% had done so in other countries in the previous year (see Table 21.2).

Perceptions Related to HIV and Condom Use

Individual item responses and means (SD) of the scales are described in Table 21.3. Cronbach's alpha values of the Perceived Susceptibility for HIV Scale, Perceived Barriers against Condom Use Scale, Perceived Self-Efficacy of Consistent Condom Use Scale, and Transgender Identity's Impact on Condomless Sex Scale were acceptable (0.85, 0.82, 0.70, and 0.70, respectively). Single factors were identified for these four scales by using exploratory factor analysis (EFA) and explained 58.5–71.8% of the total variances.

Factors Associated with CRAIMC in the Previous Month

In the bivariate analysis, only one of the background factors (education level) was significantly associated with CRAIMC, while two (i.e., use of HIV prevention services in the preceding six months [$p = .062$] and unknown HIV serostatus [$p = .089$]) were of marginal statistical significance (i.e., $.05 < p < .1$) (odds ratios are shown in Table 21.4). Adjusted for these three background variables, the three other variables that were significantly and positively associated with CRAIMC were (1) feminizing medical interventions (AOR: 2.22, 95% CI 1.03, 5.11), (2) male sex clients most often recruited at hotels (AOR: 5.02, 95% CI 1.97, 12.79), and (3) the Transgender Identity's Impact on Condomless Sex Scale score (AOR: 1.20, 95% CI 1.09, 1.32). The two significantly and negatively associated variables were: (1) charge per episode of sex practice with clients (201–400 RMB: AOR: 0.27, 95% CI 0.11, 0.67; reference group: ≤100 RMB) and (2) perceived self-efficacy of consistent condom use with male clients (AOR: 0.56, 95% CI 0.45, 0.70). Perceived susceptibility of HIV transmission was positively associated with a marginal p value of .052 (AOR: 1.12, 95% CI 1.00, 1.26) (Table 21.5).

Testing the Mediation Hypotheses

Perceived self-efficacy of consistent condom use with male clients was significantly correlated with the Transgender Identity's Impact on Condomless Sex Scale (Spearman $r = -0.422$, $p < .001$). Furthermore, the significant association between this scale on perceived transgender identity's impact on condomless sex and CRAIMC became nonsignifi-

TABLE 21.4

Associations between Background Variables and CRAIMC in the Previous Month

	%	OR (95%CI)
Education level		
Primary or below	44.0	Reference
Junior secondary	26.6	0.46 (0.18, 1.17)
Senior secondary	22.0	0.36 (0.14, 0.91)*
Tertiary	29.2	0.52 (0.16, 1.71)
HIV prevention services use in the previous six months		
No	44.4	Reference
Yes	25.2	0.42 (0.16, 1.13)**
HIV serostatus		
Self-reported as being HIV-positive	22.0	Reference
Tested as positive in rapid HIV testing	32.4	1.92 (0.78, 4.74)
Tested as negative in rapid HIV testing	15.0	0.71 (0.18, 2.75)
Self-reported HIV-negative or unknown HIV serostatus but refused to take up HIV testing	32.3	1.91 (0.92, 3.95)**

OR: univariate odds ratios.
NOTE: Variables that were considered but were nonsignificant are not listed in this table; they included age group, monthly income, resident of Shenyang, and duration of stay in Shenyang.
*$p < 0.05$. **$p < 0.10$.

cant (AOR: 1.09; 95% CI 0.98, 1.22) after perceived self-efficacy was added to the multiple logistic regression model; the variable of self-efficacy remained strongly associated with CRAIMC in that model. The results suggest a full mediation effect. Feminizing medical intervention was not significantly associated with perceived self-efficacy (Spearman r: −0.005, $p = .642$); therefore, the second mediation hypothesis was not tested.

TABLE 21.5

Associations between Feminizing Medical Interventions, Sexual Practice with Male Clients, Perceptions on HIV and Condom Use, and CRAIMC in the Previous Month

	OR (95%CI)	AOR (95%CI)
Feminizing medical interventions		
Had undertaken such intervention(s)	2.71 (1.26, 5.81)*	2.22 (1.03, 5.11)*
Sexual practice with male clients		
Channel most often used to recruit clients		
Internet	Reference	Reference
Park	2.16 (1.07, 4.37)*	1.85 (0.86, 3.97)
Hotel	4.47 (1.84, 10.87)**	5.02 (1.97, 12.79)**
Engaged in sexual practice with clients in other Chinese cities in the previous year		
No	Reference	
Yes	1.78 (0.98, 3.25)†	NS
Average charge per episode of sex with clients (in RMB)		
≤ 100 RMB	Reference	Reference
101–200 RMB	1.26 (0.54, 2.90)	1.22 (0.50, 2.98)
201–400 RMB	0.28 (0.12, 0.65)**	0.27 (0.11, 0.67)**
≥ 401 RMB	0.41 (0.17, 0.99)*	0.42 (0.16, 1.12)†
Perceptions on HIV and condom use		
Perceived Susceptibility for HIV Scale	1.13 (1.02, 1.26)*	1.12 (1.00, 1.26)†
Perceived Self-Efficacy of Consistent Condom Use Scale	0.54 (0.43, 0.67)***	0.56 (0.45, 0.70)***
Transgender Identity's Impact on Condomless Sex Scale	1.19 (1.09, 1.31)***	1.20 (1.09, 1.32)***

OR: univariate odds ratios.

AOR: adjusted odds ratios; odds ratios adjusted by significant background variables (educational level, HIV prevention services use in the preceding six months, and HIV serostatus).

NOTE: Variables that were considered but were nonsignificant are not listed in this table; they included anal intercourse with noncommercial male sex partner(s) in the previous month, venues where sexual practices with clients took place, engagement in sexual practices with clients in other countries, number of male clients and female clients, use of alcohol or drugs before or during sexual practices with clients, the Perceived Barrier of Condom Use Scale, and perceived cue to action of condom use.

*$p < 0.05$. **$p < 0.01$. ***$p < 0.001$. NS: $p > 0.10$, †$p < 0.10$.

DISCUSSION

Transwomen sex workers in China are likely to be at high risk of HIV, which is indicated by the 25.9% HIV prevalence according to self-reported and testing data. Moreover, more than 40% of all participants self-reported negative or unknown HIV status and refused free HIV testing offered by this study. These participants were more likely to report CRAIMC, although this was marginally statistically significant. Some participants may have felt uncomfortable disclosing their HIV-positive status to interviewers. Disclosure of HIV status is not a norm in China and is highly stigmatized. Therefore, the self-reported HIV prevalence was probably understated. Further research on HIV prevalence and incidence among transwomen sex workers is required to inform policy makers and health workers.

Over 25% of all participants and one-third of those who self-reported being HIV-positive had engaged in CRAIMC, suggesting that we need to develop more effective and tailor-made HIV prevention interventions for transwomen sex workers. There is a dearth of NGOs serving transwomen sex workers in China. Establishment of transgender-friendly NGOs is needed. The majority of transwomen sex workers also had sex with men who were nonclients, and such occasions frequently involved condomless anal intercourse. HIV interventions should take into account the different types of partner that transwomen sex workers have.

Importantly, nearly 5% of the participants also served female clients. Because we focused on male clients of transwomen sex workers, we did not investigate condom use related to female clients. More research is required to understand the implications for HIV prevention. Mobility of transwomen sex workers is a concern, as this is a known risk factor for HIV transmission (McGrath et al., 2015). The majority of the participants came to Shenyang from other parts of China, and half had traveled to other Chinese cities or to other countries for sex work in the previous year. Prevalence of CRAIMC while working in other cities was also high. Mobility may have created additional challenges for designing HIV interventions for transwomen sex workers in China.

We need to understand factors associated with CRAIMC in order to design effective HIV prevention programs. As was the case in previous studies on condomless anal intercourse among MSM (Lau et al., 2014), education level was negatively associated with CRAIMC. Unlike MSM studies that found 40.7–69.6% in Chinese cities had attained university education (Xu et al., 2014; Wang et al., 2015, Liu et al., 2016), our study of transwomen sex workers found that only 10.9% had a university education. The lower educational level may create additional challenges for HIV prevention efforts targeting transwomen sex workers. As in previous studies involving female sex workers (Tucker et al., 2011) and two that surveyed transwomen sex workers (Nemoto et al., 2012; Michie et al., 2008), we found that a lower price for sexual practices with clients was associated with CRAIMC. About one-third of our participants charged 100 RMB or less per episode of sex. The lower income might result in financial difficulty and lower negotiation power over condom use with male clients. Attention should be given to those with low educational level and those who charge less for their sex work.

Only 15% of study participants had taken up at least one type of feminizing medical intervention (mostly cosmetic surgeries: 13.2%), and only one had received sex reassignment surgery. It is unknown whether that participant had vaginal sex with male clients. In China, cosmetic surgeries are available at most plastic surgery hospitals nationwide. Sex-reassignment surgery is, however, costly (about 30,000 RMB, or 4,838 USD) and is unaffordable for many transwomen. Accessibility is extremely low, as the surgery can be performed only by senior plastic surgeons of major hospitals (Jiang et al., 2014), endorsement must be obtained from the applicant's next of kin, and an official proof of being free from any past criminal offenses has to be issued by a local public security office. Meanwhile, sex work remains illegal in China (Ren, 1999). We found that participants who underwent feminizing medical interventions were at higher risk of CRAIMC. These interventions were not associated with self-efficacy in condom use with male clients, and their association with CRAIMC was hence not mediated by self-efficacy.

Though perceptions related to condom use, including those derived from HBM, were associated with condomless anal intercourse in research among male sex workers (Lau, Cai, et al., 2012), such factors had not been studied among transwomen sex workers. We found that self-efficacy for consistent condom use with male clients was a protective factor against CRAIMC. Concern about transgender identity's impact on condomless sex was significantly correlated with both self-efficacy and CRAIMC. Furthermore, its association with CRAIMC was fully mediated by self-efficacy. This suggests that being transgender may have created additional difficulties for condom use with male clients. This finding is consistent with results obtained from qualitative studies that found being transgender and worrying about exposure of transgender identity to male clients were obstacles to negotiating condom use with male clients (Nemoto, Operario, Keatley, & Villega, 2004; Bockting et al., 1998; Bianchi et al., 2014). Skills training to increase self-efficacy for condom use and address concerns about exposing one's status as a transwoman may be important components of HIV prevention.

Another factor, perceived susceptibility to HIV transmission, was of marginal statistical significance; however, it still may be important to increase perception of HIV transmission risk among transwomen sex workers. Perceived barriers and cue to action (e.g., display of prevention messages at sex venues) were not significant, and strategies based on these factors may not be useful for HIV prevention targeting this population in China.

Although over 90% had received HIV-related services in the preceding six months, prevalence of CRAIMC was high. Half of all participants did not know their HIV status, which indicates there is much room for improvement in HIV testing and condom-promotion strategies. Tailored HIV prevention services for transwomen sex workers are virtually unavailable in mainland China. They may be treated as MSM in the eyes of workers of the CDC, which would neglect their unique prevention needs. Barriers to condom use, however, differ between transwomen sex workers and male sex workers. For instance, some circumstances during sex work linked to their transgender identity (e.g., worry about disclosure of transgender status) may create additional risks of CRAIMC. Needs assessments for developing tailored HIV prevention services for transwomen sex workers and their male clients are urgently warranted. Segmentation is a key to success in HIV prevention, according to social marketing principles (Valente & Fosados, 2006). We strongly advocate a policy review and training for CDC workers about gender identity and the special needs of transwomen sex workers.

CONCLUSIONS

This study, for the first time, describes the complex high-risk situations of transwomen sex workers in mainland China, including high prevalence of HIV and CRAIMC, high intercity mobility involving sex work, and involvement in sexual networks consisting of multiple types of sex partners. Interventions are urgently needed and should target transwomen sex workers with lower education levels and who charge less for sex work services. Factors unique to transwomen sex workers further increase risk of CRAIMC, such as feminizing medical intervention and perceived transgender identity's impact on condomless sex. Skills training should be provided to increase self-efficacy in condom use. Further research is warranted to better understand the determinants of CRAIMC and to develop effective intervention programs.

NOTE

This chapter originally appeared in the *Journal of the International AIDS Society*, 19 (Suppl. 2), July 2016. In the original article, the authors were listed as "Yong Cai, Zixin Wang, Joseph TF Lau, Jinghua Li, Tiecheng Ma, and Yan Liu." The authorship is revised here at the joint request of the authors.

ACKNOWLEDGMENTS

The authors would like to thank all the participants in the study. Funding: This study is supported by internal funding of the Centre for Health Behaviours Research, the Chinese University of Hong Kong.

AUTHORS' CONTRIBUTIONS

Yong Cai participated in conceptualizing the study, designing the protocol and questionnaires, managing the data collection, and revising the manuscript critically. Zixin Wang participated in designing the questionnaires, analyzing and interpreting the data, reviewing literature, and drafting and revising the manuscript. Joseph T. F. Lau participated in conceptualizing the study, designing the protocol and questionnaires, providing scientific and management leadership, interpreting the data, and drafting and revising the manuscript. Jinghua Li participated in conceptualizing the study, designing the protocol and questionnaires, and managing the data collection. Tiecheng Ma and Yan Liu participated in conceptualizing the study, commented on the questionnaire, and coordinated the data collection.

REFERENCES

Baral, S. D., Poteat, T., Strömdahl, S., Wirtz, A. L., Guadamuz, T. E., & Beyrer, C. (2013). Worldwide burden of HIV in transgender women: A systematic review and meta-analysis. *Lancet Infectious Diseases, 13* (3), 214–222.

Baron, R. M., & Kenny, D. A. (1986). The moderator-mediator variable distinction in social psychological research: Conceptual, strategic, and statistical considerations. *Journal of Personality and Social Psychology, 51*, 1173–1182.

Best, J., Tang, W., Zhang, Y., Han, L., Liu, F., & Huang, S. (2015). Sexual behaviors and HIV/syphilis testing among transgender individuals in China: Implications for expanding HIV testing services. *Sexually Transmitted Diseases, 42* (5), 281–285.

Bianchi, F. T., Reisen, C. A., Zea, M. C., Vidal-Ortiz, S., Gonzales, F. A., & Betancourt, F. (2014). Sex work among men who have sex with men and transgender women in Bogotá. *Archives of Sexual Behavior, 43* (8), 1637–1650.

Bockting, W. O., Robinson, B. E., & Rosser, B. R. (1998). Transgender HIV prevention: A qualitative needs assessment. *AIDS Care, 10* (4), 505–525.

Centers for Disease Control and Prevention. (2006). HIV prevalence among populations of men who have sex with men—Thailand, 2003 and 2005. *Morbidity and Mortality Weekly Report, 55* (31), 844–848.

Chew, S., Tham, K. F., & Ratnam, S. S. (1997). Sexual behaviour and prevalence of HIV antibodies in transsexuals. *Journal of Obstetrics and Gynaecology Research, 23* (1), 33–36.

Hawkes., S., Collumbien, M., Platt, L., Lalji, N., Rizvi, N., & Andreasen, A. (2009). HIV and other sexually transmitted infections among men, transgenders, and women selling sex in two cities in Pakistan: A cross-sectional prevalence survey. *Sexually Transmitted Infections, 85* (Suppl. 2), ii8–16.

Herbst, J. H., Jacobs, E. D., Finlayson, T. J., McKleroy, V. S., Neumann, M. S., & Crepaz, N. (2008). Estimating HIV prevalence and risk behaviors of transgender persons in the United States: A systematic review. *AIDS and Behavior, 12* (1), 1–17.

Janz, N. K., & Becker, M. H. (1984). The Health Belief Model: A decade later. *Health Education Quarterly, 11* (1), 1–47.

Jiang, H., Wei, X., Zhu, X., Wang, H., & Li, Q. (2014). Transgender patients need better protection in China. *Lancet, 384*, 2109–2110.

Keatley, J., & Clements-Nolle, K. (2001). What are the prevention needs of male-to-female transgender persons (MTFs)? Center for AIDS Prevention Studies, University of California, San Francisco. Retrieved from www.caps.ucsf.edu/pubs/FS/MTF.php.

Lau, J. T., Cai, W., Tsui, H. Y., Chen, L., Cheng, J., & Lin, C. (2012). Unprotected anal intercourse behavior and intention among male sex workers in Shenzhen serving cross-boundary male clients coming from Hong Kong, China: Prevalence and associated factors. *AIDS Care, 24* (1), 59–70.

Lau, J. T., Gu, J., Tsui, H.Y., Chen, H., Holroyd, E., & Wang, R. (2012). Prevalence and associated factors of condom use during commercial sex by female sex workers who were or were not injecting drug users in China. *Sexual Health, 9* (4), 368–376.

Lau, J. T., Ho, S. P., Yang, X., Wong, E., Tsui, H. Y, & Ho, K. M. (2007). Prevalence of HIV and factors associated with risk behaviours among Chinese female sex workers in Hong Kong. *AIDS Care, 19* (6), 721–732.

Lau, J. T., Wang, Z., Lau, M., & Lai, C. H. (2014). Perceptions of HPV, genital warts, and penile/anal cancer and high-risk sexual behaviors among men who have sex with men in Hong Kong. *Archives of Sexual Behavior, 43* (4), 789–800.

Liu, Y. Y., Tao, H. D., Liu, J., Fan, Y. G., Zhang, C., & Li, P. (2016). Prevalence and associated factors of HIV infection among men who have sex with men in Hefei, China, 2013–2014: A cross-sectional study. *International Journal of STD & AIDS, 27* (4), 305–312.

McGrath, N., Eaton, J. W., Newell, M. L., & Hosegood, V. (2015). Migration, sexual behaviour, and HIV risk: A general population cohort in rural South Africa. *Lancet HIV, 2* (6), e252–259.

Michie, S., Johnston, M., Francis, J., Hardeman, W., & Eccle, M. (2008). From theory to intervention: Mapping theoretically derived behavioural determinants to behaviour change techniques. *Applied Psychology, 57,* 660–680.

Nemoto, T., Iwamoto, M., Perngparn, U., Areesantichai, C., Kamitani, E., & Sakata, M. (2012). HIV-related risk behaviors among kathoey (male-to-female transgender) sex workers in Bangkok, Thailand. *AIDS Care, 24* (2), 2101–2109.

Nemoto, T., Operario, D., Keatley, J., Han, L., & Soma, T. G. (2004). HIV risk behaviors among male-to-female transgender persons of color in San Francisco. *American Journal of Public Health, 94* (7), 1193–1199.

Nemoto, T., Operario, D., Keatley, J., & Villegas, D. (2004). Social context of HIV risk behaviours among male-to-female transgenders of colour. *AIDS Care, 16* (6), 724–735.

Operario, D., Soma, T., & Underhill, K. (2008). Sex work and HIV status among transgender women: Systematic review and meta-analysis. *Journal of Acquired Immune Deficiency Syndrome, 48* (1), 97–103.

Poteat, T., Wirtz, A. L., Radix, A., Borquez, A., Silva-Santisteban, A., & Deutsch, M. B. (2015). HIV risk and preventive interventions in transgender women sex workers. *Lancet, 385,* 274–286.

Ren, X. (1999). Prostitution and economic modernization in China. *Violence against Women, 5* (12), 1411–1436.

Richter, M. L., Chersich, M., Temmerman, M., & Luchters, S. (2013). Characteristics, sexual behaviour and risk factors of female, male and transgender sex workers in South Africa. *South African Medical Journal = Suid-Afrikaanse tydskrif vir geneeskunde, 103* (4), 246–251.

Roche, K., & Keith, C. (2014). How stigma affects healthcare access for transgender sex workers. *British Journal of Nursing, 3* (2), 1147–1152.

Spizzichino, L., Zaccarelli, M., Rezza, G., Ippolito, G., Antinori, A., & Gattari, P. (2001). HIV infection among foreign transsexual sex workers in Rome: Prevalence, behavior patterns, and seroconversion rates. *Sexually Transmitted Diseases, 28* (7), 405–411.

Sutmoller, F., Penna, T. L., de Souza, C. T., Lambert, J., & Oswaldo Cruz Foundation. (2002). Human immunodeficiency virus incidence and risk behavior in the "Projeto Rio": Results of the first 5 years of the Rio de Janeiro open cohort of homosexual and bisexual men, 1994–98. *International Journal of Infectious Diseases, 6* (4), 259–265.

Tucker, J. D., Yin, Y. P., Wang, B., Chen, X. S., & Cohen, M. S. (2011). An expanding syphilis epidemic in China: Epidemiology, behavioural risk, and control strategies with a focus on low-tier female sex workers and men who have sex with men. *Sexually Transmitted Infections, 87* (Suppl. 2), ii16–18.

Valente, T. W., & Fosados, R. (2006). Diffusion of innovations and network segmentation: The part played by people in promoting health. *Sexually Transmitted Diseases, 33* (7) (Suppl.), S23–31.

Vinoles, J., Serra, M., Russi, J. C., Ruchansky, D., Sosa-Estani, S., & Montano, S. M. (2005). Seroincidence and phylogeny of human immunodeficiency virus infections in a cohort of commercial sex workers in Montevideo, Uruguay. *American Journal of Tropical Medicine and Hygiene, 72* (4), 495–500.

Wang, Z., Li, D., Lau, J. T., Yang, X., Shen, H., & Cao, W. (2015). Prevalence and associated factors of inhaled nitrites use among men who have sex with men in Beijing, China. *Drug and Alcohol Dependence, 149*, 93–99.

Xu, J. J., Qian, H. Z., Chu, Z. X., Zhang, J., Hu, Q. H., & Jiang, Y. J. (2014). Recreational drug use among Chinese men who have sex with men: A risky combination with unprotected sex for acquiring HIV infection. *BioMed Research International, 72*, 361–366.

SECTION VII

CARE AND TREATMENT OF TRANSGENDER SEX WORKERS

The proper assessment and treatment of transgender sex workers involves an understanding of the issues bearing on the lives of these individuals. In this section, Radix and Goldstein provide a current and much-needed review of these issues that will interest anyone involved with caring for transgender sex workers.

CHAPTER 22

Issues in the Care and Treatment of Transwomen Sex Workers

Asa Radix[1]
Zil Goldstein[2]

[1] Director of research and education at the Callen-Lorde Community Health Center and a doctoral student in the Department of Epidemiology at Columbia University.
[2] Nurse practitioner and transgender activist who also serves as program director at the Center for Transgender Medicine and Surgery in the Mount Sinai Hospital System.

SUMMARY

In this article, we present and discuss basic principles for the care and treatment of transgender sex workers. These individuals have typically experienced an array of difficulties and life challenges, including different forms of abuse, aspects of discrimination, and family problems, and caring for them requires a holistic understanding of these issues as they may relate to substance use and mental health issues. Better care and treatment of transgender sex workers are sorely needed, and we hope this chapter will assist practitioners in better serving this population.

KEY TERMS

aspects of abuse; holistic and comprehensive treatment; substance use; transgender sex workers

Transgender sex workers may require healthcare services for many reasons, including sexual health (prevention, screening, and treatment of sexually transmitted infections [STIs]), injuries resulting from harm or violence, mental health concerns, urgent care needs, and routine primary healthcare (Abel, 2014; Harcourt et al., 2001; Rekart, 2015; Sausa,

Nuttbrock, Larry, *Transgender Sex Work and Society*
dx.doi.org/10.17312/harringtonparkpress/2017.11.tsws.022
© 2018 by Harrington Park Press

Keatley, & Operario, 2007). Transwomen additionally may want to access transition-related services (hormones and gender-affirming surgeries). Studies have indicated that transgender individuals often avoid or delay needed healthcare services (Grant, Mottet, & Tanis, 2010; Jaffee, Shires, & Strousma, 2016; Lombardi, 2007; Nemoto et al., 2015; Reisner, Hughto, et al., 2015) because of experiences of discrimination, including denial of care, verbal and physical violence, and encountering providers who are not knowledgeable about transgender health issues (Carabez, Eliason, & Martinson, 2016; Dy et al., 2016; Grant et al., 2010; Irwig, 2016; Kenagy, 2005; Marin et al., 2015; Nemoto et al., 2015; Unger, 2015). Transgender individuals may also avoid care because of a fear of disclosure of their transgender identity (Xavier et al., 2005) or discomfort with medical examinations (Rachlin, Green, & Lombardi, 2008).

Transwomen working in the sex trade face additional stigma and may be hesitant to disclose their occupation to their primary care providers because of fears or actual experiences of discrimination or judgmental attitudes (Abel, 2014; Cohan et al., 2006; Jones & Singh, 2013; Lazarus et al., 2012; Marin et al., 2015; McCullough & Patterson, 2014). Additional barriers to care may include lack of insurance or undocumented legal status (Marin et al., 2015). In addition, clinics that operate predominantly during the day may not be convenient for sex workers (Marin et al., 2015). Many people who engage in trading sex fear that their comprehensive health needs will not be addressed after disclosure, owing to provider bias against sex workers (Jones & Singh, 2013; McCullough & Patterson, 2014). The way in which questions are asked can either facilitate or impede disclosure. In one study conducted among transwomen and men who have sex with men, only 6.2% identified as sex workers even though 52.1% had a personal history of being paid for sex. Compared to those who had never been paid for sex, those who had engaged in transactional sex had significantly higher rates of STIs (Solomon et al., 2015), which underscores the importance of disclosure for meeting their specific health needs.

Delivering care in gender-affirming settings that build rapport and support frank discussions about sexual practices and behaviors and caregivers who are knowledgeable about the diverse healthcare needs of sex workers are therefore essential to providing comprehensive healthcare to transwomen in the sex trade. Examples of healthcare settings that demonstrate best practices for gender-affirming care include centers such as Fenway Health in Boston, Massachusetts, and the Callen Lorde Community Health Center in New York (Reisner, Bradford, et al., 2015; Reisner, Radix, & Deutsch, 2016). In both centers, care is taken to use the names and pronouns that patients request, regardless of whether legal name and gender marker changes have occurred. Registration forms collect information on gender identity using a two-step question that asks a person's gender as well as sex assigned at birth (Deutsch et al., 2013). Attention is paid to the environment, ensuring gender-neutral or all-gender restrooms, signage and materials inclusive of transgender identities, employment of transgender and gender-nonconforming clinic staff, and training providers in transgender medicine, including provision of hormone therapy.

Improving disclosure of patients who trade sex requires a certain set of interpersonal skills to convey nonjudgmental attitudes while a patient may be discussing what providers are taught to think of as risky behavior. And, though sex work is often seen as an inevitable matter of fact in some transgender people's lives, it can often shock providers who have not been sensitized to both sex work and transgender-specific issues (McCullough & Patterson, 2014; Sausa et al., 2007).

Providers are taught to ask questions like "Have you ever traded sex for money, drugs, or a place to stay?" But these questions can suggest to patients that the provider is not familiar with the nuances of trading sex, and is therefore not a safe person with whom to discuss these activities (McCullough & Patterson, 2014).

Providers should recognize that there are a variety of experiences that people may have in trading sex. In preparing to have more frank, and less scripted, conversations, it is important to treat whatever form of trading sex someone is engaged in as a legitimate choice. Sex work includes varied roles (e.g., escort, dancer, pornographic film actor) and may be performed in different locations (e.g., indoors in clubs or clients' locations, outdoors on the street, web-based, or on the telephone). Understanding these differences allows the provider to appropriately assess and counsel for risk. Someone who engages in bondage, discipline, sadism, and masochism (BDSM) work without having sexual intercourse, called "not doing full-service," might answer "no" if asked, "Have you ever traded sex for money, drugs, or a place to stay?" but shares a lot of the same stressors as a professional escort who would answer "yes" to the same question.

Asking instead, "What do you do to support yourself?" will elicit far more information in terms of what types of sex work a consumer is engaged in, and if that person has other means of financial support. In the same vein, questions such as "How do you get your drugs?" and "What is your housing situation?" can assist in eliciting a broader range of responses and better understanding of how to best work with a patient. These questions also allow patients to bring up their concerns with trading sex. They can help frame the discussion in terms of occupational health and safety rather than risky behavior, which will create more buy-in among transwomen who have historically failed to access safer sex interventions such as pre-exposure prophylaxis (PrEP) to prevent HIV infection (Sevelius et al., 2016).

Further assessment of workplace safety is also easier to integrate into a healthcare visit when asking these questions. It is important to assess where patients are working, how they are working, how they are finding their clients, what happens to the money they earn, and if they feel forced to do sex work, in addition to finding out how much of the time they are using condoms. Getting a holistic picture of a client's work life will help to assess his or her overall safety.

SEXUAL HEALTH

Providers should be competent in obtaining a comprehensive sexual health history that includes information on sexual practices and behaviors, past STIs, sexual partners, HIV/STI prevention tools, and sexual satisfaction.

Transgender sex workers are more likely to be HIV-infected than cisgender male or female sex workers (Baral et al., 2013) and have a higher prevalence of other sexually transmitted diseases, such as gonorrhea, chlamydia, syphilis, hepatitis B, and human papillomavirus, compared to cisgender male sex workers or transwomen who are not engaged in sex work (Cohan et al., 2006; dos Ramos Farías, Garcia, et al., 2011; dos Ramos Farías, Picconi et al., 2011; Gupte et al., 2011; Nemoto et al., 2015; Operario, Soma, & Underhill, 2008; Poteat et al., 2015; Solomon et al., 2015; Toibaro et al., 2009).

Transwomen preferentially engage in receptive anal sex over insertive anal sex (Nemoto et al., 2014) in part because being the receptive partner may be perceived as more aligned with a female identity (Bockting, Robinson, & Rosser, 1998; Sevelius, 2013) and also because the use of androgen blockers and estrogens, as part of feminizing hormonal therapy, reduces erectile function (Hembree et al., 2009). This places them at increased risk for extragenital (anal and pharyngeal) STIs, which are more likely to be asymptomatic and therefore less likely to be treated (Lutz, 2015; Workowski & Bolan, 2015). For transwomen who have undergone vaginoplasty, less is known about HIV and STI risk; however, case reports indicate that it is possible to acquire STIs, including gonorrhea, genital warts, and bacterial vaginosis (Bodsworth, Price, & Davies, 1994; Jain & Bradbeer, 2007; Matsuki et al., 2015; van der Sluis, et al., 2015; Yang et al., 2009). Providers should assess the pattern of condom use for primary, casual, and transactional partners. Transwomen may not use condoms when experiencing financial pressures, as clients may offer more money for sex without condoms. In addition, alcohol and substance use as well as the need for gender validation may undermine the use of condoms in this setting (Operario et al., 2011; Reisner et al., 2009; Sausa et al., 2007; Sevelius, 2013). Transwomen, even when using condoms for work, may not use them for sex with a primary partner (Nemoto et al., 2014), and therefore the risk of HIV/STIs is still a concern.

The CDC guidelines for sexually transmitted infections advise that screening for transgender persons should occur on the basis of anatomic considerations and sexual behaviors. Current recommendations are to screen for pharyngeal, rectal, and urethral infections caused by *Neisseria gonorrhoeae* and *Chlamydia trachomatis* using nucleic acid amplification testing (NAAT) (Workowski & Bolan, 2015). Screening for STIs in persons at highest risk should be conducted every three months. There are no guidelines regarding the types of screening for transwomen who have undergone vaginoplasty; however, visual inspection using a small vaginal speculum or anoscope for visualization and STI testing is suggested for symptoms (Deutsch, 2016; Weyers et al., 2010). Routine testing should also occur for syphilis and HIV every three to six months. Patients should be assessed for infection or immunity to hepatitis B and vaccinated against hepatitis A and B, HPV, and meningococcal infections if indicated. Those living with HIV infection should be tested for hepatitis C yearly. Transwomen who have a negative HIV screen should be given information about HIV prevention, including condoms and biomedical interventions, such as PrEP and post-exposure prophylaxis (PEP). Pre-exposure chemoprophylaxis for HIV should be offered to all patients who trade sex, regardless of history of condom use, as some evidence suggests certain sex workers are more at risk in their personal sex lives than in their professional lives (Choudhury, 2010). This assertion may or may not be true when it comes to transwomen, particularly outdoor workers, who are pressured to offer more services at a lower price because of many workers congregating in a small geographic area and pushing prices down.

VIOLENCE

Transwomen sex workers are at heightened risk for violence (both from their intimate partners and from their pimps, clients, and police) (Clements-Nolle, Guzman, & Harris, 2008; Cohan et al., 2006; Reisner et al., 2009). Cohan and colleagues (2006), studying sex workers who accessed care at a San Francisco clinic, reported that 53.2% of transgender sex workers experienced sex-work-related violence, and 57.9% experienced violence from a partner or family member. These rates of violence were higher than those faced by cisgender male and female sex workers. Transgender sex workers may present with acute injuries as well as chronic health issues related to physical trauma. Providers should screen for violence at intake and during routine visits and learn where to refer clients for forensic examination in the instance of sexual assault. Providers should become familiar with resources, such as safe houses or shelters and legal services that are inclusive of transgender people. Because of the extremely high rates of trauma experienced by transwomen, implementation of trauma-aware and trauma-informed care may create environments that foster engagement in care, as well as disclosure of gender identity and of participation in sex work.

GENDER-AFFIRMATION CARE

Transgender people may decide to use hormonal or surgical intervention (or both) to align their physical appearance with their gender identity. Protocols for the provision of hormone therapy include those from the World Professional Association of Transgender Health—WPATH (Coleman et al., 2011) and the Endocrine Society (Hembree et al., 2009). Feminizing hormonal therapy usually consists of a combination of estrogens and androgen blockers. Estrogens are available in oral, transdermal, and injectable forms. Different androgen blockers are used around the world; however, spironolactone is most frequently used in the United States. Although feminizing therapy is generally considered safe, it may result in increased risk of venous thrombosis, dyslipidemias, and cardiovascular disease, especially if there are concurrent issues such as tobacco use or HIV infection (Asscheman et al., 2011; Asscheman et al., 2014; Deutsch, 2016). Transwomen may also decide to undergo gender-affirming surgeries, including breast augmentation, tracheal shave, brow lift, orchiectomy (removal of testes), and vaginoplasty (creation of a vagina most commonly using penile and scrotal tissue) (Schechter, 2016). When transwomen do not have access to gender-affirming care in medical settings, they may self-medicate with hormones or inject soft-tissue fillers (silicone) into the breasts, hips, buttocks, and face to feminize their appearance (Garafalo et al., 2006; Sanchez, Sanchez, & Danoff, 2009; Wiessing et al., 1999; Wilson et al., 2014).

PRIMARY CARE NEEDS

In addition to health needs that are specific to their occupation, transgender sex workers have routine primary care needs. The commonly used guidelines from the US Preventive Services Task Force are gender-specific, and providers need to consider their applications to transgender people, especially those who have undergone hormonal therapy or gender-affirming surgeries. In general, providers are advised to perform an anatomic inventory and screen according to the organs that are present (Deutsch, 2016; Unger, 2014). Providers should address known disparities—for example, higher rates of tobacco use (Cohan et al., 2006) and substance use (Clements-Nolle et al., 2001; Nemoto et al., 2004), including injection drug use (Cohan et al., 2006). Transwomen on hormones experience higher rates of osteoporosis and should undergo screening for this; they should also receive advice on diet and exercise (Deutsch, 2016; Van Caenegem & T'Sjoen, 2015).

ACCESS TO MENTAL HEALTH SERVICES

Multiple studies have shown that transwomen have high rates of mood disorders, including depression and suicidality; this is true especially among those who face discrimination that is due to their gender identity (Bockting et al., 2013; Clements-Nolle et al., 2001; Nuttbrock et al., 2014). Programs that provide primary care services to transwomen should include robust and trans-affirming mental health services.

SUMMARY

To provide comprehensive and holistic care to transwomen sex workers, healthcare providers need to be skilled in providing fully competent and nonstigmatizing care that affirms gender identity and supports disclosure of work in the sex trade. Health services need to be comprehensive—that is, not focusing just on sexual health but also addressing access to gender-transition services, mental health services, and primary care. Sexual health should include prevention, screening, and treatment of HIV/STIs, as well as behavioral and biomedical prevention (PrEP and PEP) interventions. Clinical settings should provide care during times that are convenient and assist patients in accessing health insurance. Other considerations include having access to or timely referrals to legal services.

REFERENCES

Abel, G. (2014). Sex workers' utilisation of health services in a decriminalised environment. *New Zealand Medical Journal, 127* (1390), 30–37.

Asscheman, H., Giltay, E. J., Megens, J. A., de Ronde, W. P., van Trotsenburg, M. A., & Gooren, L. J. (2011). A long-term follow-up study of mortality in transsexuals receiving treatment with cross-sex hormones. *European Journal of Endocrinology, 164* (4), 635–642. doi:10.1530/EJE-10-1038; 10.1530/EJE-10-1038.

Asscheman, H., T'Sjoen, G., Lemaire, A., Mas, M., Meriggiola, M. C., Mueller, A., . . . & Gooren, L. J. (2014). Venous thrombo-embolism as a complication of cross-sex hormone treatment of male-to-female transsexual subjects: A review. *Andrologia, 46* (7), 791–795. doi:10.1111/and.12150.

Baral, S. D., Poteat, T., Strömdahl, S., Wirtz, A. L., Guadamuz, T. E., & Beyrer, C. (2013). Worldwide burden of HIV in transgender women: A systematic review and meta-analysis. *Lancet Infectious Diseases, 13* (3), 214–222. doi:10.1016/S1473-3099(12)70315-8; 10.1016/S1473-3099(12)70315-8.

Bockting, W. O., Miner, M. H., Swinburne Romine, R. E., Hamilton, A., & Coleman, E. (2013). Stigma, mental health, and resilience in an online sample of the U.S. transgender population. *American Journal of Public Health, 103* (5), 943–951. doi:10.2105/AJPH.2013.301241; 10.2105/AJPH.2013.301241.

Bockting, W. O., Robinson, B. E., & Rosser, B. R. (1998). Transgender HIV prevention: A qualitative needs assessment. *AIDS Care, 10* (4), 505–525. doi:10.1080/09540129850124028.

Bodsworth, N. J., Price, R., & Davies, S. C. (1994). Gonococcal infection of the neovagina in a male-to-female transsexual. *Sexually Transmitted Diseases, 21* (4), 211–212.

Carabez, R. M., Eliason, M. J., & Martinson, M. (2016). Nurses' knowledge about transgender patient care: A qualitative study. *Advances in Nursing Science, 39* (3), 257–271. doi:10.1097/ans.0000000000000128.

Choudhury, S. M. (2010). "As prostitutes, we control our bodies": Perceptions of health and body in the lives of establishment-based female sex workers in Tijuana, Mexico. *Culture, Health & Sexuality, 12* (6), 677–689. doi:10.1080/1369105100 3797263.

Clements-Nolle, K., Guzman, R., & Harris, S. G. (2008). Sex trade in a male-to-female transgender population: Psychosocial correlates of inconsistent condom use. *Sexual Health, 5* (1), 49–54.

Clements-Nolle, K., Marx, R., Guzman, R., & Katz, M. (2001). HIV prevalence, risk behaviors, health care use, and mental health status of transgender persons: Implications for public health intervention. *American Journal of Public Health, 91* (6), 915–921.

Cohan, D., Lutnick, A., Davidson, P., Cloniger, C., Herlyn, A., Breyer, J., . . . & Klausner, J. (2006). Sex worker health: San Francisco style. *Sexually Transmitted Infections, 82* (5), 418–422. doi:10.1136/sti.2006.020628.

Coleman, E., Bockting, W., Botzer, M., Cohen-Kettenis, P., DeCuypere, G., Feldman, J., . . . & Zucker, K. (2011). Standards of care for the health of transsexual, transgender, and gender-nonconforming people, version 7. *International Journal of Transgenderism, 13*, 165. doi:10.1080/15532739.2011.700873.

Deutsch, M. B. (ed.). (2016, June 17). *Guidelines for the primary and gender-affirming care of transgender and gender nonbinary people.* San Francisco: Center of Excellence for Transgender Health. Retrieved from www.transhealth.ucsf.edu/guidelines.

Deutsch, M. B., Green, J., Keatley, J., Mayer, G., Hastings, J., Hall, A. M., & World Professional Association for Transgender Health, EMR Working Group. (2013). Electronic medical records and the transgender patient: Recommendations from the World Professional Association for Transgender Health EMR Working Group. *Journal of the American Medical Informatics Association, 20* (4), 700–703. doi:10.1136/amiajnl-2012-001472.

dos Ramos Farías, M. S., Garcia, M. N., Reynaga, E., Romero, M., Gallo Vaulet, M. L., Fermepín, M. R., . . . & Avila, M. M. (2011). First report on sexually transmitted infections among trans (male to female transvestites, transsexuals, or transgender) and male sex workers in Argentina: High HIV, HPV, HBV, and syphilis prevalence. *International Journal of Infectious Diseases, 15* (9), e635–e640. doi: 10.1016/j.ijid.2011.05.007.

dos Ramos Farías, M. S., Picconi, M. A., Garcia, M. N., González, J. V., Basiletti, J., Pando, M., & Avila, M. M. (2011). Human papilloma virus genotype diversity of anal infection among trans (male to female transvestites, transsexuals or transgender) sex workers in Argentina. *Journal of Clinical Virology, 51* (2), 96–99. doi:10.1016/j.jcv.2011.03.008.

Dy, G. W., Osbun, N. C., Morrison, S. D., Grant, D. W., & Merguerian, P. A. (2016). Exposure to and attitudes regarding transgender education among urology residents. *Journal of Sexual Medicine, 13* (10), 1466–1472. doi:10.1016/j.jsxm.2016.07.017.

Garofalo, R., Deleon, J., Osmer, E., Doll, M., & Harper, G. W. (2006). Overlooked, misunderstood and at-risk: Exploring the lives and HIV risk of ethnic minority male-to-female transgender youth. *Journal of Adolescent Health, 38* (3), 230–236. doi:10.1016/j.jadohealth.2005.03.023.

Grant, J. M., Mottet, L. A., & Tanis, J. (2010). *National Transgender Discrimination Survey Report on Health and Health Care.* Washington, DC: National Center for Transgender Equality and the National Gay and Lesbian Task Force.

Gupte, S., Daly, C., Agarwal, V., Gaikwad, S. B., & George, B. (2011). Introduction of rapid tests for large-scale syphilis screening among female, male, and transgender sex workers in Mumbai, India. *Sexually Transmitted Diseases, 38* (6), 499–502. doi:10.1097/OLQ.0b013e318205e45d.

Harcourt, C., van Beek, I., Heslop, J., McMahon, M., & Donovan, B. (2001). The health and welfare needs of female and transgender street sex workers in New South Wales. *Australian and New Zealand Journal of Public Health, 25* (1), 84–89.

Hembree, W. C., Cohen-Kettenis, P., Delemarre–van de Waal, H. A., Gooren, L. J., Meyer, W. J., Spack, N. P., . . . & Endocrine Society. (2009). Endocrine treatment of transsexual persons: An Endocrine Society clinical practice guideline. *Journal of Clinincal Endocrinology & Metabolism, 94* (9), 3132–3154. doi: 10.1210/jc.2009-0345; 10.1210/jc.2009-0345.

Irwig, M. S. (2016). Transgender care by endocrinologists in the United States. *Endocrine Practice, 22* (7), 832–836. doi:10.4158/ep151185.or.

Jaffee, K. D., Shires, D. A., & Stroumsa, D. (2016). Discrimination and delayed health care among transgender women and men: Implications for improving medical education and health care delivery. *Medical Care.* doi:10.1097/mlr.0000000000000583.

Jain, A., & Bradbeer, C. (2007). A case of successful management of recurrent bacterial vaginosis of neovagina after male to female gender reassignment surgery. *International Journal of STD & AIDS, 18* (2), 140–141. doi:10.1258/095646207779949790.

Jones, H. T., & Singh, S. (2013). How can healthcare services for female sex workers be better tailored to meet their health needs? *Sexually Transmitted Infections, 89* (5), 414. doi:10.1136/sextrans-2013-051134.

Kenagy, G. P. (2005). Transgender health: Findings from two needs assessment studies in Philadelphia. *Health & Social Work, 30* (1), 19–26.

Lazarus, L., Deering, K. N., Nabess, R., Gibson, K., Tyndall, M. W., & Shannon, K. (2012). Occupational stigma as a primary barrier to health care for street-based sex workers in Canada. *Culture, Health & Sexuality, 14* (2), 139–150. doi: 10.1080/13691058.2011.628411.

Lombardi, E. (2007). Public health and trans-people: Barriers to care and strategies to improve treatment. *In* I. N. Meyer, (ed.), *The health of sexual minorities: Public health perspectives on lesbian, gay, bisexual, and transgender populations* (pp. 638–652). New York: Springer.

Lutz, A. R. (2015). Screening for asymptomatic extragenital gonorrhea and chlamydia in men who have sex with men: Significance, recommendations, and options for overcoming barriers to testing. *LGBT Health, 2* (1), 27–34. doi:10.1089/lgbt.2014.0056.

Marin, G., Silberman, M., Martinez, S., & Sanguinetti, C. (2015). Healthcare program for sex workers: A public health priority. *International Journal of Health Planning and Management, 30* (3), 276–284. doi:10.1002/hpm.2234.

Matsuki, S., Kusatake, K., Hein, K. Z., Anraku, K., & Morita, E. (2015). Condylomata acuminata in the neovagina after male-to-female reassignment treated with CO_2 laser and imiquimod. *International Journal of STD & AIDS, 26* (7), 509–511. doi:10.1177/0956462414542476.

McCullough, E. P., and Patterson, S. E. (2014). "No lectures or stink-eye": The healthcare needs of people in the sex trade in New York City. New York: Persist Health Project.

Nemoto, T., Bödeker, B., Iwamoto, M., & Sakata, M. (2014). Practices of receptive and insertive anal sex among transgender women in relation to partner types, sociocultural factors, and background variables. *AIDS Care, 26* (4), 434–440. doi:10.1080/09540121.2013.841832.

Nemoto, T., Cruz, T. M., Iwamoto, M., & Sakata, M. (2015). A tale of two cities: Access to care and services among African-American transgender women in Oakland and San Francisco. *LGBT Health, 2* (3), 235–242. doi:10.1089/lgbt.2014.0046.

Nemoto, T., Operario, D., Keatley, J., & Villegas, D. (2004). Social context of HIV risk behaviours among male-to-female transgenders of colour. *AIDS Care, 16* (6), 724–735. doi:10.1080/09540120413331269567.

Nuttbrock, L., Bockting, W., Rosenblum, A., Hwahng, S., Mason, M., Macri, M., & Becker, J. (2014). Gender abuse and major depression among transgender women: A prospective study of vulnerability and resilience. *American Journal of Public Health, 104* (11), 2191–2198. doi:10.2105/AJPH.2013.301545.

Operario, D., Nemoto, T., Iwamoto, M., & Moore, T. (2011). Risk for HIV and unprotected sexual behavior in male primary partners of transgender women. *Archives of Sexual Behavior, 40* (6), 1255–1261. doi:10.1007/s10508-011-9781-x.

Operario, D., Soma, T., & Underhill, K. (2008). Sex work and HIV status among transgender women: Systematic review and meta-analysis. *Journal of Acquired Immune Deficiency Syndrome, 48* (1), 97–103. doi:10.1097/QAI.0b013e31816e3971.

Poteat, T., Wirtz, A. L., Radix, A., Borquez, A., Silva-Santisteban, A., Deutsch, M. B., . . . & Operario, D. (2015). HIV risk and preventive interventions in transgender women sex workers. *Lancet, 385* (9964), 274–286. doi:10.1016/s0140-6736(14)60833-3.

Rachlin, K., Green, J., & Lombardi, E. (2008). Utilization of health care among female-to-male transgender individuals in the United States. *Journal of Homosexuality*, 54 (3), 243–258. doi:10.1080/00918360801982124.

Reisner, S. L., Bradford, J., Hopwood, R., Gonzalez, A., Makadon, H., Todisco, D., . . . & Mayer, K. (2015). Comprehensive transgender healthcare: The gender affirming clinical and public health model of Fenway Health. *Journal of Urban Health*, 92 (3), 584–592. doi:10.1007/s11524-015-9947-2.

Reisner, S. L., Hughto, J. M., Dunham, E. E., Heflin, K. J., Begenyi, J. B., Coffey-Esquivel, J., & Cahill, S. (2015). Legal protections in public accommodations settings: A critical public health issue for transgender and gender-nonconforming people. *Milbank Quarterly*, 93 (3), 484–515. doi:10.1111/1468-0009.12127.

Reisner, S. L., Mimiaga, M. J., Bland, S., Mayer, K. H., Perkovich, B., & Safren, S. A. (2009). HIV risk and social networks among male-to-female transgender sex workers in Boston, Massachusetts. *Journal of the Association of Nurses in AIDS Care*, 20 (5), 373–386. doi:10.1016/j.jana.2009.06.003.

Reisner, S. L., Radix, A., & Deutsch, M. B. (2016). Integrated and gender-affirming transgender clinical care and research. *Journal of Acquired Immune Deficiency Syndrome*, 72 (Suppl. 3), S235–242. doi:10.1097/qai.0000000000001088.

Rekart, M. L. (2015). Caring for sex workers. *BMJ*, 351, h4011. doi:10.1136/bmj.h4011.

Sanchez, N. F., Sanchez, J. P., & Danoff, A. (2009). Health care utilization, barriers to care, and hormone usage among male-to-female transgender persons in New York City. *American Journal of Public Health*, 99 (4), 713–719. doi:10.2105/ajph.2007.132035.

Sausa, L., Keatley, J., & Operario, D. (2007). Perceived risks and benefits of sex work among transgender women of color in San Francisco. *Archives of Sexual Behavior*, 36 (6), 768–777. doi:10.1007/s10508-007-9210-3.

Schechter, L. S. (2016). Gender confirmation surgery: An update for the primary care provider. *Transgender Health*, 1 (1), 32–40. doi:10.1089/trgh.2015.0006.

Sevelius, J. M. (2013). Gender affirmation: A framework for conceptualizing risk behavior among transgender women of color. *Sex Roles*, 68 (11–12), 675–689. doi: 10.1007/s11199-012-0216-5.

Sevelius, J. M., Keatley, J., Calma, N., & Arnold, E. (2016). "I am not a man": Trans-specific barriers and facilitators to PrEP acceptability among transgender women. *Global Public Health*, 11 (7–8), 1060–1075. doi:10.1080/17441692.2016.1154085.

Solomon, M. M., Nureña, C. R., Tanur, J. M., Montoya, O., Grant, R. M., & McConnell, J. J. (2015). Transactional sex and prevalence of STIs: A cross-sectional study of MSM and transwomen screened for an HIV prevention trial. *International Journal of STD & AIDS*, 26 (12), 879–886. doi:10.1177/0956462414562049.

Toibaro, J. J., Ebensrtejin, J. E., Parlante, A., Burgoa, P., Freyre, A., Romero, M., & Losso, M. H. (2009). [Sexually transmitted infections among transgender individuals and other sexual identities]. *Medicina*, 69 (3), 327–330.

Unger, C. A. (2015). Care of the transgender patient: A survey of gynecologists' current knowledge and practice. *Journal of Women's Health, 24* (2), 114–118. doi:10.1089/jwh.2014.4918.

———. (2014). Care of the transgender patient: The role of the gynecologist. *American Journal of Obstetrics & Gynecology, 210* (1), 16–26. doi:10.1016/j.ajog.2013.05.035.

Van Caenegem, E., & T'Sjoen, G. (2015). Bone in trans persons. *Current Opinion in Endocrinology, Diabetes, and Obesity, 22* (6), 459–466. doi:10.1097/med.0000000000 0000202.

van der Sluis, W. B., Bouman, M. B., Gijs, L., & van Bodegraven, A. A. (2015). Gonorrhoea of the sigmoid neovagina in a male-to-female transgender. *International Journal of STD & AIDS, 26* (8), 595–598. doi:10.1177/0956462414544725.

Weyers, S., De Sutter, P., Hoebeke, S., Monstrey, G., T'Sjoen, G., Verstraelen, H., & Gerris, J. (2010). Gynaecological aspects of the treatment and follow-up of transsexual men and women. *Facts, Views & Visions in ObGyn, 2* (1), 35–54.

Wiessing, L. G., van Roosmalen, M. S., Koedijk, P., Bieleman, B., & Houweling, H. (1999). Silicones, hormones, and HIV in transgender street prostitutes. *AIDS, 13* (16), 2315–2316.

Wilson, E., Rapues, J., Jin, H., & Raymond, H. F. (2014). The use and correlates of illicit silicone or "fillers" in a population-based sample of transwomen, San Francisco, 2013. *Journal of Sexual Medicine, 11* (7), 1717–1724. doi:10.1111/jsm.12558.

Workowski, K. A., & Bolan, G. A. (2015, June 15). Sexually transmitted diseases treatment guidelines, 2015. *Morbidity and Mortality Weekly Report Recommendations and Reports, 64* (RR3), 1–137.

Xavier, J. M., Bobbin, M., Singer, B., & Budd, E. (2005). A needs assessment of transgendered people of color living in Washington, DC. *International Journal of Transgenderism, 8* (2–3), 31–47. doi:10.1300/J485v08n02_04.

Yang, C., Liu, S., Xu, K., Xiang, Q., Yang, S., & Zhang, X. (2009). Condylomata gigantea in a male transsexual. *International Journal of STD & AIDS, 20* (3), 211–212. doi:10.1258/ijsa.2008.008213.

CRIMINAL JUSTICE VERSUS PUBLIC HEALTH PERSPECTIVES ON TRANSGENDER SEX WORK

Because sex work is illegal in almost all areas in the United States, dealing with it has primarily been the province of the criminal justice system. In an attempt to deter this illegal activity, transgender sex workers are often arrested and occasionally jailed. Surveillance of street-based sex work occurs in conjunction with broad-based "sweeps" of stroll areas, which may include the confiscation of condoms carried by transwomen. Possession of condoms is seen as evidence of illegal activity and confiscating them is thought to deter this activity.

A different perspective looks at transgender work from the point of view of public health. Sex work is regarded, first and foremost, as a public health issue. Condoms are made available in an attempt to prevent HIV/STI, and services are made available to deal with issues of abuse and substance use (examined in previous chapters).

A public health perspective on transgender sex work should be considered in the context of the current worldwide debate regarding legalization or decriminalization of sex work. Numerous countries, including Sweden and Canada, are moving toward decriminalization of the sex trade in large part because of the health issues involved. The World Health Organization (WHO) is now advocating for sex work decriminalization as a way of slowing the HIV pandemic.

CHAPTER 23

Police Abuse, Depressive Symptoms, and High-Risk Sexual Behavior for HIV among Transwomen

Larry A. Nuttbrock[1]

1 Previously affiliated with the National Development and Research Institutes (NDRI) and now a private consultant living in New York City.

SUMMARY

Building on a previous longitudinal study describing the effects of broad measures of gender abuse on depressive symptomatology and high-risk sexual behavior for HIV among transgender women, the current analysis examined longitudinal associations of perceived psychological abuse by the police with depressive symptoms and high-risk sexual behavior for HIV in this population. The analysis suggests that psychological abuse by the police elevates depressive symptoms, which then reduce the odds of using condoms with different types of partners. These findings suggest that aggressive policing in urban areas such as New York City may be counterproductive from a public health perspective.

KEY TERMS

aggressive policing; condom use; depressive symptoms; police abuse

Adversarial relationships between the police and gender-nonconforming individuals have been described historically (Feinberg, 1997; Stryker, 2008), but it was not until the beginning of the twenty-first century that agencies promoting human rights began to document patterns of abusive police tactics directed at transgender persons and transwomen

Nuttbrock, Larry, *Transgender Sex Work and Society*
dx.doi.org/10.17312/harringtonparkpress/2017.11.tsws.023
© 2018 by Harrington Park Press

in particular (Amnesty International, 2005; Grant et al., 2011; Sex Workers Project at the Urban Justice Center, 2003). A significant proportion (25% to 75%) of transgender women included in these surveys reported intimidation and harassment by the police, and significant numbers indicated some form of physical abuse, coercive tactics (including false arrests and imprisonment), and sexual assaults (including rape) (Make the Road New York, 2012; National Coalition of Anti-Violence Programs, 2013). All these reports suggest higher levels of police abuse among transwomen in the sex trade, although transwomen in general and transwomen of color, in particular, may be profiled as sex workers (US Department of Justice, 2015).

Since the turn of this century, abusive police tactics have been framed as a public health issue (Geller et al., 2014), and studies have begun to quantify the effect of this abuse on the health of targeted populations, including sex workers and transwomen. Among transwomen with a history of sex work, exposures to violence and transphobia, perpetrated in part by the police, have been associated with depressive symptoms (Nemoto, Bödeker, & Iwamoto, 2011). In qualitative studies of transgender or transvestite sex workers, histories of violence, including police abuse, have been correlated with HIV risk behavior (Clements-Nolle, Guzman, & Harris, 2008; Rhodes et al., 2008). In surveys of transgender sex workers seeking social or medical services, previous confrontations with the police were linked to biologically determined sexually transmitted infections (Cohan et al., 2006; Hill et al., 2011). These studies are consistent with a broader literature of experienced violence and HIV risk behavior among female sex workers (Shannon & Csete, 2010).

Aggressive policing of sex workers is now understood, worldwide, as a significant driver of the HIV pandemic, and epidemiological studies have begun to quantify the effect of this abuse on the course of the epidemic (Shannon et al., 2015). Abusive police tactics and high levels of HIV typically co-occur in the context of sex work as illegal activity, and there are increasing calls to decriminalize sex work as a way of slowing the HIV epidemic (World Health Organization, 2012; Shannon et al., 2015).

This literature poses the issue of police-perpetrated abuse as an issue for public health, but none of these studies specifically examined the adverse effects of such abuse on transwomen, and the methodological quality of most of these studies may be debated. Findings based on highly selective samples, such as those seeking medical services or recruited in high-crime urban areas, may not apply to all transwomen. Perceived abuse in the distant past may not be causally related to current health issues or behavior. Potential confounding in observed associations of police abuse with health issues has not been adequately evaluated.

Building on my previous work describing the effects of broad measures of gender abuse on depressive symptomatology and high-risk sexual behavior for HIV among transgender women in New York City (Nuttbrock et al., 2013), the current study examined, more specifically, longitudinal associations of perceived psychological abuse by the police (defined below) with depressive symptoms and high-risk sexual behavior for HIV among transwomen. The analysis included a host of variables (age, education, ethnicity, nativity, sexual orientation, hormone therapy, sex work, and substance use) that may potentially confound these associations. Following the parent study, in an attempt to better understand why police abuse affects the health of transgender women (if it does), I examined the hypothesis that police abuse results in high-risk sexual behavior, in part, because of elevated depressive symptoms (mediation analysis). Following the four steps for assessing mediation (Baron and Kenny, 1986), four hypotheses were tested: (1) police abuse is associated with unprotected receptive anal intercourse (URAI); (2) police abuse is associated with depressive symptoms; (3) depressive symptoms are associated with URAI; and (4) the association of police abuse with URAI is reduced when depressive symptoms are controlled.

METHOD

Transgender or gender-variant individuals were actively involved in all aspects of this project. They assisted with the design of the instrument, training of the field staff, interviewing, data collection, and some of the data analysis. The Institutional Review Board (IRB) of the National Development and Research Institutes (NDRI) approved all the research protocols.

Selection of Study Participants

A total of 571 study participants were initially recruited for a community-based study of transwomen in the New York metropolitan area. Approached individuals were eligible for the study if they were assigned as male at birth but subsequently did not regard themselves as "completely male" in all situations or roles (reflecting an MTF/transgender spectrum). Eligibility criteria also included age of 19 through 59 and the absence of psychotic ideation. Study participants were broadly recruited through transgender organizations in the New York metropolitan area, the Internet, newspaper advertisements, the streets, clubs, client referrals of other clients, and assistants from transgender communities who worked on a day-to-day basis with the field staff.

From the 571 transwomen initially recruited for the retrospective component of the study, 62% (N = 354) were biologically assayed as HIV-negative, and 230 of these individuals were then randomly assigned to the prospective component of the study, which was designed to evaluate risk factors for new cases of HIV/STI. To increase efficiency of the research design, younger respondents and those reporting recent high-risk sexual behavior were oversampled.

Because of time constraints in this five-year study, there was variation in the number of years study participants could potentially be followed. The recruitment phase, which began in December 2004, was extended to September 2007 so that all participants could potentially be followed for at least one year. From the initial pool of 230 HIV-negatives included in the prospective component, 171/230 (74.3%), 92/230 (40.0%), and 56/230 (24.3%) were followed and interviewed at years one, two, and three, respectively. The percentages of potentially available study participants who were reinterviewed and biologically tested for new HIV/STI were 74.3% (171/230), 68.1% (92/135), and 75.7% (56/74) at years one, two, and three, respectively.

Measurements

At baseline, and 6, 12, 24, and 36 months thereafter, study participants completed face-to-face interviews in conjunction with the Life Review of Transgender Experiences (LRTE), an instrument designed to collect a broad range of information about transgender experiences, including HIV risks. The English version of the LRTE was translated to Spanish, and 19% (44/230) were interviewed in Spanish by a fluent interviewer. Study participants were compensated $40 for completing all the protocols associated with a given assessment period.

Age was coded as a continuous variable from 19 through 59. *Education* was classified as less than high school, high school graduate, some college, and college graduate or higher. Preestablished census categories were used to classify *ethnicity*. It was grouped as non-Hispanic white as compared to all other categories (coded high). *Nativity* was defined as a birthplace outside the United States as compared to those US born. *Sexual orientation* was based on reports of sexual attraction to men only, women only, men and women, and neither men nor women. This variable was grouped as sexual attraction to men only (androphilic) versus all other categories. *Hormone therapy*, defined as using any type of female hormone supplements during the previous six months, was assessed at all points.

Respondents were asked at all assessment points if they traded sex for money, drugs, or gifts during the preceding sex months. For the current analysis, *sex work* was coded as none versus any. Respondents were asked at all assessment times about the use of alcohol (five or more drinks on a given occasion), cannabis (marijuana or hashish); cocaine (crack or powder); heroin; amphetamines or methamphetamines; downers or tranquilizers; phencyclidine, or PCP; LSD or other hallucinogens; ecstasy, or XTC; poppers, nitrates, or other inhalants; misused prescription drugs; or any other drug during the previous month. *Substance use* was quantified for this report as an overall summary of days using a particular drug added across all drugs that were used (capped at 15 to reduce skewing and outliers).

Depressive symptoms were evaluated with the 20-item CES-D (Center for Epidemiologic Studies Depression) scale. This scale reflects experiences of depression during the previous week with a theoretical range of 0 through 60 (Radloff, 1977).

Respondents were asked at all assessment points about the number of episodes of receptive anal intercourse with committed, casual, or commercial partners during the preceding six months, and whether any of these episodes was unprotected (URAI). The current report uses an overall measure of any URAI with committed, casual, or commercial partners (coded as none or any).

Study participants were queried at all assessment points about whether they were "verbally abused or harassed" during the previous six months and thought it was because of their gender identity or presentation. If they reported any such abuse, they were further queried about the identity of the perpetrator. Psychological abuse by the police was coded if the perpetrator was identified as the police or a sheriff.

This variable was coded as no abuse versus any abuse. Participants were likewise asked about whether they were "physically abused or beaten" as a result of gender nonconformity. Physical abuse by the police was coded if the perpetrator was identified as the police or a sheriff and coded as no abuse versus abuse. Because of the low frequency, physical abuse by the police was described but not fully analyzed.

Statistical Techniques

Generalized estimating equations (GEE) with a binomial link were used for dichotomous outcomes, and the effects were expressed as odds ratios (OR) (Hardin & Hilbe, 2012). GEE with an identity link were used for continuous outcomes, and the effects were expressed as unstandardized betas. Clustering within individuals across time was modeled with an exchangeable working correlation structure. The longitudinal GEE modeling used five time points (baseline and 6, 12, 24, and 36 months thereafter). All the data analysis was conducted with version 9 of Stata. The background variables (except hormone therapy) were analyzed using baseline measurements only. Hormone therapy and all the other variables were assessed across follow-ups and included in the analysis as time-varying covariates or end points.

Mediation was assessed using the four-step approach originally proposed by Baron and Kenny (1986). Mediation was claimed if an initial effect was reduced by 10% or more with controls for hypothesized mediators (Selvin, 2004). Estimates of mediation may be biased if the initial association is confounded by other variables (MacKinnon et al., 2002). To reduce this problem, background variables associated with both predictor and outcome variables were controlled, as appropriate.

RESULTS

Study Attrition

Attrition included those who were not followed at a given point because of study time constraints (administrative attrition) and the potentially available participants at given points who were not located and interviewed (client-related attrition). The subsets of the 230 study participants followed at years one, two, and three were compared to those not so followed with regard to baseline measurements of background variables, gender abuse, depressive symptoms, and other variables (combined administrative and client-related attrition). Only older age with study completion at years one ($r = .15$; $p < .05$) and three ($r = .16$; $p < .05$) was significant. Because study attrition was, for the most part, not predicted from variables included in the analysis, the data may likely be analyzed without a significant bias as a result of missing data.

Study Participants

Study participants were by design between 19 to 59 years of age (mean = 34.0; SD = 12.4). Less than half (42.2%) did not graduate from high school; 6.1% were college graduates or higher. Ethnicity was 35.7% Hispanic; 35.2% non-Hispanic white; 17.4% non-Hispanic black; and 11.7% any other identification. Less than one-fourth (22.4%) were foreign-born. Most (58.9%) were attracted to men only (androphilic); 25.4% to women only; 13.8% to men and women; and 1.8% to neither men nor women. At baseline, 52.2% reported hormone therapy during the previous six months.

At baseline, 40% reported sex work during the preceding six months; 10.9% reported police abuse; the mean score for depressive symptoms was 24.0 (SD = 12.0); 70.0% had used some type of drug at least one day during the previous month; and URAI with any type of partner was 38.6%. Perceived psychological abuse by the police varied from 10.9% at baseline to 8.7% at the 36-month follow-up. Perceived physical abuse by the police varied from 2.1% at baseline to 0.0 at the 24-month follow-up.

Background Variables with Police Abuse, Depressive Symptoms, and URAI

For descriptive purposes, and to evaluate potential confounders, the background variables were associated with police abuse, depressive symptoms, and URAI (Table 23.1). In a multivariate analysis, with all variables simultaneously included, sex work (OR = 4.66) and substance use (OR = 1.35) were associated with police abuse. Sex work ($b = 7.33$) and substance use ($b = 2.96$) were likewise associated with depressive symptoms. Education (OR = 1.36), nativity (OR = 1.74), androphilic sexual orientation (OR = 2.62), hormone therapy (OR = 1.98), sex work (OR = 1.43), and substance use (OR = 1.21) were associated with URAI. Two variables—sex work and substance use—are common predictors across all these outcomes. As I suggested above, these variables are potential con-

TABLE 23.1

Background Variables with Police Abuse, Depressive Symptoms, and URAI

	POLICE ABUSE (OR)	DEPRESSIVE SYMPTOMS (*b*)	URAI (OR)
Age	.97	.02	.99
Education	.94	.24	1.36*
Ethnicity[a]	3.32	–.07	1.10
Nativity[b]	.48	.06	1.74*
Sexual orientation[c]	.68	.39	2.62**
Hormone therapy	2.19	8.60	1.98**
Sex work	4.66**	7.33**	1.43**
Substance use[d]	1.35**	2.96**	1.21**

NOTE: Generalized estimating equations with a binomial link (police abuse and URAI) and an identity link (depressive symptoms).
[a] Nonwhite as compared to white.
[b] Those born outside the United States as compared to US born.
[c] Androphilic as compared to non-androphilic.
[d] Cumulative measurement of number of drugs and the number of days each was used during the previous month, with a range of 0 through 15.
*$p < .05$. **$p < .01$.

founders in associations among police abuse, depressive symptoms, and URAI, and they will be controlled, as appropriate, in the analysis below.

Effect of Police Abuse on URAI

The overall association of police abuse with URAI was moderately strong and statistically significant (OR = 2.51). (Note: Associations are statistically significant at $p = .05$ if the 95% confidence intervals exclude the null value of 1.00.) This association was reduced by approximately 40%, but was still statistically significant, with sex work (OR = 1.63) and substance use (OR = 1.68) controlled (Table 23.2).

TABLE 23.2

Police Abuse with URAI

	URAI OR	(95% CI)
Police abuse	2.51	(1.56, 4.06)
Controls		
Sex work	1.63	(1.02, 2.74)
Substance use[a]	1.68	(1.03, 2.92)

NOTE. Generalized estimating equations with a binomial link.

[a] Cumulative measurement of number of drugs and the number of days each was used during the previous month, with a range of 0 through 15.

Effect of Police Abuse on Depressive Symptoms

The overall association of police abuse with depressive symptoms was statistically significant and strong in magnitude (unstandardized beta = 16.72). This association was reduced by approximately 40%, but was still statistically significant and strong, with sex work (b = 9.82) and substance use (b = 9.15) controlled (Table 23.3).

TABLE 23.3

Police Abuse with Depressive Symptoms

	DEPRESSIVE SYMPTOMS b	(95% CI)
Police abuse	16.72	(12.73, 20.70)
Controls		
Sex work	9.82	(6.12, 13.52)
Substance use[a]	9.15	(4.74, 13.43)

NOTE. Generalized estimating equations with an identity link.

[a] Cumulative measurement of number of drugs and the number of days each was used during the previous month, with a range of 0 through 15.

Effect of Depressive Symptoms on URAI

The overall association of depressive symptoms and URAI was statistically significant and strong ($b = 1.04$). This association was little changed and remained statistically significant with sex work ($b = 1.03$) and substance use ($b = 1.03$) controlled. This association was reduced by approximately 40%, but was still statistically significant and strong, with sex work ($b = 9.82$) and substance use ($b = 9.15$) controlled (Table 23.4).

TABLE 23.4

Depressive Symptoms with URAI

	URAI OR	(95% CI)
Depressive symptoms	1.04	(1.03, 1.05)
Controls		
Sex work	1.03	(1.02, 1.04)
Substance use [a]	1.03	(1.02, 1.04)

NOTE. Generalized estimating equations with an identity link.

[a] Cumulative measurement of number of drugs and the number of days each was used during the previous month, with a range of 0 through 15.

Effect of Police Abuse on URAI Controlling for Depressive Symptoms

With controls for the potential confounders (sex work and substance use) and the hypothesized mediator (depressive symptoms), the association of police abuse and URAI was substantially reduced (OR = 1.19) and no longer statistically significant. This suggests a mediation model whereby police abuse leads to depressive symptoms, which then lead to URAI (Table 23.5).

TABLE 23.5

Police Abuse with URAI Controlled for Potential Confounders and Depressive Symptoms

	URAI OR	(95% CI)
Police abuse Sex work, substance use, and depressive symptoms controlled	1.19	(.70, 2.03)

NOTE. Generalized estimating equations with an identity link.

DISCUSSION

During three years of follow-ups, about 10% of the transwomen included in this study reported psychological abuse by the police that stemmed from their gender nonconformity. This abuse was longitudinally associated with a ten-point increase in depressive symptoms as measured by the CES-D and a 70% increase in the likelihood of unprotected receptive anal intercourse (URAI). Emotional turmoil associated with depressed affect and identity threat may lead to lapses in judgment about condom use and URAI. All the variables in this analysis—police abuse, depressive symptoms, and URAI—were associated with both sex work and substance use (which suggests confounding) and the above findings were obtained with these variables controlled.

These findings suggest that an adversarial relationship between the police and transwomen, examined here as psychological abuse, directly affects the mental health of these women and, by promoting high-risk sexual behavior, ultimately contributes to the HIV epidemic in this population. These findings should be part of a conversation about the necessity of reducing abusive police tactics aimed at transwomen; they should also inform a broader conversation about decriminalizing sex work as a long-term strategy to promote better relationships between the police and transgender persons.

NOTE

This research was supported by a grant from the National Institute on Drug Abuse (NIDA) (1 R01 DA018080) (Larry Nuttbrock, principal investigator).

REFERENCES

Amnesty International. (2005). *USA: Stonewalled: Police abuse and misconduct against lesbian, gay, bisexual and transgender people in the U.S.* New York: Amnesty International Publications.

Baron, R. M. & Kenny, D. S. (1986). The moderator-mediator variable distinction in social psychological research: Conceptual, strategic, and statistical issues. *Journal of Personality and Social Psychology, 51,* 1173–1182.

Clements-Nolle, K., Guzman, R., & Harris, S. G. (2008). Sex trade in a male-to-female transgender population: Psychosocial correlates of inconsistent condom use. *Sexual Health, 5,* 49–54.

Cohan, D., Lutnick, A., Davidson, P., Cloniger, C., Herlyn, A., Breyer, J., . . . & Klausner, J. (2006). Sex worker health: San Francisco style. *Sexually Transmitted Infections, 82,* 418–422.

Cooper, H., Moore, L., Graskin, S., & Krieger, N. (2008). Characterizing perceived police violence: Implications for public health. *American Journal of Public Health, 94,* 1109–1118.

Deering, K. N., Armin, A., Shoveller, J., Nesbitt, A., . . . & Shannon, K. (2014). A systematic review of correlates of violence against sex workers. *American Journal of Public Health, 104,* 42–44.

Feinberg, L. (1997). *Transgender Warriors: From Joan of Act to Dennis Rodman.* Boston: Beacon Press.

Geller, A., Fagan, J., Tyler, T., & Link, B. G. (2014). Aggressive policing and the mental health of young urban men. *American Journal of Public Health, 104* (12), 2321–2327.

Grant J. M., Mottet, L. A., Janis, J., Harrison, J., Herman, J. L., & Keisling, M. (2011). *Injustice at every turn: A report of the National Transgender Discrimination Survey.* Washington, D.C.: National Center for Transgender Equality and National Gay and Lesbian Task Force.

Hardin, J. R., & Hilbe, J. R. (2012). *Generalized estimating equations* (2nd ed.). New York: CRC Press.

Hill, S. C., Daniel, J., Benzie, A., Ayres, J., King, G., & Smith, A. (2011). Sexual health of transgender sex workers attending an inner-city genitourinary medical clinic. *International Journal of STD and AIDS, 22,* 686–687.

MacKinnon, D. P., Lockwood, C. M., Hoffman J. M., West, S. G., & Sheets, V. (2002). A comparison of methods to test mediation and other intervening variable effects. *Psychological Methods, 7,* 83–104.

Make the Road New York. (2012). *Transgressive policing: Police abuse of LGBTQ communities of color in Jackson Heights.* New York: Make the Road New York.

National Coalition of Anti-Violence Programs (NCAVP). (2013). *Lesbian, gay, bisexual, transgender, queer, and HIV-affected hate violence in 2012.* New York: Gay and Lesbian Anti-Violence Programs.

Nemoto, T., Bödeker, B., & Iwamoto, M. (2011). Social support, exposure to violence and transphobia, and correlates of depression among male-to-female transgender women with a history of sex work. *American Journal of Public Health, 101,* 818–823.

Nuttbrock, L. (2012). Culturally competent substance abuse treatment with transgender persons. *Journal of Addictive Diseases, 31,* 236–241.

Nuttbrock, L., Bockting, W., Rosenblum, A., Hwahng, S., Mason, M., Macri, M., and Becker, J. (2013). Gender abuse, depressive symptoms, and HIV and sexually transmitted infections among male-to-female transgender persons: A three-year prospective study. *American Journal of Public Health, 103,* 300–307.

Poteat, T., Wirtz, A., Radix, A., Borques, A., Silva-Santisteban, A., Deutsch, M. B., . . . & Operario, D. (2015). HIV risk and prevention interventions in transgender women sex workers. *Lancet, 385,* 274–286.

Radloff, L. S. (1977). The CES-D scale: A self-report depression scale for research in the general population. *Applied Psychological Measurement, 1,* 385–401.

Rhodes, T., Simic, M., Baros, S., Platt, L., & Zikic, B. (2008). Police violence and sexual risk among female and transvestite sex workers in Serbia: Qualitative study. *BMJ, 337,* 560–563.

Selvin, S. (2004). *Statistical analysis of epidemiologic data* (3rd ed.). New York: Oxford University Press.

Sex Workers Project at the Urban Justice Center. (2003). *Revolving door: An analysis of street-based prostitution in New York City.* New York: Urban Justice Center.

Shannon, D., & Csete, J., (2010). Violence, condom negotiation, and HIV/STI risk among sex workers. *Journal of the American Medical Association, 304,* 573–574.

Shannon, D., Strathdee, S. A., Goldenberg, S. M., Duff, P., Mwangi, M. A., Rusakova, M., . . . & Boily, M.-C. (2015). Global epidemiology of HIV among female sex workers: Influence of structural determinants. *Lancet, 385* (9962), 55–71.

Stotzer, R. L. (2009). Violence against transgender people: A review of United States data. *Aggression and Violent Behavior, 14,* 170–179.

———. (2008). Gender identity and hate crimes: Violence against transgender people in Los Angeles County. *Sex Research and Social Policy, 5,* 43–52.

Stryker, S. (2008). *Transgender history.* Berkeley, CA: Seal Press.

US Department of Justice. (2015). *President's task force on 21st century policing.* Washington, DC: US Department of Justice.

Valera, R. J., Sawyer, R. G., & Schiraldi, G. R. (2000). Violence and post traumatic stress disorder in a sample of inner city street prostitutes. *American Journal of Health Studies, 16,* 149–155.

World Health Organization. (2012). *Prevention and treatment of HIV and other sexually transmitted infections in low- and middle-income countries.* Geneva: World Health Organization.

CHAPTER 24

Criminal Justice versus Health and Human Rights Perspectives on Transgender Sex Work

Tara Lyons[1]
Leslie Pierre[2]
Andrea Krüsi[3]
Kate Shannon[4]

[1] Faculty member in the Department of Criminology at Kwantlen Polytechnic University, Surrey, BC, and a research scientist with the Gender and Sexual Health Initiative at the BC Centre for Excellence in HIV/AIDS, Vancouver, BC.

[2] Research assistant with the Gender and Sexual Health Initiative of the BC Centre for Excellence in HIV/AIDS, Vancouver, BC.

[3] Post-doctoral fellow at the School of Population and Public Health at the University of British Columbia and a research associate with the Gender and Sexual Health Initiative of the BC Centre for Excellence in HIV/AIDS, Vancouver, BC.

[4] Associate professor of medicine at the University of British Columbia and director of the BC Centre for Excellence in HIV/AIDS, Vancouver, BC.

SUMMARY

In this chapter we systematically present the array of factors and issues associated with a criminal justice as compared to a public health perspective on sex work. Focusing on transgender sex workers, we discuss and summarize the different perspectives and controversies involved in this ongoing debate.

KEY TERMS

criminal justice perspective; public health perspective; transgender sex work

Nuttbrock, Larry, *Transgender Sex Work and Society*
dx.doi.org/10.17312/harringtonparkpress/2017.11.tsws.024
© 2018 by Harrington Park Press

In most places in North America, as in most countries, activities surrounding sex work are legally prohibited because of the state's overarching goal to eliminate sex work. This strategy is largely ineffective and is imposed through criminal sanctions (Open Society Foundations, 2012). It is well documented that this approach of criminalizing sex work harms sex workers. Specifically, sex workers routinely face violence owing to their being conceived of as deserving of criminal punishments and violence because of the stigmatized and criminalized character of buying and selling sex (Shannon et al., 2015; World Health Organization, 2005, 2012).

Criminalization also increases sex workers' vulnerability to HIV infection (Bhattacharjya et al., 2015; Shannon & Csete, 2010). For example, sex workers who face violence are less able to engage in HIV prevention, such as condom negotiation with clients (Deering et al., 2013; Shannon, Strathdee, et al., 2009). Criminalization of sex work also affects sex workers' working conditions, particularly where they are able to work. For example, it has been documented that criminalization and policing practices result in sex workers being pushed to work in areas that are isolated and less safe (Shannon et al., 2008; Shannon, Kerr, et al., 2009).

Over the past two decades there has been increased interest by a number of higher-income countries in attempting to eradicate prostitution through "end-demand criminalization," which criminalizes the purchase, but not the selling, of sexual services. Sweden, Norway, Iceland, Northern Ireland, France, and, since December 2014, Canada have implemented end-demand criminalization, also known as the Nordic Model approach. Similarly, there have been recent calls for the United States to implement sex work legislation along the lines of a Nordic Model approach (Peters, 2016). The Nordic Model approach to regulating sex work has been implemented in the absence of scientific evidence substantiating its supporters' claims that this approach will eliminate sex work and end the exploitation of sex workers. Indeed, evaluations of Nordic Model approaches have indicated that the criminalization and policing of sex workers' clients reproduce the harms created by the criminalization of sex workers, in particular risks for violence and continued stigmatization of sex workers (Global Commission on HIV and the Law, 2012; Krüsi et al., 2016; Krüsi et al., 2014).

The literature has noted that the negative effects of criminalizing any aspect of sex work may be more pronounced for some trans sex workers, given their intersecting structural vulnerabilities. For example, transwomen sex workers are more likely to be living with HIV than cisgender sex workers owing to a variety of factors, including criminalization and stigma (Poteat et al., 2015). Research has also documented how trans sex workers may be particularly vulnerable to violence because of a complex interplay of social-structural contexts of racism and economic barriers (Hwahng & Nuttbrock, 2007). In addition, transwomen sex workers report significantly higher rates of physical and sexual violence by clients than cisgender sex workers (Cohan et al., 2006; Nemoto, Bödeker, & Iwamoto, 2011). Additionally, trans sex workers have reported police violence (Rhodes et al., 2008). Thus, criminalization shapes trans sex workers' vulnerability to violence as well as to police abuse, as demonstrated by the work of Nuttbrock in Chapters 2 and 3 of this book.

METHODS

Data from this chapter have been drawn from in-depth interviews examining the lived experiences of violence of trans sex workers in Vancouver, Canada (Lyons et al., 2017). This research is situated within an ongoing community-based longitudinal qualitative and ethnographic examination of the physical, social, and policy factors that influence violence, HIV, and access to care among sex workers, which runs alongside a parallel longitudinal epidemiological cohort of street and off-street sex workers (An Evaluation of Sex Workers Health Access), details of which have been published elsewhere (Shannon et al., 2015).

Between June 2012 and May 2013, the first author (TL) conducted in-depth, semistructured interviews with 33 trans sex workers. The interviews were conducted before the change in sex work laws in Canada. Though the buying and selling of sex itself was legal, the Criminal Code of Canada prohibited the operation of a "bawdy house," "living off the avails of prostitution," and "communication" for the purposes of selling sex (Goodyear & Cusick, 2007; Shannon, Strathdee, et al., 2009). Interviews lasted approximately one hour, and participants were paid CND$20 to compensate them for their time. Interview and ethnographic data were analyzed using a theory- and data-driven approach (DeCuir-Gunby, Marshall, & McCulloch, 2011) that was guided by a framework that positions health as an outcome of social-structural contexts (Rhodes et al., 2005; Shannon et al., 2008). TL conducted the first-level open coding. Additional data and thematic-driven codes and subcodes were created during second- and third-level coding using a participatory analysis approach developed by TL with two experiential peer research associates, including the second author (LP). This study received ethical approval through the Providence Health Care/University of British Columbia Research Ethics Board. Pseudonyms are used to protect the identity of participants.

STUDY PARTICIPANTS

Participants reported a range of gender identities and expressions, and some of these varied over time and with sex work. All participants had been assigned the male sex at birth; however, not all identified as women. Participants most often described themselves as transgender (N = 16), as women (N = 8), and as transsexual (N = 7). Six participants identified as two-spirit; three participants reported dressing as a woman for sex work; and one identified as androgynous.

Participants ranged in age from 23 to 52 years, with an average age of 39 years. There was an overrepresentation of indigenous persons in our sample: 23 (69.7%) participants identified as such. Seven (21.2%) participants identified as white, and three identified as Filipino, Asian, and "Other" visible minority. Just over half of the sample (54.5%, or N = 18) reported current use of illicit drugs, and the majority (78.8%, or N = 26) were currently engaged in sex work. Of those currently working, 19 (73.1%) solicited in street sex work environments. Of 30 participants with known HIV status, 60% (N = 18) were living with HIV.

HOW CRIMINALIZATION SHAPED VIOLENT EXPERIENCES

As we noted, there is now a large body of social science and epidemiological research demonstrating that the criminalization of any aspect of sex work and enforcement of restrictive laws exacerbates violence against sex workers. Given the data that trans sex workers are more vulnerable to violence because of intersections of social-structural factors, we will illustrate the various ways that criminalization shaped trans sex workers' experiences of violence.

Trans sex workers in our study detailed violence that they experienced while working, and many of these experiences of violence were rooted in transphobia. In particular, violent incidents, or potential violence, were associated with the discovery of gender identity. Violent incidents often occurred as a result of a client's misreading or discovering the sex worker's gender identity while negotiating the terms of the sex work activity or during the transaction. For example, Willow described a client discovering she was trans during a date and how he physically attacked her as a result: "I gave him a blow job and he started getting mad. And he was a bigger guy and big muscles. I was scared. And he, tried to hit me—he almost hit me and he hit the car seat."

Similarly, Lydia described experiencing violence as a result of a client discovering she was trans during the date: "I got my hair pulled and [head] banged on the dash. And then he opened the door, threw me out." Participants often reported fearing for their safety and their lives if a client was to discover their gender.

These violent experiences of gender disclosure, while intertwined with transphobia, were also shaped by the criminalization of sex work and the social-structural stigmas and barriers that burdened participants. For example, under the conditions of criminalization, trans sex workers are forced to rush negotiations with clients, including the negotiation of gender disclosure when appropriate. Sex workers in our study and in other settings (Sanders, 2004) have reported that screening potential clients, including negotiating the terms of the transaction and assessing whether clients are under the influence of drugs, is a key aspect of managing potential client violence. As the findings illustrate, the criminalization of sex work heightens trans sex workers' vulnerability to client violence because they have to rush gender disclosure and sex work negotiations with potential clients. This is the case even when sex workers themselves no longer represent enforcement targets (Krüsi et al., 2016; Krüsi et al., 2014).

Additionally, trans sex workers reported negative police responses to experiences of violence. In general, participants did not report client violence to police because, as one participant explained, "It's useless. Why even report it 'cause nothing's gonna be done." There were feelings that the police would not act on the report appropriately—either by ignoring or minimizing the complaint—and in some cases there were fears that police would contribute to additional stigmatization. Participants did not feel that the police would act as protectors, and in some instances participants did not report violence to the police for fear of arrest on sex work charges. Participants discussed instances of reporting violence and sexual assaults to the police and the police not acting on the information. For example, Aron reported a sexual assault to an officer, including the license plate of the client's vehicle, and "nothing happened. . . . I trusted her and I thought she'd help." A year and a half later, after repeated attempts to contact the officer, a photo lineup of potential suspects was arranged. Aron continued: "I'm like, why do I have to do a photo lineup when I gave you a license plate number? And they had no answer. And later, a different officer said, well you know the risks that you take when you do [the] sex trade."

Police and sex work laws have historically not protected trans sex workers in Vancouver (Ross, 2012), where the police infamously ignored calls from the community to investigate missing women and sex workers (Oppal, 2012). Perhaps it is unsurprising that trans sex workers in our study and others (Namaste, 2000; Rhodes et al., 2008) are reluctance to report violence or to engage with police. Lack of police response to violence against trans sex workers is firmly rooted within a criminal justice approach, whereby sex workers are considered criminals.

As the findings illustrate, Canadian sex work laws enhance trans sex workers' vulnerability to violence and unsafe working conditions. Indigenous trans sex workers may be more vulnerable to the harms of criminalization, as evidenced by the vast overrepresentation of indigenous persons in Canadian jails and prisons (Correctional Investigator, 2014). Indigenous persons constitute approximately 4.3% of the Canadian population (Statistics Canada, 2013), yet they make up 22.8% of those incarcerated (Correctional Investigator, 2014). Therefore, it is time to investigate different approaches to sex work. Below we outline a public health approach to sex work.

AN EVIDENCE-BASED HEALTH AND HUMAN RIGHTS APPROACH TO SEX WORK

A health- and human rights–based approach conceptualizes sex work not as a criminal justice issue. Instead, this approach gives priority to the human rights, health, and safety of sex workers. Human rights are centralized within this framework, and this perspective considers social determinants of health (e.g., poverty) and the negative effects of criminalization (Canadian Public Health Association, 2014). Decriminalization of sex work—the removal of criminal sanctions associated with sex work activities—is one way to shift from a criminal justice approach toward a human rights–based approach to regulating sex work.

Decriminalization of All Aspects of Sex Work

New Zealand decriminalized sex work activities in 2003 and serves as an example of a shift to a labor- and human rights–based approach to the regulation of sex work, where workplace health and safety standards have been established in consultation with sex workers, and sex workers can take employment complaints to governing bodies (Goodyear & Weitzer, 2011). The law was established to protect the health, labor, and human rights of sex workers. Sex work is regulated like any other business, through standard employment health and safety regulations; delineating the location of commercial sex establishments through zoning bylaws; and specifying the health and safety obligations of managers and workers. Regulating sex work like any other business in the service industry has significantly reduced the structural stigma of sex work in New Zealand (Bruckert & Hannem, 2013). The use of condoms is a central aspect of the law; however, there are no criminal sanctions for sex workers who were found not to use condoms (Open Society Foundations, 2012). The Prostitution Law Review Committee, which was established to review the sex work policy as part of the legislation, found in its five-year review that sex workers "were now more likely to report incidents of violence to the police" (Government of New Zealand, 2008, p. 14). The review also found that sex workers reported better working conditions and a reduction in violent experiences since sex work was decriminalized (Government of New Zealand, 2008).

The decriminalization of sex work would also drastically improve health and human rights outcomes for trans sex workers. For example, there is statistical evidence that "decriminalisation of sex work could have the largest effect on the course of the HIV epidemic, averting 33–46% of incident infections over the next decade through combined effects on violence, police harassment, safer work environments, and HIV transmission pathways" (Shannon et al., 2015, p. 67). Also, when sex work was decriminalized in the state of Rhode Island between 2004 and 2009, there were sharp decreases in reported rape offences (31% decrease) and in gonorrhea cases among women (39% decrease) (Cunningham & Shah, 2014).

Policy Implications

A health and human rights perspective on transgender sex work should be considered in the context of the current worldwide debate regarding the decriminalization of sex work. Global policy guidelines and organizations, including the World Health Organization (WHO), UNAIDS, the Global Commission on HIV and Law, and Amnesty International, have all firmly called on decriminalization as critical to the health and human rights of sex workers (Amnesty International, 2016; Global Commission on HIV and the Law, 2012; World Health Organization, 2012). For example, a recently released UNAIDS strategy for 2016–2021 has also proposed the decriminalization of sex work in order to combat HIV and promote human rights (UNAIDS, 2015). Because there is strong support for and evidence of the necessity to decriminalize sex work, it is vital that trans sex workers are meaningfully included in all policy discussions on laws, given the historical exclusion of trans persons and sex workers in policy changes.

REFERENCES

Amnesty International. (2016, May 26). *Amnesty international policy on state obligations to respect, protect, and fufil the human rights of sex workers.* New York.

Bhattacharjya, M., Fulu, E., Murthy, L., with Saraswathi Seshu, M., Cabassi, J., & Vallejo-Mestres, M. (2015). *The right(s) evidence — sex work, violence and HIV in Asia: A multi-country qualitative study.* Bangkok: United Nations Population Fund (UNFPA), United Nations Development Programme (UNDP), and Asia Pacific Network of Sex Workers (CASAM).

Bruckert, C., & Hannem, S. (2013). Rethinking the prostitution debates: Transcending structural stigma in systemic responses to sex work. *Canadian Journal of Law and Society, 28* (1), 43–63.

Canadian Public Health Association. (2014, December). *Sex work in Canada: The public health perspective.* Ottawa, ON: Canadian Public Health Association.

Cohan, D., Lutnick, A., Davidson, P., Cloniger, C., Herlyn, A., Breyer, J., . . . & Klausner, J. (2006). Sex worker health: San Francisco style. *Sexually Transmitted Infections, 82* (5), 418–422.

Correctional Investigator. (2014). *Annual report of the Office of the Correctional Investigator, 2013–2014.* Ottawa, ON: Government of Canada.

Cunningham, S., & Shah, M. (2014). *Decriminalizing indoor prostitution: Implications for sexual violence and public health.* Cambridge, MA: National Bureau of Economic Research.

DeCuir-Gunby, J. T., Marshall, P. L., & McCulloch, A. W. (2011). Developing and using a codebook for the analysis of interview data: An example from a professional development research project. *Field Methods, 23* (2), 136–155.

Deering, K. N., Lyons, T., Feng, C. X., Nosyk, B., Strathdee, S. A., Montaner, J. S., & Shannon, K. (2013). Client demands for unsafe sex: The socioeconomic risk environment for HIV among street and off-street sex workers. *Journal of Acquired Immune Deficiency Syndrome, 63* (4), 522–531.

Global Commission on HIV and the Law. (2012). *Risks, rights & health.* New York: United Nations Development Programme, HIV/AIDS Group.

Goodyear, M. D., & Cusick, L. (2007). Protection of sex workers. *BMJ, 334* (7584), 52–53.

Goodyear, M., & Weitzer, R. (2011). International trends in the control of sexual services. *In* S. Dewey & P. Kelly (eds.), *Policing pleasure: Sex work, policy, and the state in global perspective* (pp. 16–30). New York: New York University Press.

Government of New Zealand. (2008). *Report of the Prostitution Law Review Committee on the operation of the Prostitution Reform Act of 2003.* Wellington, New Zealand: Ministry of Justice.

Hwahng, S. J., & Nuttbrock, L. (2007). Sex workers, fem queens, and cross-dressers: Differential marginalizations and HIV vulnerabilities among three ethnocultural male-to-female transgender communities in New York City. *Sexuality Research and Social Policy, 4* (4), 36–59.

Krüsi, A., Kerr, T., Taylor, C., Rhodes, T., & Shannon, K. (2016). "They won't change it back in their heads that we're trash": The intersection of sex work–related stigma and evolving policing strategies. *Sociology of Health and Illness, 38* (7), 1137–1150.

Krüsi, A., Pacey, K., Bird, L., Taylor, C., Chettiar, J., Allan, S., . . . & Shannon, K. (2014). Criminalisation of clients: Reproducing vulnerabilities for violence and poor health among street-based sex workers in Canada—Qualitative study. *BMJ Open, 4* (6).

Lyons, T., Krüsi, A., Pierre, L., Kerr, T., Small, W., & Shannon, K. (2017). Negotiating violence in the context of transphobia and criminalization: The experiences of trans sex workers in Vancouver, Canada. *Qualitative Health Research, 27* (2), 182–190.

Namaste, V. K. (2000). *Invisible lives: The erasure of transsexual and transgendered people.* Chicago: University of Chicago Press.

Nemoto, T., Bödeker, B., & Iwamoto, M. (2011). Social support, exposure to violence and transphobia, and correlates of depression among male-to-female transgender women with a history of sex work. *American Journal of Public Health, 101* (10), 1980–1988.

Open Society Foundations. (2012, July). *Laws and policies affecting sex work.* New York: Open Society Foundations.

Oppal, W. T. (2012). *Forsaken: The report of the Missing Women Commission of Inquiry.* Vancouver, BC.

Peters, M. A. (2016, April 18). Nordic Model key to beating exploitation of sex workers. CNN. Retrieved from www.cnn.com/2016/04/18/opinions/prostitution-nordic-model-peters/.

Poteat, T., Wirtz, A. L., Radix, A., Borquez, A., Silva-Santisteban, A., Deutsch, M. B., . . . & Operario, D. (2015). HIV risk and preventive interventions in transgender women sex workers. *Lancet, 385* (9964), 274–286.

Rhodes, T., Simic, M., Baros, S., Platt, L., & Zikic, B. (2008). Police violence and sexual risk among female and transvestite sex workers in Serbia: Qualitative study. *BMJ: British Medical Journal, 337,* 560–563.

Rhodes, T., Singer, M., Bourgois, P., Friedman, S. R., & Strathdee, S. A. (2005). The social structural production of HIV risk among injecting drug users. *Social Science & Medicine, 61* (5), 1026–1044.

Ross, B. L. (2012). Outdoor brothel culture: The un/making of a transsexual stroll in Vancouver's west end, 1975–1984. *Journal of Historical Sociology, 25* (1), 126–150.

Sanders, T. (2004). A continuum of risk? The management of health, physical, and emotional risks by female sex workers. *Sociology of Health & Illness, 26* (5), 557–574.

Sausa, L., Keatley, J., & Operario, D. (2007). Perceived risks and benefits of sex work among transgender women of color in San Francisco. *Archives of Sexual Behavior, 36* (6), 768–777.

Shannon, K., & Csete, J. (2010). Violence, condom negotiation, and HIV/STI risk among sex workers. *JAMA, 304* (5), 573–574.

Shannon, K., Kerr, T., Allinott, S., Chettiar, J., Shoveller, J., & Tyndall, M. W. (2008). Social and structural violence and power relations in mitigating HIV risk of drug-using women in survival sex work. *Social Science & Medicine, 66* (4), 911–921.

Shannon, K., Kerr, T., Strathdee, S. A., Shoveller, J., Montaner, J. S., & Tyndall, M. W. (2009). Prevalence and structural correlates of gender based violence among a prospective cohort of female sex workers. *BMJ: British Medical Journal, 339,* b2939.

Shannon, K., Strathdee, S. A., Goldenberg, S. M., Duff, P., Mwangi, P., Rusakova, M., . . . & Boily, M.-C. (2015). Global epidemiology of HIV among female sex workers: Influence of structural determinants. *Lancet, 385* (9962), 55–71.

Shannon, K., Strathdee, S. A., Shoveller, J., Rusch, M., Kerr, T., & Tyndall, M. W. (2009). Structural and environmental barriers to condom use negotiation with clients among female sex workers: Implications for HIV-prevention strategies and policy. *American Journal of Public Health, 99* (4), 659–665.

Statistics Canada. (2013). *Aboriginal peoples in Canada: First nations people, Métis, and Inuit: National household survey, 2011.* Ottawa, ON.

UNAIDS. (2015). *2016–2021 strategy: On the fast-track to end AIDS.* Geneva, Switzerland: UNAIDS.

World Health Organization. (2012). *Prevention and treatment of HIV and other sexually transmitted infections for sex workers in low- and middle-income countries: Recommendations for a public health approach.* Geneva, Switzerland: World Health Organization.

———. (2005). *Violence against sex workers and HIV prevention.* Retrieved from www .who.int/gender/documents/sexworkers.pdf.

SECTION IX

ANALYTIC SUMMARY AND DIRECTIONS FOR FURTHER STUDY

In this concluding chapter, we provide an analytic summary of the main findings presented in the previous chapters. Building on these findings, we suggest some directions for further study.

CHAPTER 25

Analytic Summary and Directions for Further Study

Walter Bockting[1]
Larry A. Nuttbrock[2]

[1] Professor of medical psychology (in psychiatry and nursing) at Columbia University and a research scientist with the New York State Psychiatric Institute.
[2] Formerly affiliated with the National Development and Research Institutes (NDRI) and now a private consultant working in New York City.

KEY TERMS

further study; transgender sex work

This volume has described transgender sex work, and factors associated with it, in the United States and in several countries around the world. For reasons that range from identity affirmation to economic security and survival, and in settings that range from informal liaisons to brothels to the streets, significant percentages of transwomen exchange sex for some sort of material gain (Chapter 3). Perhaps in part because of a comparative lack of demand for their sexual services, the prevalence of sex work among transmen appears to be low (Chapter 3). Some of the themes running through these chapters will be highlighted with some suggestions for further study.

HETEROGENEITY AND DIVERSITY

In the United States, transwomen sex workers are an extremely diverse population. A major differentiating factor in New York City is race or ethnicity: white transwomen engage in sex work less frequently, and for shorter periods, than their nonwhite counterparts (Chapters 1–3).

Nuttbrock, Larry, *Transgender Sex Work and Society*
dx.doi.org/10.17312/harringtonparkpress/2017.11 tsws.025
© 2018 by Harrington Park Press

The extent to which such racial or ethnic differences are found in other parts of the United States, and in other parts of the world, needs to be examined.

Around the world, transgender sex work may occur in the context of distinctive identities and sexual practices that may not be understood or practiced as such outside these cultural settings (Section VI). The special character historically associated with some of these settings may be changing as a result of globalization and the Internet (Chapters 15, 16, 19, and 20). Additional research is needed to better understand these changes.

PERVASIVENESS OF ABUSE AND DISCRIMINATION

Despite these differences, within and across countries, transgender sex workers of all types frequently encounter enactments of stigma and discrimination. These may take the form of psychological or physical abuse by family, strangers, and the police (Section VI), employment discrimination (Chapter 3 and Section VI), or discriminatory practices that exclude them from legally practicing their work (Chapter 12). Additional empirical descriptions of forms of abuse and discrimination experienced by transgender sex workers in different milieus would be revealing.

EMBEDDEDNESS WITH INTERPERSONAL AND HEALTH ISSUES

Transgender sex work is seldom a distinctive form of labor that can be separated from interpersonal or health issues that often accompany it. In the United States, family conflict has been seen as one of the factors underlying entry into sex work among transgender women (Chapter 3). In Spain, family conflict has likewise been identified as a factor that distinguishes between transwomen who do and do not engage in sex work (Chapter 20). In the United States and in other countries around the world, sex work among transwomen is frequently accompanied by substance use and depression. We need to know more about how the experience and practice of sex work among transgender persons are shaped by these issues.

THE CONTINUING SPECTER OF HIV

HIV continues to be a major health issue that confronts transwomen around the world, and sex work further increases the odds of infection (Chapter 9). Sex work elevates the likelihood of HIV among transwomen, in part because of increased levels of abuse and substance use associated with sex work in this population (Chapter 10). Among those who are HIV-positive, high levels of sex work appear to reduce the odds of successfully engaging in antiretroviral therapy (ART) (Chapter 12). Specific lifestyle factors associated with transgender sex work would appear to partially account for the alarming levels of HIV among transwomen sex workers.

Ongoing study is needed to update the prevalence and incidence of HIV among transwomen sex workers. The extent to which HIV status affects the experience and practice of sex work in this population needs to be examined.

ASSESSMENT AND CARE BY SERVICE PROVIDERS

The intertwining of sex work with other interpersonal and health issues that transwomen face underscores the need for service providers and healthcare professionals to understand and treat these individuals in a holistic manner. Basic principles for such treatment are set forth in Chapter 22 and should be read by anyone charged with the responsibility of properly assessing and treating transwomen engaged in sex work. Evaluations of the effect of incorporating transgender-sensitive protocols in practice would be useful.

LEGAL STATUS

The legal status of sex work is currently being hotly debated; there are calls for decriminalization or for allowing it to be practiced under certain conditions or in certain venues without legal jeopardy. This debate is often framed by contrasting a criminal justice perspective with a public health perspective on sex work. This debate, summarized in Chapter 24 with specific reference to transgender sex work, began with ecological studies suggesting that aggressive policing may be a factor contributing to the ongoing HIV epidemic among sex workers around the world. The validity of such studies may be questioned, however, because measurements of aggressive policing and HIV risk behavior and infection were not obtained at the individual level of analysis across time. A further analysis of the New York Transgender Project, presented in Chapter 23, provides data suggesting that perceptions of psychological abuse by police (aggressive policing) are longitudinally associated with high-risk sexual behavior for HIV among transwomen in New York City. This study has provided compelling data suggesting a need to replace or fundamentally alter the criminal justice perspective on sex work. Additional research pertaining to this complex issue, with specific reference to transgender sex work, is needed.

AFFIRMATION OF GENDER AND SEXUAL IDENTITIES AND TRANSGENDER SEX WORK

In several of the chapters, sex work among transwomen was seen as motivated in part by a need to validate gender identity. This is an important observation that needs to be better understood and, we suggest, broadened to include complex and nonbinary conceptions of both gender and sexual identity. The rationale for this novel conceptualization will be described, with a focus on transgender sex work.

Virginia Prince, who popularized the term *transgender* in the 1980s or early 1990s, argued that "gender is between my ears, not between my legs" (Prince, 2005), reflecting a discourse that lasts until today and emphasizes that transgender is about gender, not about sexuality. This discourse has led to a neglect of the role of sexuality in the identity development of transgender individuals. However, it is becoming increasingly clear that gender and sexuality, while distinct constructs, are intricately connected. Yet we know very little about the sexuality of transgender people, and the little that is known often applies a binary conceptualization of transgender identity by comparing the sexuality of transgender women to that of nontransgender women (e.g., Weyers et al., 2009), and the sexuality of transgender men to that of nontransgender men (e.g., Wierckx et al., 2011).

However, a closer look at the gender identities and sexualities of transgender people, particularly over time, reveals a more complex, richer picture. If we recognize a spectrum of gender diversity, we find that gender identity and gender expression are rarely exclusively male or female, masculine or feminine (Bockting, 2008). Moreover, sexuality plays an important role in exploring, affirming, and reaffirming gender identity. Transgender people have a heightened awareness of the stigma attached to gender nonconformity. The binary nature of gender norms creates challenges for transgender people, as their identity and sexuality are often not consistent with prevailing heteronormative or homonormative scripts (Iantaffi & Bockting, 2011).

As a result, transgender people may experience shame and isolation; actual, perceived, or expected rejection; discrimination, harassment, and violence; and fewer opportunities for affirmation of identity and relationships (Hendricks & Testa, 2012). An already heightened need for affirmation of gender identity (to overcome incongruence between gender identity and sex assigned at birth) is thus further amplified by nonconformity and stigma, increasing transgender individuals' vulnerability to sex work (Bockting, Robinson, & Rosser, 1998; Nuttbrock et al., 2009; Sevelius, 2013). One general direction for future research on transgender sex work is therefore to consider the role of sexuality in the affirmation of gender and sexual orientation identity.

Fundamental to understanding transgender identity and sexuality is the recognition that transwomen are not simply women, and transmen are not simply men (Bockting, 1999). Rather, transgender individuals are a gender minority population and, no matter where they fall on the spectrum of gender identity and gender expression, they have a unique experience. Similarly, transgender women and men are not necessarily straight in terms of their sexual orientation; they may be attracted to women, men, other transgender individuals, or any combination of the above (Iantaffi & Bockting, 2011; Kuper, Nussbaum, & Mustanski, 2012). Comparing the sexuality of transgender women and men to their nontransgender counterparts runs the risk of missing how transgender sexuality may be different altogether.

One approach to begin to understand transgender sexuality is the application of sexual script theory (Simon & Gagnon, 1969, 1984, 1986). According to this theory, gender identity and sexuality are shaped by cultural scenarios that individuals must interpret to create their own intrapsychic scripts, which are enacted in social and sexual relationships and result in interpersonal scripts that serve as additional sources of information used to revise subsequent intrapsychic scripts. The sexual scripts of transgender individuals have not been examined before (Wiederman, 2015). Such an examination could provide a wealth of information with regard to how transgender individuals are affected by prevailing gender norms and sexual scripts in society, how these scripts are internalized and enacted, and how they are part of changing (or maintaining) gender and sexual scripts over time. Such an approach has the potential to uncover transgender sexuality as distinct from both male and female sexuality, and inform our understanding of the sexual interactions and experiences of transgender individuals and their partners, within and outside the context of sex work. With a better understanding of transgender sexuality and its enactment in sex work comes the responsibility to empower transgender individuals, their families, and communities; educate and train HIV prevention workers and health and social service providers; increase public awareness and reduce social stigma; and advocate for transgender and sex workers' human rights. We hope that the perspectives compiled in *Transgender Sex Work and Society* are a step toward that goal.

REFERENCES

Bockting, W. O. (2008). Psychotherapy and the real-life experience: From gender dichotomy to gender diversity. *Sexologies, 17* (4), 211–224.

———. (1999). From construction to context: Gender through the eyes of the transgendered. *Siecus Report, 28* (1), 3–7.

Bockting, W. O., Robinson, B. E., & Rosser, B. R. S. (1998). Transgender HIV prevention: A qualitative needs assessment. *AIDS Care, 10* (4), 505–525.

Hendricks, M. L., & Testa, R. J. (2012). A conceptual framework for clinical work with transgender and gender nonconforming clients: An adaptation of the Minority Stress Model. *Professional Psychology: Research and Practice, 43* (5), 460–467.

Iantaffi, A., & Bockting, W. O. (2011). Views from both sides of the bridge? Gender, sexual legitimacy, and transgender people's experiences of relationships. *Culture, Health & Sexuality, 13* (3), 355–370.

Kuper, L. E., Nussbaum, R., & Mustanski, B. (2012). Exploring the diversity of gender and sexual orientation identities in an online sample of transgender individuals. *Journal of Sex Research, 49* (2–3), 244–254.

Nuttbrock, L. A., Bockting, W. O., Hwahng, S., Rosenblum, A., Mason, M., Macri, M., & Becker, J. (2009). Gender identity affirmation among male-to-female transgender persons: A life course analysis across types of relationships and cultural/lifestyle factors. *Sexual and Relationship Therapy, 24* (2), 108–125.

Prince, V. (2005) Sex vs. gender. *International Journal of Transgenderism, 8* (4), 29–32.

Sevelius, J. M. (2013). Gender affirmation: A framework for conceptualizing risk behavior among transgender women of color. *Sex Roles, 68* (11–12), 675–689.

Simon, W., & Gagnon, J. H. (1986). Sexual scripts: Permanence and change. *Archives of Sexual Behavior, 15* (2), 97–120.

———. (1984). Sexual scripts. *Society, 22* (1), 53–60.

———. (1969). Psychosexual development. *Trans-action, 6* (5), 9–17.

Weyers, S., Elaut, E., De Sutter, P., Gerris, J., T'Sjoen, G., Heylens, G., De Cuypere, G., & Verstraelen, H. (2009). Long-term assessment of the physical, mental, and sexual health among transsexual women. *Journal of Sexual Medicine, 6* (3), 752–760. doi:10.1111/j.1743-6109.2008.01082.x.

Wiederman, M. W. (2015). Sexual script theory: Past, present, and future. *In* J. Delamater & R. F. Plante (eds.), *Handbook of the sociology of sexualities* (pp. 7–22). Heidelberg: Springer International.

Wierckx, K., Van Caenegem, E., Elaut, E., Dedecker, D., Van de Peer, F., Toye, K., . . . & T'Sjoen, G. (2011). Quality of life and sexual health after sex reassignment surgery in transsexual men. *Journal of Sexual Medicine, 8* (12), 3379–3388. doi:10.1111/j.1743-6109.2011.02348.x.

CONTRIBUTORS

Chitlada Areesantichai, PhD, works as a professor at the College of Public Health Sciences, Chulalongkorn University. She has completed a postdoctoral training fellowship in the Department of Epidemiology, College of Public Health Professions, and the College of Medicine, University of Florida. Dr. Areesantichai has experience in many research and academic areas, including alcohol, tobacco, substance use, and HIV/AIDS. She also conducts and oversees research in drug-dependent populations (IV drug users, MSM, and transgender). She has been conducting research through the Drug Dependence Research Center (DDRC), which was designated as the WHO Collaborating Centre for Research and Training in Drug Dependence (WHOCC), Bangkok, Thailand. She has conducted research as principal investigator on risk behaviors among juvenile offenders and homeless children, community action on alcohol harm reduction, and network size estimation of HIV risk groups in Thailand. Her community action research on alcohol consumption and HIV risk behaviors was recognized by the WHO Regional Office for Southeast Asia (WHO-SERO) as a good-practice project and recommended for reducing harm from alcohol use in Lop Buri province. She also works closely with the Thai government on issues related to policy matters involving control of substances.

Rafael Ballester-Arnal has been associate professor of clinical health psychology at the Universitat Jaume I in Castellón de la Plana, Spain, since 1998. He is the director of the research group Health Psychology: Prevention and Treatment and director of the Research Unit on Sexuality and AIDS (Salusex-Unisexsida). This is a health center dedicated to the sexual health promotion of university members. His scientific interest has been directed mainly toward the promotion of health and more specifically in the field of sexual health; he has written more than 30 funded research projects, 20 books, 100 papers published in prestigious journals (including *AIDS and Behavior, Journal of Health Psychology, Journal of Community Health,* and *Journal of Sex and Marital Therapy*), and 250 contributions to international conferences. Many of these studies have focused on topics such as sexual behavior of adolescents, prevention of HIV infection, homosexuality and homophobia, transgender people, male sex workers, sexual compulsivity, and sex and cybersex addiction. Since 2013 he has been dean of the Faculty of Health Sciences, which includes the degrees of medicine, nursing, and psychology.

Stefan Baral is a physician epidemiologist and an associate professor in the Department of Epidemiology at the Johns Hopkins Bloomberg School of Public Health. He completed his certification in community medicine as a fellow of the Royal College of Physicians and Surgeons of Canada and his certification in family medicine with the Canadian Council of Family Physicians. Through his role as director of the Key Populations Program at the Bloomberg School of Public Health, Baral has led HIV epidemiology and implementation research focused on characterizing the epidemiology of HIV and effective HIV prevention, treatment, and care approaches.

Lorna C. Barton is a Scottish Oral History Centre PhD candidate in the Humanities, Arts, and Social Sciences Graduate School at the University of Strathclyde in Glasgow, UK. Barton's study is an oral history of American transgender lives from the 1950s to the present. It looks at how trans individuals have historically been represented by the media, politically and socially, by means of research, archival materials, and oral history interviews she has recorded. Lorna is extremely passionate about trans rights and research that has an effect at street level and in the community. Her research interests lie in oral history, transgender studies, and sex work research. Her theoretical interests include transgender theory, social justice theory, critical theory, and intersectionality. Additionally, Barton is a researcher in residence with the Scottish Graduate School for the Arts and Humanities Sound Archives.

Trinidad Bergero-Miguel is a clinical psychologist at the Regional University Hospital in Málaga, Spain. From 1999 to December 2016, she worked in the Transgender and Gender Identity Unit at this hospital. She is one of the main scientific authorities on transsexuality in Spain. She has published several articles on transsexuality and presented papers at national and international congresses. Her main professional interest has focused on the identification of psychosocial problems such as violence, bullying, or mobbing toward transgender people.

Walter Bockting, PhD, is professor of medical psychology (in psychiatry and nursing) at Columbia University and a research scientist with the New York State Psychiatric Institute. A native of the Netherlands, Dr. Bockting received his PhD in medical psychology from the Vrije Universiteit in Amsterdam. He completed a postdoctoral fellowship at the Program in Human Sexuality, University of Minnesota Medical School, where he was a tenured professor before joining the faculty of Columbia University in 2012. Currently, Dr. Bockting is codirector of Columbia's Program for the Study of LGBT Health. Dr. Bockting is a pioneer in transgender health, and his research has been funded by AmFAR (the Foundation for AIDS Research), the National Institutes of Health, the M×A×C AIDS Fund, the New York Community Trust, and a number of other private foundations. He assisted Dr. Larry Nuttbrock with his groundbreaking study of transgender women and HIV in New York City; this study's findings are reported in this book. Dr. Bockting is currently the principal investigator of an NIH-funded multisite, longitudinal study of transgender identity development across the life span (Project AFFIRM). He served on the Institute of Medicine (IOM) committee that produced the IOM report "The Health of LGBT People: Building a Foundation for Better Understanding" (National Academy of Sciences, 2011). He is a past president of the World Professional Association for Transgender Health and a past president and fellow of the Society for the Scientific Study of Sexuality.

Charlene Bumanglag, PhD, is an assistant professor in the Department of Tropical Medicine, Medical Microbiology, and Pharmacology at the John A. Burns School of Medicine, University of Hawai'i at Manoa. Her research, teaching, and service focus on global health disparities among the disenfranchised, including LGBT communities, with an emphasis on the transgender community. She completed her NIH Global Health Fogarty Fellowship in Thailand investigating HIV health disparities among transwomen; there she also spearheaded the HIV: Qualitative Research Methods in Social and Behavioral Sciences Workshop with health professional participants from ASEAN countries. Currently, she serves on the Board of Directors for the APHA-Asian Pacific Islander Caucus.

Carlos F. Cáceres, MD, PhD, completed his medical training at Universidad Peruana Cayetano Heredia (Lima, Peru), and his masters in public health and doctorate in epidemiology at the University of California at Berkeley. In 2000 he established the Unit in Health, Sexuality, and Human Development at the School of Public Health of Universidad Peruana Cayetano Heredia, which in 2015 became the university's Center for Interdisciplinary Studies in Sexuality, AIDS, and Society (CIISSS). As professor of public health and director of CIISSS, Dr. Cáceres works with a multidisciplinary team in research on sexuality, sexual health, and human rights, and he coordinates a post-graduate program in sexuality, human rights, and policy. He is the author of numerous publications, and he participates in the advisory committees of several peer-reviewed publications. He frequently plays the role of technical adviser in activities organized by PAHO/WHO and UNAIDS.

Yong Cai, MD, is an associate professor in the School of Public Health, Shanghai Jiaotong University, China. He has engaged in teaching, research, and management for over 18 years in the field of public health. He specializes in population-based epidemiology and behavioral intervention such as HIV/AIDS prevention and tobacco control. He has been awarded 15 grants as principal investigator and 20 grants as co-investigator, including two projects from the Chinese National Natural Science Foundation and two projects from the Chinese National Ministry of Education. He was selected as Outstanding Young Talent of Public Health by the Shanghai Municipal Health Bureau in 2007 and awarded the Baosteel Prize for excellence in teaching in 2016. He has authored and coauthored 30 papers published in international peer-reviewed journals. He and his research team are now working on psychosocial syndemics associated with suicidal ideation and HIV risk behavior among MSM and transgender people in Shanghai, China.

Jesús Castro-Calvo is a clinical health psychologist who works as a researcher at the Universitat Jaume I in Castellón de la Plana, Spain. He is known for his work in sex addiction in general and cybersex addiction in particular. He is the author of more than 20 papers published in national and international peer-reviewed journals. He has also presented works on behavioral addictions among young people at important congresses.

Venkatesan Chakrapani, MD, has more than a decade of experience in conducting applied and policy-oriented health research among marginalized communities, such as men who have sex with men (MSM) and transgender people in India. He is the founder, director, and chairperson of the Centre for Sexuality and Health Research and Policy (C-SHaRP), a not-for-profit research agency in Chennai, India. Dr. Chakrapani's studies among MSM and transgender people have been on barriers to HIV prevention and treatment services; social and sexual networks and sexual risk; stigma and discrimination and structural violence; and effect of sexual minority stigma on mental health and HIV risk. He is part of the Indian National AIDS Control Organisation's Technical Resource Groups on HIV and MSM and Transgender people. He was a recipient of the NIH Fogarty Fellowship (Yale University) and the MacArthur Foundation's Fund for Leadership Development Fellowship.

Rebecca de Guzman, PhD, is a medical anthropologist who has been involved with qualitative and ethnographic public health research projects since the mid-1990s. She recently received her PhD in cultural anthropology from the Graduate Center, CUNY, where she received NIH funding to conduct an ethnographic research study that explores how public health experts construct expert knowledge about race and inequality. She lives in San Francisco with her girlfriend and their two elderly dogs.

Ceylan Engin is a doctoral student in the Department of Sociology at Texas A&M University. She is an interdisciplinary scholar of sociology, demography, and women's and gender studies. Her areas of specialization are the intersections of religion, gender, and sexuality issues; her specific focus is on Turkey. Her current research centers on the sex industry as well as women and LGBT rights in Turkey. Engin is also the author of the article "LGBT in Turkey: Policies and Experiences," in which she examines the institutional discrimination that LGBT individuals experience at a macro level and the violence and discrimination that transgender individuals experience at a micro level.

Maria Dolores Gil-Llario is associate professor at the University of Valencia, Spain. Her scientific career since 1995 has focused on health education, primarily on sexual health. She has published several articles in relevant scientific journals, as well as chapters in books, of which she has been the coordinator several times. She has participated in 17 research projects, often as principal investigator. She has directed six doctoral theses. In addition, she has contributed to national and international congresses with more than 150 works. She has received several research awards. One of them is the award given by the Government Territorial Department of the Valencian Region in scientific dissemination for SALUSEX-UNISEXSIDA group, of which she is the cofounder and director at the Valencia headquarters. She has filled various positions in academic administration, such as president of the Academic Degree Committee and subdirector (and later director) of the teacher's training college.

Tiffany R. Glynn completed her master's degree at the Brown University School of Public Health and is currently a PhD student in clinical health psychology at the University of Miami. Her research addresses biopsychosocial health disparities among sexual and gender minority populations and interventions to improve outcomes. A major focus of her work is how discrimination and stigma affect the health of transgender individuals.

Zil Goldstein is a nurse practitioner and a transgender activist working to promote better healthcare in marginalized communities. She serves as the program director at the Center for Transgender Medicine and Surgery in the Mount Sinai Hospital System, where she facilitates appropriate medical and surgical interventions for transgender people. Goldstein is an accomplished educator in transgender and sex worker health, and she has extensive experience designing programs and guidelines to best serve these communities.

José Guzmán-Parra is clinical psychologist at the Mental Health Research Unit of the Hospital Carlos Haya of Málaga, Spain. Since the beginning of his training at the University Regional Hospital of Málaga, he has been interested in such research areas as psychological difficulties and stress factors experienced by people with gender dysphoria, and the study of possible ways for reducing coercive measures in psychiatric inpatient units. At the moment, he is conducting research focusing on expression and phenotyping consequences of a genetic predisposition in families with high prevalence of bipolar and affective disorders. In addition to clinical resident training and clinical trials responsibilities, he is a member of the Biomedical Research Institute of Málaga (IBIMA), the International Society of Psychiatric Genetics (ISPG), and the GAP group (Psychosocial Andalusian Research Group), and he has received several awards for his contributions to psychology and psychiatry conferences.

Beth R. Hoffman, PhD, MPH, is an associate professor in the Public Health Department at California State University, Los Angeles. She received her MPH in 2002 and her PhD in 2005 from the University of Southern California's Institute for Prevention Research. She is an expert in social network analysis, peer influence, and high-risk behaviors, and her dissertation focused on the effects of friends' smoking on adolescent tobacco use behaviors. Her current research focuses on factors influencing and consequences of sex- and drug-related behaviors of transwomen, and she has published several articles in this area. An advocate for healthy sexuality, she created and regularly teaches an undergraduate-level course on sex and sexuality targeted for public health and child development undergraduate students.

Sel J. Hwahng, PhD, is an adjunct associate professor in the Women and Gender Studies Department at Hunter College–City University of New York. Dr. Hwahng has received numerous grants, awards, and fellowships from such organizations and institutions as the National Institute on Drug Abuse (NIDA), the National Institutes of Health, the American Public Health Association, the International AIDS Society, and the Association for Women in Psychology. Publications include over 30 sole-, first-, and coauthored articles and book chapters in peer-reviewed publications. Dr. Hwahng is on the Board of Directors of the Center for LGBTQ Studies at the City University of New York and was recently program chair for the LGBT Caucus of the American Public Health Association.

Mariko Iwamoto, MA, has a master's degree in social psychology and works as a project director at the Public Health Institute, Health Intervention Projects for Underserved Populations. She has been overseeing multiple community-based HIV and substance abuse intervention projects targeting ethnic minorities and LGBTQ populations in the United States and Asian countries. For the past ten years, she has been working to promote the health and well-being of underserved populations.

Daze Jefferies is a graduate student in gender studies at Memorial University of Newfoundland, Canada. Her work explores the intersections of folklore, health, and gender among two populations: those who are trans, and those who do sex work. Her graduate research interrogates the ways in which transwomen living in Newfoundland and Labrador narrate and navigate matters of everyday health and identity management.

Andrea Krüsi, PhD, is a postdoctoral fellow at the School of Population and Public Health at the University of British Columbia and a research associate with the Gender and Sexual Health Initiative (GSHI) of the BC Centre for Excellence in HIV/AIDS in Vancouver. Dr. Krüsi leads the community-based participatory qualitative and arts-based research program at GSHI. Dr. Krüsi's work focuses broadly on the criminalization of sexuality, with a particular focus on how intersecting social and structural contexts, including laws and policies, shape the health, safety, and well-being of sex workers and persons living with HIV.

Don Kulick is Distinguished University Professor of Anthropology at Uppsala University in Sweden, where he directs the Swedish Research Council–funded program Engaging Vulnerability. His most recent book is *Loneliness and Its Opposite: Sex, Disability, and the Ethics of Engagement* (with Jens Rydström, Duke University Press, 2015).

Joseph T. F. Lau, PhD, is a professor and the associate director of the JC School of Public Health and Primary Care, Faculty of Medicine, Chinese University of Hong Kong, and the founding president of the Hong Kong Society of Behavioral Health and convener of the Asian Network for Behavioral Health. He has a multidisciplinary research background. He is currently a director of the Centre for Medical Anthropology and Behavioral Health of Sun Yat-sen University, and he holds adjunct professorships at the Institute of Psychology, China Academic Sciences, Peking Union Medical College, Central South University, and Shantou University in China. He also serves as an overseas expert for the China Academy of Sciences. He specializes in interventions for changing risk and preventive behaviors (including HIV-related risk behaviors), psychological health, and sexual health. He has authored and coauthored over 350 papers published in international peer-reviewed journals and has been awarded 53 grants as principal investigator and 29 grants as co-investigator. He and his research team are among the first to investigate the sexual and psychological health of transwomen sex workers in China.

Jinghua Li, PhD, is currently an associate professor in the School of Public Health, Sun Yat-sen University, Guangzhou, China. She received her master's degree from the University of Tokyo and was a recipient of the University of Tokyo ASATSU-DK Scholarship. She received her PhD from the Chinese University of Hong Kong. Her interests include HIV-related behaviors, social networking and support, positive psychology, health economics, and epidemiological modeling. She has published 12 papers in international peer-reviewed journals.

Yan Liu is on staff at the Shenyang Consultation Centre of AIDS Aid and Health Service. He has rich experiences in working with the LGBT communities in China.

Tara Lyons, PhD, is a faculty member in the Department of Criminology at Kwantlen Polytechnic University in British Columbia and a research scientist with the Gender and Sexual Health Initiative of the BC Centre for Excellence in HIV/AIDS, Vancouver. Her research is situated at the intersections of health, gender, sexuality, and criminalization. Using feminist and community-based approaches, she leads research projects examining the experiences of queer and trans persons. Her research program has been developed to document the effects of criminalization on the health of marginalized populations and to shape relevant social, legal, and policy reforms.

Tiecheng Ma is the chief executive of Shenyang Consultation Centre of AIDS Aid and Health Service, a nongovernmental organization in Shenyang, China. He was awarded the Barry & Martin's Prize by the Barry & Martin's Trust in 2015. His center provides comprehensive services for the LGBT communities, such as HIV testing and counseling, social support, legal assistance, psychological counseling, and community empowerment.

Zack Marshall is an assistant professor at Renison University College, University of Waterloo, in Ontario, and colead of the Canadian Institutes of Health Research Centre for REACH in HIV/AIDS Trans Priorities Project.

Julia Moore, MS, is an assistant researcher with the Health Intervention Projects for Underserved Populations at the Public Health Institute, specializing in biostatistical analysis. Her research focus is on exploring the relationship between health and economic disparities in underserved LGBQT communities, with an emphasis on transgender populations. She completed her master's degree in biostatistics at California State University, East Bay.

Angélica Motta received her PhD in collective health from the Institute of Social Medicine (Rio de Janeiro State University) and her MA in gender studies from the Institute of Social Studies (Erasmus University, Rotterdam). She has committed her career to the fields of sexuality, gender, and reproductive health and rights; as a researcher and lecturer, she has experience in Peru, Brazil, and Germany. Currently, she is a researcher at the Center for Interdisciplinary Research in Sexuality, AIDS, and Society at Cayetano Heredia Peruvian University, where she coordinates the diploma in sexuality, human rights, and public policies in education and health.

Tooru Nemoto, PhD, is research program director at the Public Health Institute (PHI). Before joining PHI, Dr. Nemoto was an associate professor, Department of Medicine, University of California–San Francisco (UCSF). He started his research career as an epidemiologist at the Addiction Research and Treatment Corporation, New York City, in 1988. His background as a community psychologist enabled him to conduct patient-outcomes research at the largest methadone maintenance program in New York City. He completed his postdoctoral fellowship at the Institute for Health Policy Studies, UCSF, in 1993. Since then, he has been engaged mainly in substance abuse and HIV prevention studies and service projects as principal investigator for underserved and stigmatized populations, such as transwomen, men who have sex with men (MSM), female sex workers, and substance users. He has been awarded a number of grants and service contracts from NIH, SAMHSA, CDC, HRSA, and private foundations. His research has focused on understanding sociocultural contexts of substance use and HIV risk behaviors for health promotion among underserved populations in the United States and Asian countries, such as Thailand, Vietnam, Cambodia, and Malaysia. He has published a number of research papers in peer-reviewed journals and presented study findings at national and international scientific conferences. His project team has been working closely with community members to develop, implement, and evaluate community-based interventions to improve health and well-being and advocate for human rights for LBGT populations.

Peter A. Newman, PhD, is professor, University of Toronto, Factor-Inwentash Faculty of Social Work, and Canada Research Chair in Health and Social Justice. He has received substantial external funding for his transdisciplinary, global research program on social-structural and behavioral challenges of new HIV prevention technologies, and community stakeholder engagement in biomedical HIV prevention trials, with a focus on sexual and gender minorities in resource-limited settings. Dr. Newman is engaged in ongoing research and training collaborations with investigators in Canada, India, South Africa, and Thailand to promote health and human rights for sexual minority populations. He has authored or coauthored articles in more than 100 peer-reviewed publications, including *AIDS*, the *Lancet*, and the *American Journal of Public Health*. His work on HIV vaccine acceptability has been widely profiled in venues such as *Nature Medicine*, American Association for the Advancement of Science, and the media.

Ernest Noronha, MBA, is a policy analyst for human rights at the United Nations Development Program Bangkok Regional Hub, providing technical support and input to the program (South and Southeast Asia) and focusing on HIV, human rights, sexual orientation, gender identity, intersex issues, civil society, and community systems strengthening.

Aron Núnez-Curto, MA, an anthropologist, graduated from Universidad Nacional Mayor de San Marcos at Lima, Peru. He wrote his thesis on death, illness, and healthcare narratives and trajectories among transgender women in Lima for a master's degree in anthropology at Pontificia Universidad Católica del Perú. He is a researcher for Centro de Investigación Interdisciplinaria en Sexualidad, Sida, y Sociedad—CIISSS—at Universidad Peruana Cayetano Heredia, where he has participated in several research projects and coauthored publications. He is an LGBTI and feminist activist, working on sexual and reproductive issues.

Larry A. Nuttbrock, PhD, was previously affiliated with the National Development and Research Institutes (NDRI) in New York City and is now a private consultant living in New York City. In 2011 he completed a major longitudinal study of transwomen in New York City and is currently pursuing research in the field of transgender health.

Don Operario is professor of public health in the Department of Behavior and Social Sciences at Brown University. His research addresses the social psychological determinants of HIV, sexual health, substance use, and mental health among sexual and gender minority populations.

Usaneya Perngparn, PhD, works as an assistant professor at the College of Public Health Sciences, Chulalongkorn University. She completed a doctoral degree in research for health development at Chulalongkorn University and received master's degrees, one in demography and one in population research, at the University of Exeter in the United Kingdom, where she had training at the Addiction Centre. Collaborating closely at the national and international levels, she has given counseling and training in drug and alcohol addiction treatment, training analysis needs, and data management. She has been a longtime contributor to the Ministry of Public Health in compiling and processing national drug dependence treatment records. Her research areas are the sociocultural context of risk-taking behaviors among women and transgender sex workers, evaluation of drug dependence treatment systems, and multisector community development projects. She conducts and oversees research in alcohol and substance use, HIV risk, and prevention. Her works have been published in many international journals.

Leslie Pierre works as a research assistant with the Gender and Sexual Health Initiative of the BC Centre for Excellence in HIV/AIDS, Vancouver. For four years she worked at the PACE Society, a sex-worker-led organization, doing outreach, office coordination, and program development. She is an aboriginal transwoman from the Dakelh Nation.

Asa Radix, MD, MPH, is the director of research and education at the Callen-Lorde Community Health Center and a doctoral student in the Department of Epidemiology at Columbia University. Originally from the West Indies, Dr. Radix completed postgraduate training in internal medicine and infectious diseases at the University of Connecticut. Dr. Radix has over 20 years of experience providing primary care to transgender and gender nonbinary people and has contributed to national and international guidelines in transgender medicine.

Ximena Salazar, PhD, is an anthropologist who graduated from Universidad Nacional Mayor de San Marcos at Lima, Peru. She obtained her degree in cultural anthropology with a specialization in political science and Latin American studies at the Johann

Wolfgang Goethe University, Academic Program of Cultural Anthropology in Frankfurt, Germany, and her PhD in anthropology from Universidad Católica del Perú. She currently holds the position of executive coordinator of Centro de Investigación Interdisciplinaria en Sexualidad, Sida y Sociedad—CIISSS (Center of Interdisciplinary Research in Sexuality, AIDS, and Society)—at Universidad Peruana Cayetano Heredia, where she participates in substantial qualitative or mixed-methods studies in the areas of health, sexuality, gender, and public policy. Her dissertation was focused on the gender identity of transwomen. Dr. Salazar has been the author and coauthor of numerous publications, both local and international.

Ayden I. Scheim is a social epidemiologist whose research focuses on reducing health inequities related to stigma and social exclusion, particularly in the areas of HIV, substance use, and transgender health. He was a Pierre Elliott Trudeau Foundation Scholar in Epidemiology and Biostatistics at Western University in London, Canada, where he completed his PhD in summer 2017. In addition to his scientific research, Scheim has 15 years of experience in monitoring and evaluation, health provider education, and direct service provision related to trans health and HIV prevention.

Kate Shannon, PhD, MPH, is an associate professor of medicine at the University of British Columbia and director of the Gender and Sexual Health Initiative (www.gshi .cfenet.ubc.ca) of the BC Centre for Excellence in HIV/AIDS, Vancouver. She is principal investigator of the AESHA (An Evaluation of Sex Workers' Health Access) Project, within which this research is nested, and she has worked with community partners on this research since 2004. She currently holds a Canada research chair in global sexual health and HIV/AIDS, and her research focuses on structural, gender, and policy determinants shaping sexual health, violence, and access to care for marginalized populations, including women and trans persons living with HIV, sex workers, youths, and migrant communities both in Canada and globally. She is strongly committed to community-based research that promotes evidence-based sexual health policies and practice and health and social equity for marginalized communities. She has regularly acted as an expert consultant on HIV, sexual health, and human rights guidelines, including WHO/UNAIDS/NSWP guidelines on sex work and HIV, and the Global Commission on HIV and the Law.

Yik Koon Teh, PhD, is a professor of criminology and sociology at the Department of Strategic Studies, and a senior research fellow at the Centre for Defence and International Security Studies, National Defence University of Malaysia. She received her PhD in sociology (criminology) from the London School of Economics and Political Science and was a Fulbright Scholar at the University of California–Los Angeles in 2002. She was attached to the Rajaratnam School of International Studies, Nanyang Technological University, Singapore, as a visiting fellow for nine months beginning in October 2015. Her main focus at the university is on nontraditional security, particularly HIV/AIDS and health security. Her other research interests are rehabilitation of offenders, crime prevention strategies, fraud and corruption, marginalized communities, social and welfare issues of the military, and gender and sexuality.

Karen Trocki, PhD, is a social psychologist and research program director at the Alcohol Research Group (ARG) in Emeryville, CA. She has expertise in both qualitative and quantitative research. For more than two decades she has done epidemiological research on the relationship between substance use (alcohol, marijuana, and tobacco) and a variety of topics that include sexual risk taking, religion, contexts of drinking, women, psychophysiology, and LGBT populations. She has done international research in Tunisia, Goa, India, Malaysia, and Thailand. She has been the principal investigator (or one of several principal investigators) on numerous NIH R01 and R21 grants as well as Center for Substance Abuse Prevention– and California State–funded grants. She has been a co-investigator on the ARG Center's grant and has served for 20 years as a project director on the National Alcohol Survey, which is conducted at five-year intervals. Dr. Trocki's theoretical focus of interest has been on biological vulnerabilities, and the social, cognitive, and temperament factors associated with risk behavior.

Zixin Wang, PhD, is a research assistant professor in the JC School of Public Health and Primary Care, Faculty of Medicine, Chinese University of Hong Kong. He specializes in interdisciplinary behavioral health research, including sexual risk behaviors and substance use among at-risk populations and applying health behavioral theories in promoting preventive behaviors as well as biomedical HIV/STD intervention. He was awarded the Early Career Award by the International Society of Behavioral Medicine in 2016. He has authored and coauthored over 30 papers published in international peer-reviewed journals and has been awarded five grants as principal investigator and eight grants as co-investigator.

Laura Winters is a community worker and activist, as well as a grad student near completion of a PhD in sociology at the University of New Brunswick. She lives, works, and researches in Newfoundland and Labrador, and she has conducted extensive interviews with adults who work in the sex industry in Newfoundland. She also founded and runs SHOP (Safe Harbour Outreach Project), a support service whose mandate is to advocate for the human rights of women who do sex work. SHOP operates from a harm-reduction, human rights framework that is based on the understanding that sex workers are the experts on their own lives. Winters is constantly inspired by the strength, tenacity, and resistance displayed by people who do sex work in Newfoundland and across Canada, in their fight for better laws, better working conditions, and a better society free from stigma and discrimination.

Barry M. Wolfe is an international lawyer, criminologist, and human rights activist. Born in Scotland, he graduated with First Class Honours in jurisprudence and criminology at Edinburgh University, was a graduate fellow at Yale Law School, and received an LLM in public international law from Magdalene College, Cambridge University. He has lived in Brazil since 1986. Wolfe is considered an authority on the investigation of financial crime, corruption, and money laundering in Brazil. He is a specialist in criminal organizations and subcultures, human trafficking, and international immigration law. He is a practicing English solicitor and consultant in foreign law at the Brazilian bar. As a lawyer, he is known for his readiness to take on polemical and often unpopular cases involving injustice against those in a position of disadvantage or unable to protect themselves. Wolfe has worked with transgender sex workers since 2005. He founded SOS Dignity, a nongovernmental human rights project that defends and protects victims of discriminate and indiscriminate violence, torture, abuse of power, human trafficking and slavery, AIDS, and clandestine medical practices. SOS Dignity provides individual, direct support to victims and to potential victims so that they will not fall prey to, and will become independent of, exploiters.

GLOSSARY

affective disorder: a psychiatric mood disorder such as depression, anxiety, or bipolar disorder

affective relation: a relationship involving emotional connections

agency: a person's ability to act freely and independently

AKP: Justice and Development Party (Turkey)

alpha coefficient ( ): *(statistics)* the probability of a false positive result

anchored questions: survey questions used to create a reference point

Andean region: an area of South America comprising Peru, Ecuador, Colombia, and Bolivia

androgen blocker: a hormone or drug that blocks the production of androgens

androgynous: *adj.* having both male and female traits

androphilic: *adj.* being sexually attracted to men only

anoscope: a medical instrument used to inspect the anal canal

antecedent factor *or* variable: *(statistics)* an independent variable that precedes other variables in time and may or may not affect a later variable

antisocial personality disorder: a psychiatric condition characterized by a history of manipulative, exploitative, and often criminal behavior

antiviral *or* antiretroviral therapy (ART): a regimen of drugs used to slow the progression of HIV infection

AOR: adjusted odds ratio

aravani: a term of self-identification used by transgender people (parts of India)

ART: antiretroviral therapy

assay: *v.* to test for the presence of a drug or pathogen

assortativity: *(sociology)* the tendency for members of a network to affiliate with similar members

autogynephilia: *(psychology)* a theory positing that some male-to-female transgender individuals are attracted to the image of themselves as women

avant la lettre: "before the letter"; describes scholarship about a subject before a term for it had been coined

Axis I psychiatric disorder: in *DSM-IV*, a primary acute psychiatric diagnosis for which a person requires or seeks help

Axis II personality disorder: in *DSM-IV*, an underlying mental health issue usually characterized by an enduring pattern of maladaptive behavior

background variable: *(statistics)* a variable that is present and may be controlled for, but is not the variable being studied, e.g., demographic information

Badhai: the blessing of newborn babies and newlywed couples, traditionally performed by *hijras*

baht: Thai unit of currency

BDI-II: Beck Depression Inventory II

BDSM: bondage/discipline *or* dominance/submission *or* sadism/masochism

behavioral health: the branch of healthcare aimed at implementing changes in behavior to combat chronic disease, mental disorders, drug abuse, or addiction

berdache: a Native American transgender person (often considered offensive)

beta (b or): *(statistics)* the probability of a false negative result

bicha: a slang term for a transwoman, male homosexual, or effeminate man (Latin America)

binarism: a philosophical division into exactly two parts, as in the traditional division of gender as male and female

binomial link: *(statistics)* a function that makes linear the relationship between the mean of the dependent variable and two independent variables

biopsychosocial: *adj. (public health)* taking into consideration biological, psychological, and social factors

biphobia: unreasonable hostility toward, aversion to, or discrimination against bisexual people

bivariate: *adj. (statistics)* involving two variables, as in an analysis or logistic regression

black market: a marketplace for illicit substances or activities, such as drug sales or sex work

borderline personality disorder: a psychiatric condition characterized by emotional instability and usually self-injury

cafetão (plural cafetões): male pimp (Brazil)

cafetina (plural cafetinas): female and transvestite pimps (Brazil)

Candomblé: Afro-Brazilian religious tradition

Carnival: (in Portuguese, *Carnaval do Brasil*) pre-Lenten festival in Brazil

categorical variable: *(statistics)* a variable that represents an idea or category rather than a number

CDC: Centers (*or* Center) for Disease Control and Prevention (United States and China)

CD4 cell: a type of white blood cell used as an indicator of immune-system function

CES-D: Center for Epidemiologic Studies —Depression (scale); used to measure recent experiences of depression

chela: a junior member of a *hijra* community

chi-square: *(statistics)* a test for significance, used for a nonnormal distribution

CI: *(statistics)* confidence interval

cisgender: *adj.* having a gender identity that corresponds to one's biological sex assigned at birth

club drugs: illegal drugs often used by young adults at parties and in nightclubs or bars

cluster sampling: *(statistics)* a probability sampling method in which a population is divided into groups, and all members of each randomly selected group constitute the sample

cocaine base paste: an extract of the coca leaf, used as a psychoactive drug primarily in the Andean region of South America

cochón: a slang term for a transwoman, male homosexual, or effeminate man (Latin America)

cochones: a slang term for a transwoman, male homosexual, or effeminate man (Nicaragua)

coding: *n.* the process of breaking down interview data into categories for analysis

comorbid: *adj.* occurring along with another medical condition

confidence interval (CI): *(statistics)* the area under the sample distribution curve in which the true mean is most likely to fall

confound: *v. (statistics)* to affect data or variables in a way that cannot be controlled for and may introduce error or bias

contextualize: *v.* to place within a social or cultural context

continuous variable: *(statistics)* a variable that is measured along a continuum, as with time

convenience sampling: *(statistics)* a non-probability sampling method based on easily available research subjects

coolie: an epithet for an unskilled laborer (parts of Asia)

coping theory: *(psychology)* the study of the mechanisms by which people manage or minimize stress

covariate: *n. (statistics)* a variable that can be measured and may affect the outcome of a study, but is usually not the primary variable being studied

Cox proportional hazards analysis: *(statistics)* a regression model used to calculate the difference in survival or hazardous occurrence probabilities between two or more groups

CRAIMC: condomless receptive anal intercourse with male clients

Cronbach's alpha: *(statistics)* a measure of the internal consistency and therefore the reliability of a scale or test

cross-dress: *v.* to dress in clothing typically worn by members of the opposite sex

cross-sectional: *adj.* describes a small segment of a population that is intended to reflect the composition of the population at large

cross-tabulation: *(statistics)* a table displaying the frequency distribution of multiple variables, used in multivariate analysis

cue to action: *(public health)* in the Health Belief Model, a stimulus used to trigger a specific behavior

cultural intelligibility: in Judith Butler's writings, the extent to which an individual is recognized as having value, on the basis of cultural norms

cut score: the defined point on a scale at which something is presumed diagnostic; *also* the point at which a test score is considered passing

dai amma or daima: a senior *hijra* who performs ritual castrations

debt bondage: a form of servitude in which one person is required to work for another in order to pay off a debt

decriminalize: *v.* to legally abolish penalties for behavior that was previously considered criminal

dependent variable: *(statistics)* the variable that is expected to change

destructive sociality: *n.* a negative or damaging system of interactions within a social group

determinant: a factor that determines or influences an outcome

diagnostic symptoms: the symptoms of a disease or disorder that are considered central to a diagnosis

dichotomous: *adj.* having two mutually exclusive parts or outcomes

discourse: *(sociology)* the values held and communicated by a specific culture or institution; discursive: *adj.*, discursively, *adv.*

distal: *adj. (public health)* factors which are external to an individual, such as structural discrimination or stigma

downstream: *adj.* resulting from an earlier action, decision, or condition

DSM: *Diagnostic and Statistical Manual of Mental Disorders,* usually distinguished by edition number (e.g., *DSM-IV*)

duality: division into exactly two parts

dummy variable: a variable that equals 0 or 1, used to indicate the presence or absence of a categorical variable

dyad: *(sociology)* two individuals engaged in an ongoing emotionally or socially significant relationship

dyslipidemia: a medical condition characterized by abnormal levels of lipids or lipoproteins in the bloodstream

ecstasy (XTC): a synthetic amphetamine used recreationally for its hallucinogenic effects

EFA: *(statistics)* exploratory factor analysis

effect size: *(statistics)* a measure of the strength of a statistical correlation

EIA: enzyme immunoassay (screen); HIV test

embodiment: *(sociology)* the interaction between the physical body and one's perception, identity, culture, and so on

emotional dysregulation: the process of becoming less regulated or adapted emotionally

empirical: *adj.* based on observed and usually quantifiable data; empirically, *adv.*

empowerment paradigm: a scholarly theory holding that sex work can be freely chosen employment rather than the result of oppression

end-demand criminalization: a legal pol-

icy in which the purchase of sex is prohibited by law, but the sale of sex is not; *also called* Nordic model

enzyme immunoassay screen: a test for the presence of HIV

epidemiology: *(public health)* the study of health conditions and diseases within a population; epidemiological, *adj.*

estrogen: any of several hormones that promote the development of female sex characteristics

ethnographic: *adj.* based on the direct study of a culture or subculture

eunuch: a surgically castrated man

Euro-America: non-Latin America; i.e., Canada and the United States

EUROPOL: the European Union's law enforcement agency

exchangeable working correlation structure: *(statistics)* an equation used in modeling, making the assumption that all data points from an individual subject are equally correlated with each other

exogenous variable: *(statistics)* a fixed variable that is independent of other variables and affects but is not affected by them

experiential research: a research paradigm in which the subjects are involved in the design, management, and interpretation of the study along with the investigator

exploratory factor analysis (EFA): *(statistics)* a technique in which a data set is reduced to a smaller set of summary variables in order to study the underlying structure

exteriorize: *v.* to manifest externally

fairy: a slang term for a transwoman or effeminate homosexual

fatwa: in Islam, a religious ruling or law

FELGTB: Federación Estatal de Lesbianas, Gais, Transexuales y Bisexuales (Spain)

fem queen: a self-referential term used by members of New York's House Ball community

filha: "daughter" (Brazilian Portuguese); used to denote a sex worker who works under a *madrinha* (female or transgender pimp)

final test of mediation: *(statistics)* a test of whether a hypothesized association between antecedent, mediating, and outcome variables is observable in the data

fluorescent treponema antibody (FTA-TP): a test for syphilis

frango: a slang term for a transwoman, male homosexual, or effeminate man (Latin America)

FSW: female sex work *or* female sex workers

FTA-TP: fluorescent treponema antibody; syphilis test

FTM: female-to-male

gaze: *n.* a power relationship between individuals or groups of people in which the more powerful is considered to be viewing and therefore defining the image of the less powerful

GEE: *(statistics)* generalized estimating equations

gender: the social and cultural roles associated with biological sex

gender affirmation *or* validation: processes or behaviors by which a transgender person receives support for and recognition of his or her gender expression

gender binary: a historical or cultural standard in which there are exactly two genders, usually male and female

gender configuration: the cultural construct of gender within a society

gender division: the divide between two genders, usually but not always male and female

gender dysphoria: stress resulting from a perceived difference between one's gender identity and the sex assigned at birth

gender identity: an individual's inner sense of being male or female

gender inversion: stereotypically gendered behavior assigned to the opposite gender

Gender Minority Stress Model: *(psychology)* a theory positing that the effects of stigma stemming from gender or sexual identity can lead to psychological distress

genelevler: state-run brothels (Turkey)

generalized estimating equations (GEE): *(statistics)* a widely used method of analyzing clustered or longitudinal data

gharana: a social organization functioning as a clan or family of *hijra* communities

globalization: the exchange of worldviews, products, ideas, and other aspects of culture across national boundaries

GLSEN: Gay, Lesbian and Straight Education Network (United States)

GMSR: Gender Minority Stress and Resilience

granular data: highly detailed or specific data

gray literature: print or electronic literature produced by governments or industries, rather than by commercial publishers

grounded theory: a research methodology in the social sciences in which theories are developed from the analyzed data

guru: a senior member of a *hijra* community

gynandromorphophilic: *adj.* having a sexual interest in transgender women

gynephilic: *adj.* being sexually attracted to women only

hammam: a public bathing place common in many Islamic countries

hazard ratio (HR): *(statistics)* a comparison between event probability in the treatment group versus the control group

HBM: Health Belief Model

HBsAg: Hepatitis B virus surface antigen

Health Belief Model (HBM): *(public health)* a model suggesting that health-related behaviors can be explained by the beliefs and attitudes of the individuals studied

heteronormative: *adj.* reflecting an assumption of heterosexuality as the preferred and normal sexuality

heterosexism: biased beliefs and behaviors in favor of heterosexual sexuality and relationships

heterosexual imperative: the cultural and social norms underlying a heterosexist society

hijra: an individual born as male who identifies as either female or neither male nor female (Pakistan and India)

histrionic personality disorder: a psychiatric condition characterized by attention-seeking and overly emotional behavior

HIV: human immunodeficiency virus

hormone therapy: a medical regimen of hormonal drugs taken to effect a gender transition

House Ball community: a community of transgender and/or queer youths stemming from the New York City drag balls of the nineteenth and twentieth centuries

HPV: human papillomavirus

HR: hazard ratio

HS: herpes simplex

HSW: *hijra* sex worker

hukou: the household registration system in modern China, which defines an individual's official city of residence

human smuggling: the practice of arranging for or facilitating the unlawful movement of a person or persons from one country to another, usually with the consent of the person being smuggled

human trafficking: the practice of unlawfully recruiting, transporting, or restraining a person or persons for illegal purposes

hypothesized mediator: *(statistics)* a variable presumed to be part of a causal sequence between the antecedent and outcome variables

ICD-10: International Statistical Classification of Diseases and Related Health Problems, 10th revision

identity link: *(statistics)* the link function used in a standard linear regression, in which the dependent variable is not transformed

identity nonaffirmation: lack of acknowledgment of one's gender identity as a source of stress

IDU: intravenous drug use *or* injection drug user

incident: *adj.* newly acquired; used of a disease or infection

independent variable: *(statistics)* the variable that is expected to cause a change in the dependent variable

industrial silicone: nonmedical-grade silicone, normally used in manufacturing

informal economy: *see* underground economy

INR: Indian rupee (currency)

intercorrelation matrix: *(statistics)* matrix showing how groups of variables are statistically similar

internalized transphobia: self-hatred in transgender individuals

INTERPOL: International Police Organization

intersectionality: the complex ways in which multiple systems of oppression act on an individual or group

intersex *or* intersexed: *adj.* having both male and female sexual organs, or having indeterminate genitalia

intervening variable: *(statistics)* a variable, such as a mediating variable, used to explain relationships between other variables

IRB: Institutional Review Board

ITPA: Immoral Traffic (Prevention) Act (India); a 1956 law prohibiting prostitution

JJS: juvenile justice system

jogappa: a term of self-identification used by transgender people (parts of India)

jogta: a term of self-identification used by transgender people (parts of India)

joto or jota: a slang term for a transwoman, male homosexual, or effeminate man (Latin America)

Kama Sutra: an ancient Sanskrit text describing sexual behavior

kathoey: a transwoman (Thailand)

ketamine: an anesthetic drug used recreationally for its dissociative effects

khusra: a transwoman (Pakistan)

kinnar: a term of self-identification used by transgender people (parts of India)

kothi: a slang term for an effeminate male (India)

KSW: *kathoey* sex workers

launda dance: a folk dance performed by *hijra* or cross-dressed boys (Bihar, India)

LCR: ligase chain reaction; a DNA amplification method used to detect infections

LGB *or* LGBTQ *or* LGBTI: Lesbian, Gay, Bisexual; Lesbian, Gay, Bisexual, Transgendered, Queer; Lesbian, Gay, Bisexual, Transgendered, Intersex; many variants exist

life-course model: an approach to studying individuals by analyzing events or contexts across the life span

Likert scale: a rating scale widely used in surveys that allows for five to seven discrete responses across a symmetrical continuum of agreement

liminality: the condition of being in an intermediate state; in anthropology, a person's mid-ritual state, for example, between childhood and adulthood

limited agent: a person whose capacity for self-determination is restricted

linear regression: *(statistics)* a type of regression analysis used with a continuous dependent variable, yielding a solution that is graphed as a line

link function: *(statistics)* a statistical function that makes linear the relationship between dependent and independent variables

lira: Turkish unit of currency

loca: a slang term for a transwoman, male homosexual, or effeminate man (Latin America)

logistic regression: *(statistics)* a type of regression analysis used with a categorical dependent variable, yielding a solution that is graphed as a curve

Lok Sabha: the lower house of the Indian Parliament

longitudinal: *adj.* describes research that involves repeated observations conducted over a period of time

LRTE: Life Review of Transgender Experiences

LSD: lysergic acid diethylamide; a hallucinogenic drug

machismo: behaviors or attitudes associated with a belief in male superiority and innate aggression

Madonna-Whore complex: *(psychoanalysis)* the theory that some men categorize all females as either "saints" or "sluts"

madrinha: "godmother" (Brazilian Portuguese); used to denote a female or transgender pimp

mahu: a slur for a transwoman or feminine-appearing homosexual (Hawaii)

mak nyah: a transwoman (Malaysia)

maladaptive behaviors *or* coping: behaviors or coping mechanisms for responding to stress that result in negative outcomes

mangalmuki: a term of self-identification used by transgender people (parts of India)

marginality: the state of existing on the outer edges or lower levels of society

marica **or** *maricón:* a slang term for a transwoman, male homosexual, or effeminate man (Latin America)

marido: a live-in boyfriend (Brazilian Portuguese)

mediation: *(statistics)* the effect of a third variable interpolated between the antecedent and outcome variables

mediation analysis: *(statistics)* an analysis that determines the extent to which a mediator affects the outcome

mediator *also* **mediator variable:** *(statistics)* a variable that changes the relationship between the antecedent and outcome variables

meta-analysis: an analysis of multiple research studies

michê: a male prostitute (Brazilian Portuguese)

microaggression: a subtle and often unintended prejudicial statement or action

M.I.N.I.: Mini International Neuropsychiatric Interview; used to diagnose psychiatric disorders

Minority Stress Model: *(psychology)* a theory positing that the effects of stigma stemming from any minority identity can lead to psychological distress

moderator variable: *(statistics)* a variable that influences the strength of a relationship between variables but does not mediate the outcome

Modified Social Ecological Model (MSEM): *(public health)* a risk model for HIV infection

mollies: a slur for transwomen or feminine-appearing homosexuals

mona: a slang term for a transwoman, male homosexual, or effeminate man (Latin America)

MSEM: Modified Social Ecological Model

MSJE: Ministry of Social Justice and Empowerment (India)

MSM: men who have sex with men

MTF: male-to-female

MTSW: male and transgender sex workers

multistage sampling: *(statistics)* a sampling method in which samples for later study are chosen from within the sample populations of earlier phases

NAAT: nucleic acid amplification testing; used to detect pathogens

NACO: National AIDS Control Organisation (India)

natal sex: sex assigned at birth

nativity: place of birth

nayak: the leader of a *hijra gharana*

NDP: New Development Policy (Malaysia)

NDRI: National Development and Research Institutes (United States)

neovagina: a surgically created vagina

NEP: New Economic Policy (Malaysia)

network-based sampling: *(statistics)* snowball sampling within a cohort of hard-to-reach subjects

Network Scale Up Method: *(statistics)* a technique used to estimate the size of a hard-to-count population

New Economic Policy: a policy designed to facilitate the transition from an agricultural to an industrial economy (Malaysia)

NGO: nongovernmental organization

NIDA: National Institute on Drug Abuse (United States)

NIE: National Institute of Epidemiology (India)

NIH: National Institutes of Health (United States)

nirvan: castration *or* castrated male (India)

nongovernmental organization (NGO): a local, national, or international nonprofit organization that operates independently of government, usually having a humanitarian purpose

non-monotonic: *adj. (statistics)* describes a function that both increases and decreases

nonprobability or nonrandom sampling: *(statistics)* any sampling method that creates a nonrepresentative sample; all subjects do not have a known or equal probability of being chosen

Nordic model: *see* end-demand criminalization

normative: *adj.* describes a cultural standard or ideal based on shared values or norms

novela: a soap opera or similar television show (Latin America)

NSW: a study subject who is not a sex worker

nucleic acid amplification testing (NAAT): a molecular test for certain pathogens

null effect: *(statistics)* an experimental outcome in which the result does not support the hypothesis

nu women: a self-referential term used by members of New York's House Ball community

odds ratio (OR): *(statistics)* a formula calculating the extent to which a particular exposure increases or decreases the odds of a given outcome

ontology: a philosophical study of being and existence; in the information sciences, a specific set of representational terms used to define a domain

open coding: the process of identifying and defining categories or concepts in a data set as preparation for analysis

oppression paradigm: a scholarly theory considering sex work to be entirely the result of male domination and exploitation of women

OR: *(statistics)* odds ratio

outcome variable: a dependent variable that shows a change

outlier: *(statistics)* a data point outside the expected range

p: *(statistics)* a value showing the likelihood that results are statistically significant

PAHO: Pan-American Health Organization

pairwise correlations: *(statistics)* a correlation calculated between two chosen variables, disregarding other effects

pajara: a slang term for a transwoman, male homosexual, or effeminate man (Latin America)

pandemic: an epidemic that occurs across a wide geographical range

participatory analysis: in experiential research, an evaluation developed with input from both the subjects and the researchers

patriarchal imperative: the cultural and social norms underlying a male-dominated society

PCP: phencyclidine; a psychoactive drug

PEP: post-exposure prophylaxis

perceived barrier: *(public health)* in the Health Belief Model, an individual's reasons for avoiding healthy behavior

perceived benefit: *(public health)* in the Health Belief Model, an individual's understanding of the likelihood that a behavior will result in a positive outcome

perceived self-efficacy: *(public health)* in the Health Belief Model, an individual's belief that he or she is able to speak or act in his or her own self-interest

perceived severity: *(public health)* in the Health Belief Model, an individual's understanding of the hazards of certain behaviors

perceived susceptibility: *(public health)* in the Health Belief Model, an individual's understanding of his or her likelihood of coming to harm

perineum: the area of the body between the anus and the external genitalia

pharmacology: the science or study of drugs

pharyngeal: *adj.* having to do with or affecting the pharynx or throat

phi: *(statistics)* a measure of association for binary variables

polydrug use: taking multiple illicit drugs at the same or nearly the same time

polymorphous paradigm: a scholarly theory exploring the many variables that contribute to prostitution, including victimization and exploitation, but also choice, job satisfaction, and self-esteem

pondan: a slang term for a transwoman, male homosexual, or effeminate man (Malaysia)

post-exposure prophylaxis (PEP): medical treatment administered following exposure to a pathogen in order to reduce the chances of infection

postmodern: *adj.* of or relating to critical theories that radically challenge traditional cultural assumptions

potentiate: *v.* to make more effective or more likely

precultural: *adj.* before the development of culture

predictor variable: *(public health)* the variable that is being manipulated or measured

prediscursive: *adj.* before the codification of cultural norms

pre-exposure prophylaxis *or* chemoprophylaxis (PrEP): medical treatment administered before exposure to a pathogen in order to reduce the chances of infection

PrEP: pre-exposure prophylaxis

Preventrans: an HIV prevention program (Spain)

probability *or* random sampling: *(statistics)* any sampling method that creates a representative sample; all subjects have a known or equal probability of being chosen

Proluton Depot (hydroxyprogesterone hexanoate): a synthetic form of progesterone

proximal: *adj. (public health)* factors which are internal to an individual, such as the fear of prejudice

psychometrically validated: of a survey or research questionnaire, tested and shown to reliably measure what it was designed to measure

psychopathology: the study of mental illnesses

psychosocial: *adj.* involving or stemming from the interaction between one's psychological processes and the wider social world

psychotic ideation: a loss of contact with reality, such as delusions or hallucinations

PUCL-K: People's Union for Civil Liberties, Karnataka (India); a human rights organization

purposive sampling: *(statistics)* a nonprobability sampling method in which the researcher chooses subjects to fit a particular purpose or profile

quack: an unqualified medical practitioner

qualitative: *adj.* using a research approach that focuses on in-depth, nonnumerical information collected from a small or contained sample

quantitative: *adj.* using a research approach that focuses on employing mathematical and statistical techniques to measure phenomena, often across very large samples

queer theory: a school of cultural criticism challenging traditional ideas of fixed gender and sexuality

Quimbanda: Afro-Brazilian religious tradition

r: *(statistics)* the coefficient of correlation, a value showing the degree of relationship between two variables

rapid plasma reagin screen (RPR): a test for syphilis

recreational sex work: sex work engaged in primarily for the purpose of sexual experimentation

regime: *(sociology)* the principles or norms defining an area of behavior

regression analysis: *(statistics)* a mathematical analysis yielding an equation that describes the statistical relationship between two or more variables

relationship stigma: stigma stemming from a person's primary social or sexual relationship

relative risk ratio: *(statistics)* the proportional risk of an event in a control group versus a treatment group, or in different treatment groups

renminbi (RMB): Chinese unit of currency

respondent-driven sampling: *(statistics)* a modified snowball sampling method that weights the responses mathematically to make the sample more probabilistic

RMB: Chinese renminbi (currency)

robust association: *(statistics)* a strong statistical association not likely to be affected by outliers

role strain: stress resulting from conflicting expectations or demands within a single social role

RPR: rapid plasma reagin screen; syphilis test

RRR: relative risk ratio

rupee (INR): Indian unit of currency

salient cultural category: a visible and easily definable group of people within a culture

SAMHSA: Substance Abuse and Mental Health Services Administration (United States)

sampling: *n. (statistics)* the process by which a set of subjects is chosen from a larger population for a research study

sampling frame: *(statistics)* the entire population from which a sample can be chosen

sanitary control: regulation of safety and health issues

SAVA syndemic: the epidemics of substance use, violence, and HIV/AIDS taken as a whole

schizoid personality disorder: a psychiatric condition characterized by social and emotional detachment from others

schizotypal personality disorder: a psychiatric condition characterized by eccentric beliefs or behaviors and a distorted perception of reality

SCID-II: Structured Clinical Interview for *DSM-IV* Axis II Personality Disorders

sclerosis: a hardening of soft tissues of the body

SD: *(statistics)* standard deviation

SE: *(statistics)* standard error

SEED: Malaysian social services organization (Pertubuhan Pembangunan Kebajikan Dan Persekitaran Positif Malaysia)

segmentation: *(public health)* clustering people for the purposes of research methodology and outreach

self-efficacy: the ability to speak or act in one's own self-interest

sero-: *(combining form)* having to do with a person's perceived or actual HIV status, as in *seroconversion, seroprevalence,* or *serostatus*

sexual division: the divide between two sexes, usually but not always male and female

sex worker: an individual who provides sexual services or erotic performances for material compensation

shabu: street name for methamphetamine (Southeast Asia)

shadow economy: *see* underground economy

shivshakti: a term of self-identification used by trans people (parts of India)

silicone pumping: the practice of injecting nonmedical silicone into the body to modify one's appearance

skewing: *n. (statistics)* the extent to which data distribution is asymmetrical

snowball sampling: *(statistics)* a nonprobability sampling method in which research participants recommend other people as subjects

social marketing principles: business advertising methods used to encourage social or behavioral change

social-structural: *adj.* having to do with the organizational social structure of a society

socio-: *(combining form)* involving or related to society or to social interaction, as in *sociocultural, sociodemographic,* or *socioeconomic*

soft-tissue filler: a substance such as silicone used for nonmedically regulated body modification

spironolactone: an androgen blocker

SPSS: Statistical Package for the Social Sciences; software

standard deviation: *(statistics)* a measure of the average difference of data points from the mean

standard error: *(statistics)* a measure of the standard deviation for all possible samples

Stata: a statistical software package

STI *or* **STD:** sexually transmitted infection *or* disease

stigma: shame or discredit that is based on one's identity or personal characteristics

street economy: *see* underground economy

street hormones: illegal or unregulated

hormones used for body modification

Stress Process Model: *(psychology)* a model positing that increased stress leads to increased maladaptive behavior

strolling: the act of walking around a community or neighborhood in search of sex work clients

structural: *adj.* resulting from economic or political factors that are beyond an individual's control

structural vulnerability: marginalization due to membership in a stigmatized or vulnerable group

subsistence: the minimum means needed for survival, such as food, water, or housing

suicidal ideation: a preoccupation with or desire to commit suicide

surface antigen: a substance that provokes an immune response, used as a diagnostic marker for some infections

survival sex: the exchange of sex for food, shelter, drugs, or other necessary commodities

SW: sex worker

Syariah: Islamic law; sharia (Malay)

symptomatology: the symptoms of a disease taken as a whole

syndemic: *n.* a system of linked diseases within a population

synergistic: *adj.* creating a cumulative effect that is greater than the sum of the individual effects; synergistically, *adv.*

temporal: *adj.* having to do with the sequence of time

tertiary education: education beyond high school

TGSW *also* TSW: transgender sex work *or* workers

theoretical framework: the ideas or concepts underlying a research study

theory-based intervention: an intervention based on research or on a specific theoretical framework

theory of reasoned action: *(sociology)* the idea that actions are driven by the beliefs, norms, and attitudes of the individual

thirunangai: a term of self-identification used by transgender people (parts of India)

time-location sampling: *(statistics)* a venue-based sampling method for hard-to-reach populations, in which venues where prospective subjects might congregate are chosen, and subjects are sampled at chosen times at each location

time-varying covariate: *(statistics)* a variable whose value changes over time

transactional sex: sex for pay or barter

transdermal: *adj.* of a medication, formulated to be applied to and absorbed through the skin

transfeminine *or* transgender spectrum: the variety of self-definition in gender identity

transgender: *adj.* having a gender identity at odds with the sex one was assigned at birth

transgender man: an individual assigned female at birth who later experiences or expresses himself as male

transgender woman: an individual assigned male at birth who later experiences or expresses herself as female

transnational: *adj.* involving or occurring in multiple countries

transphobia: unreasonable hostility toward, aversion to, or discrimination against transgender people

transsexual: an older term for a transgender person, usually implying that the person has considered or undergone medical transition

transvestite: a person who assumes the dress and manner usually associated with the opposite sex

travesti: biologically male sex workers who present themselves as female (South America)

Tri-ESS: the Society for the Second Self; a social and support group for cross-dressers (United States)

t-test (*t*): *(statistics)* a test for significance comparing the means of two populations

two-spirit: a Native American transgender person

two-tailed: *adj. (statistics)* describes a test measuring both ends of a probability curve

Umbanda: Afro-Brazilian religious tradition

UNAIDS: Joint United Nations Programme on HIV/AIDS

uncontrolled variable: a variable that is not or cannot be controlled for

underground economy: an economic sphere in which individuals earn money primarily from illegal or illegitimate pursuits; *also* informal *or* shadow *or* street economy

UNDP: United Nations Development Programme

unstandardized beta: *(statistics)* a beta value calculated from raw data

UNTOC: United Nations Convention against Transnational Organized Crime

upstream: *adj.* describes a variable that affects individuals or outcomes

URAI: unprotected receptive anal intercourse

USD: US dollar (currency)

vaginal speculum: a medical instrument used to inspect the vaginal canal

vaginoplasty: plastic surgery to create or modify a vagina

variance: *(statistics)* a measure of the range of the differences among data points

venous thrombosis: a blood clot that has formed inside a blood vessel

venue-based sampling: *(statistics)* a sampling method for hard-to-reach populations, in which locations where prospective subjects might congregate are chosen, and subjects are chosen from those locations

venue-day-time sampling: *(statistics)* a more probabilistic time-location sampling method, in which subjects are chosen at random days and times from the nonrandom list of venues

viado: a slang term for a homosexual (Brazil)

vício: literally "vice"; a *travesti*'s non-client sex partner (Brazil)

viral load: a measure of the severity of an HIV infection

Western blot: a test for the presence of certain proteins, used to detect pathogens

WHO: World Health Organization

xanith: a slang term for a transwoman, male homosexual, or effeminate man (Oman)

XTC: ecstasy; a psychoactive drug

yaba: street name for methamphetamine (Thailand)

yearly incidence: the rate of occurrence (as of a disease or infection) within one year

INDEX

and substance use, 165, *174, 175, 175, 176*
and URAI, 165, *175, 175, 176,* 412, *413, 415, 415,* 416
violence and, 80, 81
See also major depression
desirability, 68–69, 246, 252–253, 256–257
discrimination
healthcare services and, 306–307, 393
pervasiveness of, 433
relationship stigma and, 66–67, 82, 85
and sexual identity, 79
social services and, 52
and transwomen in Brazil, 268
displacement, 49
distal stressors, 82–83
diversity, racial, 432–433
dress codes, 57
drug use. *See* substance use
dyslipidemias, 398

economic globalization, 291, 292, 299–300
economic hardship, health risk behaviors and, 70–71, 297–298, 330–331
Ecuador. *See* Andean region
education
in China, 384
discrimination and, 57, 341
and HIV risk, 168
and India, 227, 229
and major depression, 93
and police abuse, 409
as sex work factor, 20, 24, 27, *27*
elephant feet, 272
El Salvador, HIV prevalence in, 120
employment discrimination, 20–21, 24, 28, *28*, 93, 168
empowerment, 80, 81, 83, 84–85, 198
end-demand criminalization, 421
Endocrine Society, 397
enslavement, and human trafficking, 267
estrogen, 397

ethnicity
and antiretroviral therapy (ART), 186–194
diversity and, 432–433
and HIV risk, 125–126, 168
and police abuse, 410
sex work involvement and, 19, 23, 39–43, *40, 41, 42*
Europe
gender concepts in, 242, 250, 258
HIV prevalence in, 119, 123, *124–125,* 126
human trafficking and, 273–275, 276–281
migration to, 268, 340, 351–352, 354, 363
murder rates in, 54, 201
See also Spain; Turkey; United Kingdom
exploitation, 53, 267
extortion, 131, 132, 273–274, 339

families
mental health and, 356–357, *357*
rejection by, 22, 49, 276–277, 363–364
Federación Estatal de Lesbianas, Gais, Transexuales, y Bisexuales (FELGTB), 352
Federal Constitution of Malaysia, 290
female-to-male (FTM) transgender persons, and Spain, 352
femininity
cultural beauty and, 8–9, 245–246, 252–253, 256–257
and gender affirmation, 68–69, 71
gender roles and, 241–242, 245–246, 250–252, 258n8, 258n11, 259n16, 259n17
medical interventions and, 372, 375–376, 379, 380, 382, 384, 397–398
role strain and, 71
Fenway Health, 394
filha (daughter) sex workers, 274
France, end-demand criminalization in, 421